Epigenetic Contributions in Autoimmune Disease

Epigenetic Contributions in Autoimmune Disease

Edited by

Esteban Ballestar, PhD
Bellvitge Biomedical Research Institute (IDIBELL), Barcelona, Spain

Springer Science+Business Media, LLC

Landes Bioscience

Springer Science+Business Media, LLC
Landes Bioscience

Printed in the USA.

Springer Science+Business Media, LLC, 233 Spring Street, New York, New York 10013, USA
http://www.springer.com

Please address all inquiries to the publishers:
Landes Bioscience, 1806 Rio Grande, Austin, Texas 78701, USA
Phone: 512/ 637 6050; FAX: 512/ 637 6079
http://www.landesbioscience.com

The chapters in this book are available in the Madame Curie Bioscience Database.
http://www.landesbioscience.com/curie

Epigenetic Contributions in Autoimmune Disease, edited by Esteban Ballestar. Landes Bioscience/ Springer Science+Business Media, LLC dual imprint / Springer series: Advances in Experimental Medicine and Biology.

ISBN: 978-1-4419-8215-5

While the authors, editors and publisher believe that drug selection and dosage and the specifications and usage of equipment and devices, as set forth in this book, are in accord with current recommendations and practice at the time of publication, they make no warranty, expressed or implied, with respect to material described in this book. In view of the ongoing research, equipment development, changes in governmental regulations and the rapid accumulation of information relating to the biomedical sciences, the reader is urged to carefully review and evaluate the information provided herein.

Library of Congress Cataloging-in-Publication Data

Epigenetic contributions in autoimmune disease / edited by Esteban Ballestar.
     p. ; cm. -- (Advances in experimental medicine and biology ; v. 711)
Includes bibliographical references and index.
ISBN 978-1-4419-8215-5
1. Autoimmune diseases--Genetic aspects. 2. Epigenesis. I. Ballestar, Esteban, 1969- II. Series: Advances in experimental medicine and biology ; v. 711. 0065-2598
[DNLM: 1. Autoimmune Diseases--genetics. 2. Epigenesis, Genetic--immunology. W1 AD559 v.711 2010 / WD 305]
RC600.E65 2010
616.97'8042--dc22
                        2010045801

PREFACE

During the past few years, attention towards epigenetics has experienced an unprecedented growth. Interestingly, despite that epigenetics has become a very popular term in molecular biology and biomedicine, its definition still is in evolution, perhaps because the boundaries of epigenetic regulation and epigenetic phenomena are still unkown. Recently, Adrian Bird has proposed a unifying definition of epigenetic events as the structural adaptation of chromosomal regions so as to register, signal or perpetuate altered activity states. Both geneticists and epigeneticists study the gene; however, whereas the former focus on the gene sequence, the latter see gene function as not merely dependent on the DNA sequence but rather depending on the way in which the gene is packaged, signalized and used by transcription factors to become functional or silent, and ready to respond to external stimuli.

Epigenetic modifications have direct impact on cell function and identity, and the generation of aberrant patterns of epigenetic marks is associated with disease. Identification of epigenetic alterations in cancer has been the motor force for the development of strategies and technologies. However, whereas the field of cancer epigenetics is reaching a degree of maturity, the study of epigenetic alterations in most genetically complex diseases still remains relatively unexplored. The possibility of using compounds that can reverse epigenetic modification patterns has also opened new prospects and resulted in further attraction not only to the research community but also to the pharmaceutical industry.

This volume focuses on the relevance of epigenetic mechanisms in autoimmune disease. An overview of some of the key concepts in epigenetics, chromatin and the interaction with transcription factors will be introduced in the first two chapters. Then, general aspects of lymphocyte biology and immune function that are susceptible of modulation by epigenetic modifications will be presented in subsequent chapters. A chapter specifically focused on DNA methylation and autoreactivity has also been included. The role of the environment in the development of autoimmune diseases has been recognized for years, and it is evidenced by the high discordance rate of monozygotic twins for most autoimmune diseases. The specific influence of environmental factors, particularly infectious agents such as the Epstein-Barr virus, has been shown to influence or trigger the autoimmune response. These aspects will also be represented in the book. Also, the possibility that imprinting, a well studied mechanism of epigenetic control, could participate in autoimmune disease will be discussed.

In subsequent chapters, two autoimmune diseases for which the best examples of epigenetic defects have been reported will be extensively discussed, specifically systemic lupus erythematosus and rheumatoid arthritis. Factors influencing the generation epigenetic changes for these and other autoimmune diseases will be presented in different chapters of the book.

Finally, the possibilities of using epigenetics-based therapies in the context of autoimmune diseases will be discussed. We have witnessed the approval of some of these epigenetic compounds for the treatment of another group of hematological system diseases, including acute myeloid leukemia, myelodysplastic syndromes and specific types of lymphomas. Finally, the application of novel methods to characterize the epigenetic profile will be presented.

I hope that this volume provides some new directions for future research in autoimmune disease. Finally, I would like to thank not only all contributors of this volume but also researchers in the epigenetics and chromatin field who have pushed forward this area with their excellent contributions.

Esteban Ballestar, PhD
Bellvitge Biomedical Research Institute (IDIBELL), Barcelona, Spain

ABOUT THE EDITOR...

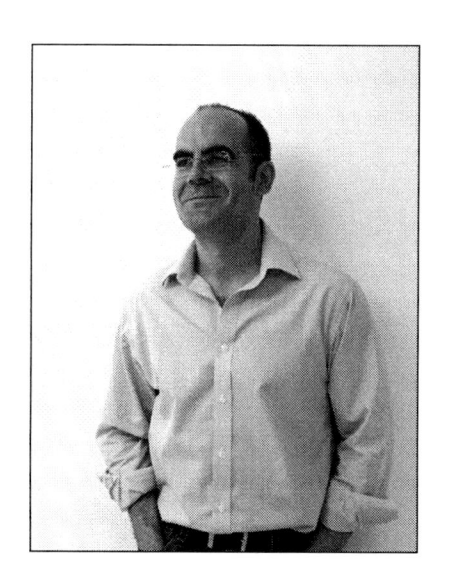

ESTEBAN BALLESTAR is head of the Chromatin and Disease Group at the Cancer Epigenetics and Biology Programme (PEBC) of the Bellvitge Biomedical Research Institute (IDIBELL) in Barcelona, Spain. Ballestar obtained his PhD degree from the University of Valencia under the supervision of Prof. Luis Franco, specialising in chromatin and histone modifications (1997). He then worked as a Postdoctoral Fellow at the National Institutes of Health, (Bethesda, MD, USA) in the laboratory of Dr. Alan Wolffe where he investigated associations between elements of the chromatin machinery and methylated DNA. From 2001 to 2008, Esteban Ballestar has worked at the CNIO Cancer Epigenetics Laboratory, in association with Dr. Manel Esteller, where his principal area of research has been the study of the implication of chromatin factors in epigenetic alterations in human cancer. His current research is devoted to the establishment of different mechanisms of epigenetic deregulation in the context of the hematopoietic system in both autoimmune diseases and hematological malignancies.

PARTICIPANTS

Eva Ay
Microbiological Research Group
National Center for Epidemiology
Budapest
Hungary

Esteban Ballestar
Cancer Epigenetics and Biology
    Programme (PEBC)
Bellvitge Biomedical Research Institute
    (IDIBELL)
Barcelona
Spain

Constanze Bonifer
Leeds Institute of Molecular Medicine
University of Leeds
St. James's University Hospital
Leeds
UK

Robert Brown
Department of Oncology
Hammersmith Hospital Campus
Imperial College London
London
UK

Cristina Camprubí
Cancer Epigenetics and Biology
    Programme (PEBC)
Bellvitge Biomedical Research Institute
    (IDIBELL)
Barcelona
Spain

Nadine Chapman-Rothe
Department of Oncology
Hammersmith Hospital Campus
Imperial College London
London
UK

Peter N. Cockerill
Leeds Institute of Molecular Medicine
University of Leeds
St. James's University Hospital
Leeds
UK

Manel Esteller
Cancer Epigenetics and Biology
    Programme (PEBC)
Bellvitge Biomedical Research Institute
    (IDIBELL)
Barcelona
Spain

Soizic Garaud
Laboratory of Immunology
University of Brest
Brest
France

Renate E. Gay
Department of Rheumatology
University Hospital Zurich
Zurich
Switzerland

Steffen Gay
Department of Rheumatology
University Hospital Zurich
Zurich
Switzerland

Biola M. Javierre
Cancer Epigenetics and Biology
    Programme (PEBC)
Bellvitge Biomedical Research Institute
    (IDIBELL)
Barcelona
Spain

Emmanuel Karouzakis
Department of Rheumatology
University Hospital Zurich
Zurich
Switzerland

Eduardo Lopez-Granados
Clinical Immunology Department
University Hospital La Paz
Madrid
Spain

José Ignacio Martín-Subero
Cancer Epigenetics and Biology
    Programme (PEBC)
Bellvitge Biomedical Research Institute
    (IDIBELL)
Barcelona
Spain

Frederick W. Miller
Environmental Autoimmunity Group
National Institutes of Health
Bethesda, Maryland
USA

Janos Minarovits
Microbiological Research Group
National Center for Epidemiology
Budapest
Hungary

David Monk
Cancer Epigenetics and Biology
    Programme (PEBC)
Bellvitge Biomedical Research Institute
    (IDIBELL)
Barcelona
Spain

Michel Neidhart
Department of Rheumatology
University Hospital Zurich
Zurich
Switzerland

Hans Helmut Niller
Institute for Medical Microbiology
    and Hygiene
University of Regensburg
Regensburg
Germany

Yves Renaudineau
Laboratory of Immunology
University of Brest
Brest
France

Bruce C. Richardson
Department of Medicine
University of Michigan
Ann Arbor, Michigan
USA

Marja C.J.A. van Eggermond
Department of Immunohematology
    and Blood Transfusion
Leiden University Medical Center
Leiden
The Netherlands

Peter J. van den Elsen
Department of Immunohematology
    and Blood Transfusion
Leiden University Medical Center
Leiden
The Netherlands

Rutger J. Wierda
Department of Immunohematology
    and Blood Transfusion
Leiden University Medical Center
Leiden
The Netherlands

Hans Wolf
Institute for Medical Microbiology
  and Hygiene
University of Regensburg
Regensburg
Germany

Pierre Youinou
Laboratory of Immunology
University of Brest
Brest
France

CONTENTS

8. DOES GENOMIC IMPRINTING PLAY A ROLE IN AUTOIMMUNITY? 103

Cristina Camprubí and David Monk

9. A NEW EPIGENETIC CHALLENGE: SYSTEMIC LUPUS ERYTHEMATOSUS 117

Biola M. Javierre and Bruce C. Richardson

10. EPIGENETIC DEREGULATION IN RHEUMATOID ARTHRITIS 137

Emmanuel Karouzakis, Renate E. Gay, Steffen Gay and Michel Neidhart

11. PROSPECTS FOR EPIGENETIC COMPOUNDS IN THE TREATMENT OF AUTOIMMUNE DISEASE 150

Nadine Chapman-Rothe and Robert Brown

12. PROFILING EPIGENETIC ALTERATIONS IN DISEASE 162

José Ignacio Martín-Subero and Manel Esteller

CHAPTER 1

AN INTRODUCTION TO EPIGENETICS

Esteban Ballestar

Chromatin and Disease Group, Cancer Epigenetics and Biology Programme (PEBC), IDIBELL, Barcelona, Spain
Email: eballestar@idibell.org

Abstract: Eukaryotic genomic information is modulated by a variety of epigenetic modifications that play both a direct role in establishing transcription profiles, modulation of DNA replication and repair processes and also indirect effects on the aforementioned processes through the organization of DNA architecture within the cell nucleus. Nowadays, the role of epigenetic modifications in regulating tissue-specific expression, genomic imprinting or X-chromosome inactivation is widely recognized. In addition, the key role of epigenetic modifications during cell differentiation and development has been highlighted by the identification of a variety of epigenetic alterations in human disease. Particular attention has been focused on the study of epigenetic alterations in cancer, which is the subject of intense multidisciplinary efforts and has an impact not only in understanding the mechanisms of epigenetic regulation but also in guiding the development of novel therapies for cancer treatment. In addition, a number of genetic disorders such as Immunodeficiency-Centromere Instability-Facial anomalies (ICF) or Rett syndromes are directly associated with defects in elements of the epigenetic machinery. More recently, epigenetic changes in cardiovascular, neurological and autoimmune disorders as well as in other genetically complex diseases have also started to emerge. All these examples illustrate the widespread association of epigenetic alterations with disease and highlight the need of characterizing the range and extension of epigenetic changes to understand their contribution to fundamental human biological processes.

INTRODUCTION

The size and complexity of eukaryotic genomes has evolved in association with the generation of mechanisms that are able to manage the genetic information that is needed at different specific physiological situations. Considering that a 10 μm-diameter eukaryotic nucleus has to accommodate an enormous length of DNA (in the order of magnitude of centimeter/meter), cells have to face two major challenges: firstly, how to optimize folding of DNA in such a tiny compartment and secondly, how to make accessible DNA sequences that will be needed at specific situations throughout their lifetime. Folding of DNA within the cell nucleus is achieved through its interaction with histones and other types of proteins, characteristic of chromatin. Regarding the second aspect, i.e., how DNA sequences retain the ability to stay functional despite their folding within chromatin, it is now obvious that the mere availability of transcription factors or DNA repair machinery cannot simply overcome the repressive effect of chromatin without additional help. Epigenetic marks provide cells with a dynamic signaling system that compartimentalizes the genome and allows the specific regulation of gene expression and accurate tuning of DNA replication and repair processes, as well as the appropriate nuclear organization in a manner adapted to particular physiological situations. These epigenetic marks are established and maintained by different groups of enzymes which are specifically targeted to their correct genomic locations through different nuclear factors, some of which directly respond to environmental signals or constitute the final step of a cell signaling cascade.

EPIGENETIC MODIFICATIONS ARE ESSENTIAL FOR CELL IDENTITY AND FUNCTION

Basically, cells encode their epigenetic information through the modification of two different groups of macromolecules: DNA and histones. DNA methylation is a major epigenetic modification with a direct contribution in the establishment of expression patterns in multicellular organisms.[1] In mammals, DNA methylation is restricted to cytosines in the context of CpG dinucleotide sequences, whose presence in the genome is much lower than expected based on GC content and exhibit a non uniform distribution. CpG sites can be present in the genome at high density in regions known as CpG islands, that are 0.4-3 kb in length, are relatively rich in G + C (>55%) and are enriched in the CpG dinucleotide relative to the remainder of the genome regions.[2] In the human genome, CpG islands are in and near approximately 76% of promoters of genes.[3,4] It has been proposed that methylation occurring at CpGs located in repetitive and parasitic elements plays a role in their stabilization.[5] Also, methylation of repetitive elements appears to contribute in the maintenance of nuclear architecture and organization of heterochromatic domains.[6] On the other hand, the majority of promoter CpG islands remain unmethylated under physiological conditions.[7] Methylation and subsequent transcriptional repression are confined to a relatively small set of genes, including some tissue-specific[8,9] and imprinted genes,[10] as well as those in the inactive X-chromosome of females.[11] The fact that promoter CpG islands can be unmethylated in both expressing and nonexpressing tissues indicates that the activity of the associated genes is not controlled by methylation. It is nonetheless widely believed that cytosine methylation regulates development. Many of the expression-methylation studies involve non-CpG island genes, which tend to have light and variable cytosine methylation that may be less in cells that express the gene. A standard method to map the methylation status of CpGs is based on the treatment of DNA with sodium bisulfite, that results in conversion of unmethylated cytosines into uracil whereas methylated cytosines remains unmodified, followed by genomic sequencing (BS).[12]

DNA methylation is a postreplicative process. The methyl group is transferred from S-adenosyl methionine to cytosines in DNA by DNA methyltransferases (DNMT) in a reaction that involves base flipping, whereby a cytosine base is swung completely out of the DNA helix into an extrahelical position so that the enzyme can access and methylate the cytosine.[13] The mammalian family of DNMTs is composed of five members [see for a review Goll and Bestor].[14] DNMT1 has been considered to be devoted to the maintenance of methylation patterns across DNA replication cycles, however whether faithful maintenance methylation is enforced by other factors that inhibit the de novo activity of DNMT1 in vivo (no such factors have been described) or the protein has de novo activity in vivo remains an unresolved issue. DNMT3A and DNMT3B have been proposed to be implicated in de novo methylation. They have a close homologue, DNMT3L, that lacks a conserved PWWP domain present in DNMT3a/b, is essential for establishment of maternal genomic imprints in the growing oocyte and at dispersed repeated sequences in the prospermatogonia. Finally, DNMT2 is an enigmatic DNMT that, despite its conservation across species and its expression in all sort of tissues, appears to lack catalytic activity.

In general, DNA methylation is considered to be a stable epigenetic mark, although mechanisms of active DNA demethylation have been reported to occur in specific physiological contexts, including development and cell differentiation.[15,16] In contrast with the precise identification of the machinery involved in promoting or maintaining DNA methylation, there is some controversy with respect to the enzymatic activities involved in active demethylation. Genetic and biochemical studies in *Arabidopsis* demonstrated that a subfamily of DNA glycosylases function to promote DNA demethylation through a base excision-repair pathway. These specialized bifunctional DNA glycosylases remove the 5-methylcytosine base and then cleave the DNA backbone at the abasic site, resulting in a gap that is then filled with an unmethylated cytosine nucleotide by as yet unknown DNA polymerase and ligase enzymes. Evidence suggests that active DNA demethylation in mammalian cells is also mediated at least in part by a base excision repair pathway where activation-induced cytosine deaminases (AID) convert 5-methylcytosine to thymine followed by G/T mismatch repair by the DNA glycosylase MBD4 or TDG.[17-19] However other possible mechanisms of active DNA demethylation have also been proposed.

In parallel with DNA methylation, histone modifications constitute a fundamental source of epigenetic information. Core histones are the building elements of the octameric complex around which the DNA is wrapped within chromatin. Histones can be modified at different amino acid residues. There are over sixty different sites on histones where modifications have been detected either by mass spectrometry or by specific antibodies, but not all these modifications will be on the same histone at the same time. However, this represents a huge underestimate of the number of modifications that could potentially take place on histones. Additional complexity comes also from the fact that methylation at lysines or arginines may be one of three different forms: mono-, di-, or trimethyl for lysines and mono- or di- (asymmetric or symmetric) for arginines. This vast array of modifications confers enormous potential for functional responses. The timing of the appearance of a modification will depend on the signaling conditions within the cell. The use of modification-specific antibodies in chromatin immunoprecipitation assays (ChIP) coupled to gene array technology (ChIP-on-chip) has revolutionized our ability to monitor the global incidence of histone modifications. Such global analysis has only been done on a subset of modifications (acetylation and lysine methylation), but the results clearly show that modifications are not uniformly distributed. Combinations or sequential addition of different histone modifications have different functional consequences for gene activity and chromatin organization.[20] For instance, reversible acetylation of histone lysines at their N-terminal tails is generally associated with transcriptional activation,[21] although there are some particularities on the functional consequences that depend on the specific lysine that it is acetylated (see for example refs. 22 and 23). On the other hand, methylation of histones can occur in lysine and arginine residues; the functional consequences depend on the type of residue and specific site that is modified.[24-26] For instance, methylation of H3 at K4[27] and R17[28] is closely linked to transcriptional competence, whereas methylation of H3 at K9, or H4 at K20, is associated with transcriptional repression.[29,30] The identification of the enzymes that direct modification has been the focus of intense activity over the last 10 years. Enzymes have been identified for acetylation,[31] methylation,[32] phosphorylation,[33] ubiquitination,[34] ADP-ribosylation,[35] sumoylation,[36] deimination[37,38] and proline isomerization.[39]

Histone modifications have been implicated in a number of epigenetic phenomena. The classic definition of epigenetics is the study of heritable phenotype changes that do not involve alterations in DNA sequence. The use of the term "heritable" has been eliminated in more recent definitions, allowing the term epigenetic to mean the information carried by the genome (e.g., on chromatin) that is not coded by DNA. However the classic term, that includes heritability, is important to maintain as it defines a nongenetic memory of function that is transmitted from generation to generation. A number of cellular phenotypes are transmitted in this way, including imprinting (discussed in Chapter 8), X chromosome inactivation, aging, heterochromatin formation, reprogramming and gene silencing. In addition there are environmentally induced changes, which are passed on from generation to generation, without the need for the original stimulus.

Several mechanisms link DNA methylation with specific histone modifications. However, not every posttranslational modification at the core histone tails depends on the methylation status of the DNA. The mechanisms by which promoter CpG island methylation leads to gene silencing involve changes in the modification of profile of histones. This process has been reported to occur place through the direct recruitment of histone modification enzymes by DNMTs[40] and other nuclear factors such as methyl-CpG binding domain (MBD) proteins.[41,42] Additional mechanistic connections between elements of the histone modification and DNA methylation machineries exist. For instance, Polycomb group (PcG) protein EZH2, which catalyzes methylation of K27 of histone H3, associates and targets DNA methylation to specific sites.[43-45]

Therefore, histone modification patterns can be established through DNA methylation-associated mechanisms or, alternatively, in a DNA methylation-independent fashion. In the latter case, recruitment of histone modification enzymes at specific genomic loci depends on the availability of particular transcription factors or through the ligand-dependent response of nuclear receptors which in turn recruit histone modification enzymes.

In multicellular organisms, cells usually respond to environmental or intracellular signals in a manner that depends on the participation of transcription factors which often recruit epigenetic enzymes.[46] Within any particular organism, different cell lineages share a common genome although available sets of transcription factors and epigenetic marks are cell type specific and functionally interconnected. The balance between epigenetic modifications, transcription factors and their ability to respond to environmental stimuli is delicate and guarantees proper cell function. Epigenetic modifications and the required sets of transcription factors are also transmitted through successive rounds of DNA replication and cell division. However, disruption of a variety of pathways results in different types of epigenetic alterations, some of which have already been associated with disease.

EPIGENETIC DEREGULATION MECHANISMS IN HUMAN DISEASE

The recognition of the widespread occurrence and significance of epigenetic alterations in cancer has been essential in attracting the attention of the Biomedicine field towards Epigenetics. Cells from most cancer types suffer dramatic changes in their DNA methylation and histone modification content and distribution. Tumor cells undergo a decrease in the global content of 5-methylcytosine, which can be mainly attributed to loss of methylation at repetitive sequences.[47,48] However, the promoter CpG islands of many tumor suppressor genes become hypermethylated and this process represents an important mechanism by which these genes are inactivated.[49] Early analysis of the profile of promoter CpG island hypermethylation of candidate genes encouraged the view that the profiles of promoter methylation are tumor-type specific.[50,51] This notion has been reinforced with more recent genome-wide analysis that evidence the specificity of the DNA hypermethylation profiles in different tumor types.[52,53]

Several lines of evidence indicate that hypermethylation of tumor-suppressor genes plays an active role in the development and progression of cancer. In the first place, hypermethylation occurs early in cancer. This is the case of p14ARF in colorectal adenomas[54] and hMLH1 in endometrial hyperplasias[55] and gastric adenomas.[56] A second observation highlighting the functional relevance of promoter CpG island hypermethylation in tumorigenesis is its occurrence in the absence of genetic mutations. Both events (genetic and epigenetic) abolish normal gene function and their coincidence in the same allele would be redundant from an evolutionary point of view. However, one of the main findings that support for a critical role for CpG island hypermethylation in the origin and progression of a tumor is the demonstration of the existence of relevant biological consequences associated with the epigenetic inactivation of a particular gene. A classical example of this statement is represented by the hypermethylation of the DNA repair gene O6-methylguanine DNA methyltransferase (MGMT).[57] The MGMT gene product removes the promutagenic O6-methylguanine, generated from the addition of a methyl group to the base guanine, which is then read as an an adenine by DNA polymerases and thus may generate G to A mutations. It has been shown that the DNA repair gene MGMT is transcriptionally silenced by promoter hypermethylation in primary human tumors.[58] These tumors might accumulate a considerable number of G to A transitions, some of them affecting key genes, in a similar way that loss of the hMLH1 mismatch repair gene by methylation targets other genes. This information has led to the finding that the hypermethylation- associated inactivation of MGMT gives rise to the appearance of G to A transition mutations in the oncogene K-ras[59] and the universal tumor suppressor p53[60] in human colorectal tumorigenesis. These findings indicate that epigenetic lesions can cause genetic lesions in genes that are of key importance in the development of cancer.

As mentioned above, the comprehensive analysis of methylation in many different tumor types and gene promoters has provided evidence for the existence of the tumor-type-specific methylation profile indicated above. In theory, CpG islands should be the most 'attractive' substrate for DNA methylation, since, by definition, they contain a high concentration of CpG-rich sequences. However, under physiological circumstances most CpG island promoters remain unmethylated. It has been speculated on the existence of mechanisms that would normally prevent unscheduled methylation at CpG islands and for some reasons those mechanisms would lose stringency in cancer cells. Many other questions then arise including the reason why certain CpG islands (while others never do) become methylated in cancer and whether this is a targeted process or a random one.

Genome-wide analysis of DNA methylation changes in cancer cells have shed some light on these questions by revealing that tumor-specific methylated genes belong to distinct functional categories, have common sequence motifs in their promoters and are found in clusters on chromosomes.[61] These results are consistent with the hypothesis that cancer-related de novo methylation may be specifically targeted through a trans-acting mechanism. Schlesinger and colleagues[44] showed that genes methylated in colon cancer cells are specifically packaged with nucleosomes containing histone H3 trimethylated on K27. The early establishment of this chromatin mark in unmethylated promoter CpG island-containing genes early in development and then maintained in differentiated cell types by the presence of an EZH2-containing Polycomb complex suggests that PcG proteins predefines genes that are methylated in cancer. In cancer cells, as opposed to normal cells, the presence of this complex brings about the recruitment of DNMTs, leading to de novo methylation. These results suggest that tumor-specific targeting of de novo methylation is preprogrammed by an established epigenetic system that normally has a role in marking embryonic genes for repression.[44]

DNA methylation and histone modification profiles are mechanistically coupled by multiple mechanisms. In addition to PcG mediated-connections between histone modifications and DNA methylation, other factors have been implicated in DNA methylation-dependent silencing. In this context, MBD proteins have been proposed to play a pivotal role.[62] MBD proteins have the ability to bind selectively to methylated CpGs and recruit different HDAC- and HMT-containing complexes.[42] In addition to the association of MBDs, promoter CpG island hypermethylation has been found to be associated with a decrease in the acetylation levels of histones H3 and H4 and loss of 3mK4 of histone H3.[62] In contrast, hypomethylation of repetitive sequences in cancer is associated with a loss of monoacecetyl K16 and trimethyl K20 of histone H4.[63,64] It has been suggested that this change could be associated with changes in the expression levels of specific histone modification enzymes, like K16 H4-specific HAT MOF[65] or K20 H4-specific HMT Suv4-20h2.[66]

The importance of epigenetic mechanisms involved in the pathogenesis of cancer is also revealed by a mechanism frequently found in hematopoietic malignancies. In leukemias and lymphomas, in contrast to most solid tumors, an additional mechanism for epigenetic dysregulation arises from the occurrence of nonrandom chromosomal translocations that disrupt genes residing in the translocation breakpoint region. In many cases, genes residing at these breakpoint regions are epigenetic enzymes or transcription factors that can themselves recruit epigenetic enzymes and are directly involved in hematopoietic cell differentiation, apoptosis, or proliferation. Therefore, generation of fusion proteins through this mechanism is commonly associated with epigenetic dysregulation at the target sites of the enzymes involved. These chromosomal translocations indicate how disruptions of the function of the enzymes that control chromatin structure can cause alterations of the histone modification profile in a target-specific fashion, resulting in an altered chromatin structure that affects gene expression at specific loci and ultimately causes cellular transformation. Typical examples of proteins include MLL (mixed-lineage leukemia), a histone H3 K4-specific methyltransferase, RUNX1 (also known as AML1) which is associated with HATs or HDACs and PML, whose frequent fusion partner (RAR) has been described to interact with various epigenetic modifiers.[67]

Our knowledge on the importance of epigenetic alterations in cancer has greatly increased in the last few years. The contribution of DNA methylation-dependent epigenetic inactivation of tumor suppressor genes is widely recognized. More specifically in hematological malignancies, the epigenetic switch at many genomic sites is also commonly recognized. We need a better understanding on the causes that result in epigenetic deregulation in cancer. Mapping epigenomic changes, at the DNA methylation, histone modification and factor binding level, in cancer cells will surely provide a solid ground to address these issues.

Despite the enormous efforts invested in epigenetics studies, our knowledge on epigenetic alterations in other disease contexts is relatively poor. Epigenetic alterations occur in a wide range of biological scenarios, including the occurrence of genetic defects in the enzymes that regulate the epigenetic balance or epigenetic changes that result from a change in the environment. Although the best studied relationship between epigenetic alterations and disease are in the context of cancer, a number of diseases have proved to exhibit a fundamental epigenetic component. The first group of disorders for which an epigenetic component has been recognized includes diseases for which there is a genetic defect involving proteins implicated in the maintenance of epigenetic regulation. In this group are included a few rare syndromes such as Immunodeficiency-Centromere Instability-Facial anomalies (ICF) syndrome or Rett syndrome among others.

ICF syndrome, a rare autosomal recessive disorder characterized by the presence of variable immunodeficiency and a unique type of instability of pericentromeric heterochromatin, has been shown to be associated with mutations in DNMT3B. Epigenetic alterations associated with this defect include hypomethylation at various repetitive sequences[68] and chromosomal territory reorganization which may have an impact in alterations of gene expression of many genes.[69] In Rett syndrome, an X-linked dominant neurodevelopmental disorder affecting almost exclusively girls, mutations in MECP2, the archetypical member of the MBD family, have been found to be present in up to 80% of classical cases.[70] It has been proposed that loss of function of MECP2 results in the DNA methylation-dependent deregulation of genes,[71] although more recently it has been proposed that binding of MeCP2 outside gene boundaries may organize chromatin into functionally important domains or loops of imprinted regions, thereby modulating gene expression in either a positive or a negative manner.[72]

In other groups of disorders, genetic defects have been associated with clear distinctive epigenetic defects. This is for instance the cases of facioscapulohumeral muscular dystrophy (FSHD), where the deletion of a critical number of repetitive elements (D4Z4) is associated with hypomethylation,[73] or the imprinting disorders Beckwith-Wiedemann syndrome (BWS) and the Prader-Willi/Angelman syndromes (PWS/AS), where deletion of imprinting control regions results in biallelic expression of associated genes.[74]

The existence of an epigenetic component has been suggested for many other diseases for which a direct genetic defect is not obvious or complex genetic patterns have been suggested. This is for instance the case of autoimmune or neurological disorders and cardiovascular disease. The evidence for an epigenetic component in these diseases has been highlighted by the existence of discordance rates in sets of monozygotic twins.[75] Analysis of global and locus-specific differences of DNA methylation and histone modification in a cohort of identical twins has suggested the existence of an age-dependent epigenetic 'drift', which may result from the independent influence of environmental factors.[76] More recent studies have addressed the relevance of epigenetic differences between twins discordant for autoimmune diseases.[77,78]

Our knowledge on the epigenetic contribution for these diseases requires additional research efforts: firstly, a detailed description of the type and extent of epigenetic alterations needs to be addressed. In addition, identification of the upstream mechanisms that lead to the generation of epigenetic changes should be investigated.

The availability of novel technologies for the genome-wide analysis of epigenetic alterations and systematic analysis of DNA methylation changes in specific diseases will surely lead to the discovery of specific markers with both basic research an clinical implications (discussed in Chapter 12). Initial high-throughput studies looking for epigenomic changes in atutoimmune disease, such as those carried out for systemic lupus erythematosus,[77] multiple sclerosis[78] or Type 1 diabetes[79] highlight the need of defining the range and extent of epigenetic alterations in this set of complex disorders.

CONCLUSION

In eukaryotic organisms, epigenetic modifications act as a signaling system that defines, in concert with transcription factors and other nuclear elements, the functionality of the genome in each particular cell type and in specific stages of the cell cycle during differentiation and development. Histone modifications and DNA methylation are major elements of the epigenetic signaling system and have a direct impact in the cell transcriptome, as well as in DNA repair and replication. The aberrant establishment or maintenance of epigenetic profiles is directly associated with cell misfunction and ultimately disease. This has been extensively studied for cancer and various genetic syndromes. The availability of novel strategies to characterize the profile of epigenetic modifications at the genome-wide level together with the possibility of pharmacological reversion of epigenetic alterations has attracted researchers to investigate the epigenetic component of genetically complex diseases, including autoimmune disorders.

ACKNOWLEDGEMENTS

EB is supported by PI081346 (FIS) grant from the Spanish Ministry of Science and Innovation (MICINN) and 2009SGR184 grant from AGAUR (Catalan Government).

REFERENCES

1. Jaenisch R, Bird A. Epigenetic regulation of gene expression, how the genome integrates intrinsic and environmental signals. Nat Genet 2003; 33, Suppl:245-254.
2. Gardiner-Garden M, Frommer M. CpG islands in vertebrate genomes. J Mol Biol 1987; 196:261-282.
3. Davuluri RV, Grosse I, Zhang MQ. Computational identification of promoters and first exons in the human genome. Nat Genet 2001; 29:412-417.
4. Mariño-Ramirez L, Spouge JL, Kanga GC et al. Statistical analysis of over-represented words in human promoter sequences. Nucleic Acids Res 2004; 32:949-958.
5. Robertson KD, Wolffe AP. DNA methylation in health and disease. Nat Rev Genet 2000; 1:11-19.
6. Espada J, Ballestar E, Fraga MF et al. Human DNMT1 is essential to maintain the histone H3 modification pattern. J Biol Chem 2004; 279:37175-37184.
7. Siegfried Z, Cedar H. DNA methylation, a molecular lock. Curr Biol 1997; 7:R305-307.

8. Futscher BW, Oshiro MM, Wozniak RJ et al. Role for DNA methylation in the control of cell type specific maspin expression. Nature Genet 2002; 31:175-179.
9. Song F, Smith JF, Kimura MT et al. Association of tissue-specific differentially methylated regions (TDMs) with differential gene expression. Proc Natl Acad Sci USA 2005; 102:3336-3341.
10. Reik W, Collick A, Norris ML et al. Genomic imprinting determines methylation of parental alleles in transgenic mice. Nature 1987; 328:248-251.
11. Wolf SF, Migeon BR. Studies of X chromosome DNA methylation in normal human cells. Nature 1982; 295:667-671.
12. Clark SJ, Harrison J, Paul CL et al. High sensitivity mapping of methylated cytosines. Nucleic Acids Res 1994; 22:2990-2997.
13. Roberts RJ, Cheng X. Base flipping. Annu Rev Biochem 1998; 67:181-198.
14. Goll MG, Bestor TH. Eukaryotic cytosine methyltransferases. Annu Rev Biochem 2005; 74:481-514.
15. Reik W, Dean W, Walter J. Epigenetic reprogramming in mammalian development. Science 2001; 293:1089-1093.
16. Wilson CB, Merkenschlager M. Chromatin structure and gene regulation in T-cell development and function. Curr Opin Immunol 2006; 18:143-151.
17. Zhu JK. Active DNA demethylation mediated by DNA glycosylases. Annu Rev Genet 2009; 43:143-166.
18. Bhutani N, Brady JJ, Damian M et al. Reprogramming towards pluripotency requires AID-dependent DNA demethylation. Nature 2010; 463:1042-1047.
19. Popp C, Dean W, Feng S et al. Genome-wide erasure of DNA methylation in mouse primordial germ cells is affected by AID deficiency. Nature 2010; 463:1101-1105.
20. Wang Y, Fischle W, Cheung W et al. Beyond the double helix, writing and reading the histone code. Novartis Found Symp 2004; 259:3-17.
21. Chahal SS, Matthews HR, Bradbury EM. Acetylation of histone H4 and its role in chromatin structure and function. Nature 1980; 287:76-79.
22. Rundlett SE, Carmen AA, Suka N et al. Transcriptional repression by UME6 involves deacetylation of lysine 5 of histone H4 by RPD3. Nature 1998; 392:831-835.
23. Shogren-Knaak M, Ishii H, Sun JM et al. Histone H4-K16 acetylation controls chromatin structure and protein interactions. Science 2006; 311:844-847.
24. Rao B, Shibata Y, Strahl BD et al. Demethylation of histone H3 at lysine 36 demarcates regulatory and nonregulatory chromatin genome-wide. Mol Cell Biol 2005; 25:9447-9459.
25. Lachner M, O'Carroll D, Rea S et al. Methylation of histone H3 lysine 9 creates a binding site for HP1 proteins. Nature 2001; 410:116-120.
26. Schotta G, Lachner M, Sarma K et al. A silencing pathway to induce H3-K9 and H4-K20 trimethylation at constitutive heterochromatin. Genes Dev 2004; 18:1251-1262.
27. Santos-Rosa H, Schneider R, Bannister AJ et al. Active genes are tri-methylated at K4 of histone H3. Nature 2002; 419:407-411.
28. Bauer UM, Daujat S, Nielsen SJ et al. Methylation at arginine 17 of histone H3 is linked to gene activation. EMBO Rep 2002; 3:39-44.
29. Bannister AJ, Zegerman P, Partridge JF et al. Selective recognition of methylated lysine 9 on histone H3 by the HP1 chromo domain. Nature 2001; 410(6824):120-124.
30. Karachentsev D, Sarma K, Reinberg D et al. PR-Set7-dependent methylation of histone H4 Lys 20 functions in repression of gene expression and is essential for mitosis. Genes Dev 2005; 19:431-435.
31. Sterner DE, Berger SL. Acetylation of histones and transcription-related factors. Microbiol Mol Biol Rev 2000; 64:435-459.
32. Zhang Y, Reinberg D. Transcription regulation by histone methylation, interplay between different covalent modifications of the core histone tails. Genes Dev 2006; 15:2343-2360.
33. Nowak SJ, Corces VG. Phosphorylation of histone H3, a balancing act between chromosome condensation and transcriptional activation. Trends Genet 2004; 20:214-220.
34. Shilatifard A. Chromatin modifications by methylation and ubiquitination, implications in the regulation of gene expression. Annu Rev Biochem 2006; 75:243-269.
35. Hassa PO, Haenni SS, Elser M et al. Nuclear ADP-ribosylation reactions in mammalian cells, where are we today and where are we going? Microbiol Mol Biol Rev 2006; 70:789-829.
36. Nathan D, Ingvarsdottir K, Sterner DE et al. Histone sumoylation is a negative regulator in Saccharomyces cerevisiae and shows dynamic interplay with positive-acting histone modifications. Genes Dev 2006; 20:966-976.
37. Cuthbert GL, Daujat S, Snowden AW et al. Histone deimination antagonizes arginine methylation. Cell 2004; 118:545-553.
38. Wang Y, Wysocka J, Sayegh J et al. Human PAD4 regulates histone arginine methylation levels via demethylimination. Science 2004; 306:279-283.

39. Nelson CJ, Santos-Rosa H, Kouzarides T. Proline isomerization of histone H3 regulates lysine methylation and gene expression. Cell 2006; 126:905-916.
40. Burgers WA, Fuks F, Kouzarides T. DNA methyltransferases get connected to chromatin. Trends Genet 2002; 18:275-277.
41. Hendrich B, Bird A. Identification and characterization of a family of mammalian methyl-CpG binding proteins. Mol Cell Biol 1998; 18:6538-6547.
42. Ballestar E, Wolffe AP. Methyl-CpG-binding proteins, targeting specific gene repression. Eur J Biochem 2001; 268:1-6.
43. Vire E, Brenner C, Deplus R et al. The Polycomb group protein EZH2 directly controls DNA methylation. Nature 2006; 439:871-874.
44. Schlesinger Y, Straussman R, Keshet I et al. Polycomb-mediated methylation on Lys27 of histone H3 premarks genes for de novo methylation in cancer. Nat Genet 2007; 39:232-236.
45. Mohn F, Weber M, Rebhan M et al. Lineage-specific polycomb targets and de novo DNA methylation define restriction and potential of neuronal progenitors. Mol Cell 2008; 30:755-766.
46. Feil R. Environmental and nutritional effects on the epigenetic regulation of genes. Mutat Res 2006; 600:46-57.
47. Feinberg AP, Vogelstein B. Hypomethylation distinguishes genes of some human cancers from their normal counterparts. Nature 1983; 301:89-92.
48. Ehrlich M. DNA methylation in cancer, too much, but also too little. Oncogene 2002; 21:5400-5413.
49. Jones PA, Baylin SB. The fundamental role of epigenetic events in cancer. Nat Rev Genet 2002; 3:415-428.
50. Costello JF, Frühwald MC, Smiraglia DJ et al. Aberrant CpG-island methylation has nonrandom and tumour-type-specific patterns. Nat Genet 2000; 24:132-138.
51. Esteller M, Corn PG, Baylin SB et al. A gene hypermethylation profile of human cancer. Cancer Res 2001a; 61:3225-3229.
52. Mokarram P, Kumar K, Brim H et al. Distinct high-profile methylated genes in colorectal cancer. PLoS One 2009; 4:e7012.
53. Martinez R, Martin-Subero JI, Rohde V et al. A microarray-based DNA methylation study of glioblastoma multiforme. Epigenetics 2009; 4:255-264.
54. Esteller M, Tortola S, Toyota M et al. Hypermethylation-associated inactivation of p14(ARF) is independent of p16(INK4a) methylation and p53 mutational status. Cancer Res 2000; 60:129-133.
55. Esteller M, Lluis Catasus, Matias-Guiu X et al. hMLH1 promoter hypermethylation is an early event in human endometrial tumorigenesis. Am J Pathol 1999; 155:1767-1772.
56. Fleisher AS, Esteller M, Wang S et al. Hypermethylation of the hMLH1 gene promoter in human gastric cancers with microsatellite instability. Cancer Res 1999; 59:1090-1095.
57. Pegg AE, Dolan ME, Moschel RC. Structure, function, and inhibition of O6-alkylguanine-DNA alkyltransferase. Prog Nucleic Acid Res Mol Biol 1995; 51:167-223.
58. Esteller M, Hamilton SR, Burger PC et al. Inactivation of the DNA repair gene O6-methylguanine-DNA methyltransferase by promoter hypermethylation is a common event in primary human neoplasia. Cancer Res 1999; 59:793-797.
59. Esteller M, Toyota M, Sanchez-Cespedes M et al. Inactivation of the DNA repair gene O6-methylguanine-DNA methyltransferase by promoter hypermethylation is associated with G to A mutations in K-ras in colorectal tumorigenesis. Cancer Res 2000; 60:2368-2371.
60. Esteller M, Risques RA, Toyota M et al. Promoter hypermethylation of the DNA repair gene O(6)-methylguanine-DNA methyltransferase is associated with the presence of G,C to A,T transition mutations in p53 in human colorectal tumorigenesis. Cancer Res 2001; 61:4689-4692.
61. Keshet I, Schlesinger Y, Farkash S et al. Evidence for an instructive mechanism of de novo methylation in cancer cells. Nat Genet 2006; 38:149-153.
62. Ballestar E, Paz MF, Valle L et al. Methyl-CpG binding proteins identify novel sites of epigenetic inactivation in human cancer. EMBO J 2003; 22:6335-6345.
63. Fraga MF, Ballestar E, Villar-Garea A et al. Loss of acetylation at Lys16 and trimethylation at Lys20 of histone H4 is a common hallmark of human cancer. Nat Genet 2005; 37:391-400.
64. Seligson DB, Horvath S, Shi T et al. Global histone modification patterns predict risk of prostate cancer recurrence. Nature 2005; 435:1262-1266.
65. Pfister S, Rea S, Taipale M et al. The histone acetyltransferase hMOF is frequently downregulated in primary breast carcinoma and medulloblastoma and constitutes a biomarker for clinical outcome in medulloblastoma. Int J Cancer 2008; 122:1207-1213.
66. Tryndyak VP, Kovalchuk O, Pogribny IP. Loss of DNA methylation and histone H4 lysine 20 trimethylation in human breast cancer cells is associated with aberrant expression of DNA methyltransferase 1, Suv4-20h2 histone methyltransferase and methyl-binding proteins. Cancer Biol Ther 2006; 5:65-70.

67. Di Croce L. Chromatin modifying activity of leukaemia associated fusion proteins. Hum Mol Genet 2005; 14 Spec No 1:R77-84.
68. Kondo T, Bobek MP, Kuick R et al. Whole-genome methylation scan in ICF syndrome, hypomethylation of nonsatellite DNA repeats D4Z4 and NBL2. Hum Mol Genet 2000; 9:597-604.
69. Matarazzo MR, Boyle S, D'Esposito M et al. Chromosome territory reorganization in a human disease with altered DNA methylation. Proc Natl Acad Sci USA 2007; 104:16546-16551.
70. Amir RE, Van den Veyver IB, Wan M et al. Rett syndrome is caused by mutations in X-linked MECP2, encoding methyl-CpG-binding protein 2. Nat Genet 1999; 23:185-188.
71. Ballestar E, Ropero S, Alaminos M et al. The impact of MECP2 mutations in the expression patterns of Rett syndrome patients. Hum Genet 2005; 116:91-104.
72. Yasui DH, Peddada S, Bieda MC et al. Integrated epigenomic analyses of neuronal MeCP2 reveal a role for long-range interaction with active genes. Proc Natl Acad Sci USA 2007; 104:19416-19421.
73. van Overveld PG, Lemmers RJ, Sandkuijl LA et al. Hypomethylation of D4Z4 in 4q-linked and non4q-linked facioscapulohumeral muscular dystrophy. Nat Genet 2003; 35:315-317.
74. Arnaud P, Feil R. Epigenetic deregulation of genomic imprinting in human disorders and following assisted reproduction. 2005; 75:81-97.
75. Petronis A. Epigenetics and twins, three variations on the theme. Trends Genet 2006; 22:347-350.
76. Fraga MF, Ballestar E, Paz MF et al. Epigenetic Differences Arise During the Lifetime of Monozygotic Twins. Proc Natl Acad Sci USA 2005; 102:10604-10609.
77. Javierre BM, Fernandez AF, Richter J et al. Changes in the pattern of DNA methylation associate with twin discordance in systemic lupus erythematosus. Genome Res 2010; 20:170-179.
78. Baranzini SE, Mudge J, van Velkinburgh JC et al. Genome, epigenome and RNA sequences of monozygotic twins discordant for multiple sclerosis. Nature 2010; 464:1351-1356.
79. Miao F, Smith DD, Zhang L et al. Lymphocytes from patients with type 1 diabetes display a distinct profile of chromatin histone H3 lysine 9 dimethylation: an epigenetic study in diabetes. Diabetes 2008; 57:3189-3198.

CHAPTER 2

CHROMATIN MECHANISMS REGULATING GENE EXPRESSION IN HEALTH AND DISEASE

Constanze Bonifer and Peter N. Cockerill

Section of Experimental Haematology, Leeds Institute of Molecular Medicine, University of Leeds, St James's University Hospital, Leeds, UK.
Emails: c.bonifer@leeds.ac.uk and p.n.cockerill@leeds.ac.uk

Abstract: It is now well established that the interplay of sequence-specific DNA binding proteins with chromatin components and the subsequent expression of differential genetic programs is the major determinant of developmental decisions. The last years have seen an explosion of basic research that has significantly enhanced our understanding of the basic principles of gene expression control. While many questions are still open, we are now at the stage where we can exploit this knowledge to address questions of how deregulated gene expression and aberrant chromatin programming contributes to disease processes. This chapter will give a basic introduction into the principles of epigenetics and the determinants of chromatin structure and will discuss the molecular mechanisms of aberrant gene regulation in blood cell diseases, such as inflammation and leukemia.

INTRODUCTION

The range of diseases found to have an epigenetic component responsible for aberrant gene regulation is steadily increasing and diseases of blood cells represent some of the best-defined models for studying this type of dysregulation. Many factors control the growth, differentiation and activation status of blood cells and when these are dysregulated the result can be either leukemia with aberrant growth and differentiation, or autoimmune and inflammatory diseases where the immune system is chronically active.

In this chapter we will introduce the basic concepts of chromatin structure and the processes that control gene expression by modifying chromatin. We will draw upon

Epigenetic Contributions in Autoimmune Disease, edited by Esteban Ballestar.
©2011 Landes Bioscience and Springer Science+Business Media.

examples from both our own work and the work of others to illustrate the role that chromatin and DNA modifications play in normal gene regulation and in blood cell disease. To introduce some of these concepts we will also discuss the consequences of the reprogramming of the transcriptional regulatory network in leukemic cells that result in abnormal patterns of epigenetic modifications within chromatin.

THE ROLE OF TRANSCRIPTION FACTORS AND CHROMATIN STRUCTURE IN ESTABLISHING PATTERNS OF GENE EXPRESSION

Gene expression programs are established during cell differentiation by the concerted actions of sets of transcription factors specific to each cell type and to their state of differentiation and activation. Transcription factors perform multiple functions: they recognize a specific DNA sequence, interact with other transcription factors binding to neighboring DNA-sequences or even several kilobases away,[1] respond to extracellular signals and most importantly, recruit nonDNA-binding factor complexes that cooperate to either maintain the active state, or initiate the establishment of an inactive state. These factors, in turn, exert their effects largely at the level of chromatin structure by creating permissive or nonpermissive states. The genome exists naturally in a repressed state by virtue of the fact that regulatory and coding DNA sequences are for the most part occluded by nucleosomes which assemble into highly condensed and inaccessible structures. Before a gene can be expressed, it is necessary to first create accessible sites for the binding of transcription factors required for transcription initiation and secondly, to modify the histones within nucleosomes and reorganize the higher order chromatin structure to create an environment permissive for the passage of RNA polymerases.

Gene expression programs are typically controlled by transcription factors that are expressed in a temporal sequence during differentiation. Factors such as RUNX1, GATA-2 and PU.1 play pivotal roles in enabling early stages in blood cell differentiation, whereas other factors are responsible for the differentiation of specific hematopoietic lineages. Regulators of differentiation are exemplified by factors such as GATA-3, T-bet and FoxP3 which play important roles in maintaining the balance between effector and regulatory T cells. Other specific classes of transcription factors only become transcriptional activators as a result of external signals. This is true for inducible factors such as NFAT, AP-1 and NF-κB that play essential roles in mediating responses to immune stimuli. Both the developmentally regulated and the inducible classes of transcription factors can contribute to an aberrantly active immune system.

In addition to exerting transient inducible effects, transcription factors can also introduce stably maintained chromatin alterations. In some cases, transcription factors can establish an imprint within chromatin, creating a memory of a previous stimulatory event which persists after inducible transcription has ceased. For example, we and others have evidence that immune or pro-inflammatory stimuli can induce the formation of modified chromatin structures that can persist many cell cycles after the stimulus is withdrawn and which can remain as long-lived imprints in memory T cells for example.[2,3] Alternatively, specific developmentally regulated transcription factors such as RUNX1 can initiate a cascade of events that become self-perpetuating during blood cell differentiation even after the subsequent removal of the differentiation initiating factor.[4,5]

BASIC FEATURES OF CHROMATIN STRUCTURE

The vast majority of the genome (~99%) exists as nucleosomes comprising ~146 bp of DNA wrapped around an octamer of histone proteins made up of two molecules each of histones H2A, H2B, H3 and H4.[6,7] As depicted in Figure 1, nucleosomes assemble in a step-wise manner by first loading two histone H3/H4 dimers as a tetramer onto ~80

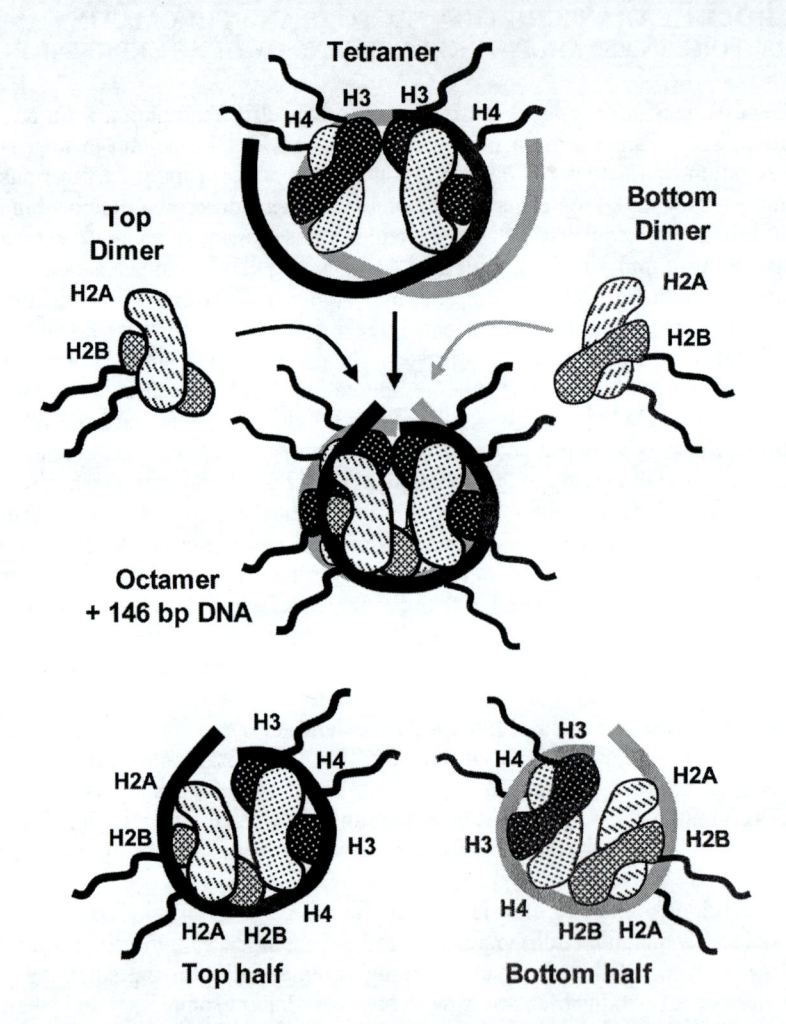

Figure 1. Nucleosome structure. Cartoon representation of the structure of the nucleosome based on the X-Ray crystal structure.[7] Nucleosomes are assembled in a stepwise manner from 146 bp of DNA which first recruits two histone H3/H4 dimers to form a tetramer and then two histone H2A/H2B dimers to form the histone octamer. In a nucleosome, the DNA makes 1.7 turns around the histone octamer. In the side-view of a nucleosome presented here, we have depicted the nearest 0.85 coil of DNA (73 bp) in black and the far-side 0.85 coil of DNA in grey. In the exploded view at the bottom, where the upper and lower faces of the nucleosome are separated, it can be seen that a nucleosome comprises two symmetrical halves. Each half contains one molecule of each of the four core histones which each make two major contacts with the DNA. The positively charged lysine-rich histone tails do not adopt a rigid structure but extend out from the nucleosome and have the potential to wrap around the DNA.

bp of DNA and then incorporating two histone H2A/H2B dimers to form a nucleosome particle comprising 146 bp of DNA coiled 1.7 times around the histone octamer core. This model illustrates the fact that nucleosome stability is maintained by multiple contacts along the entire length of the nucleosomal DNA, with each of the eight histone molecules mediating major contacts at two separate sites. It is also significant that this structure has the histone N-terminal tails protruding from the nucleosome core particle, because these tails are the sites of numerous covalent modifications that regulate the structure and function of chromatin.

Individual nucleosomes are organized into highly regular arrays where they are separated by linker regions of ~50 bp of DNA, to give an overall average repeat length of ~190-200 bp.[8-10] Chains of nucleosomes essentially never exist in a completely decondensed drawn out state, but are arranged in a zig-zag conformation within a highly complex higher order structure. Despite decades of investigation, the precise details of this structure remain elusive. At the first level of folding, nucleosomes coil into 30 nm diameter chromatin fibers (Fig. 2A),[8-11] which then assemble further as even more compact structures,[12] in which much of the DNA is inaccessible (Fig. 2). This higher order folding is mediated in part by histone H1 which occupies about 20 bp of the linker region between nucleosomes and in part by the positively charged histone tails that extend out from the nucleosome and most likely wrap around the DNA.[6]

Only about 1% of the genome exists in a decondensed accessible state in any one cell. These accessible regions exist as DNase I hypersensitive sites (DHSs)[13] where regulatory factor complexes have opened up localized regions of the chromatin fiber and in most cases this probably involves displacement or disruption of nucleosomes that would otherwise occupy these regions (Fig. 2B). It is also taken for granted that a passing polymerase must transiently create open regions of chromatin (Fig. 2C). This appears to be driven by chromatin remodeling factors and histone acetyltransferases (HATs) associated with the polymerase complex and is reversed by factors such as histone deacetylases (HDACs) recruited to chromatin that has just been transcribed (Fig. 2C).[14,15] One of the purposes of this cycle is to maintain transcribed genes in a predominantly condensed state so as to suppress cryptic promoters.[14]

The histone tails are subject to a bewildering number of posttranslational modifications. These include lysine acetylation, lysine and arginine methylation, serine and threonine phosphorylation, lysine ubiquitination, poly-ADP ribosylation, lysine sumoylation, arginine deimination and proline isomerisation.[16] Each modification is installed by different families of enzymatic activities, such as HATs, histone methyltransferases (HMTs), kinases or ubiquitin ligases. Depending on the transcriptional state, these modifications are removed by opposing enzymatic activities, such as HDACs and histone demethylases which, like the "writers" of histone modifications, belong to extended families of enzymes with different substrate specificity. Each histone modification serves a distinctive purpose to support either the maintenance of the active (e.g., histone H3 K9 acetylation and K4 methylation) or the inactive (e.g., histone H3 K9 methylation) transcriptional state.

In addition to creating binding sites for various cofactors, the modification of histones also has a direct effect on overall chromatin structure. For example, histone acetylation leads to the neutralization of the positively charged lysines in the histone tails and to a reduced level of compaction, as seen after acetylation of histone H4 K16 (Fig. 2).[17] Activation of enhancers and promoters, and the process of transcription, are also accompanied by the replacement of canonical histones with variant histones, such as H2AZ or H3.3 which

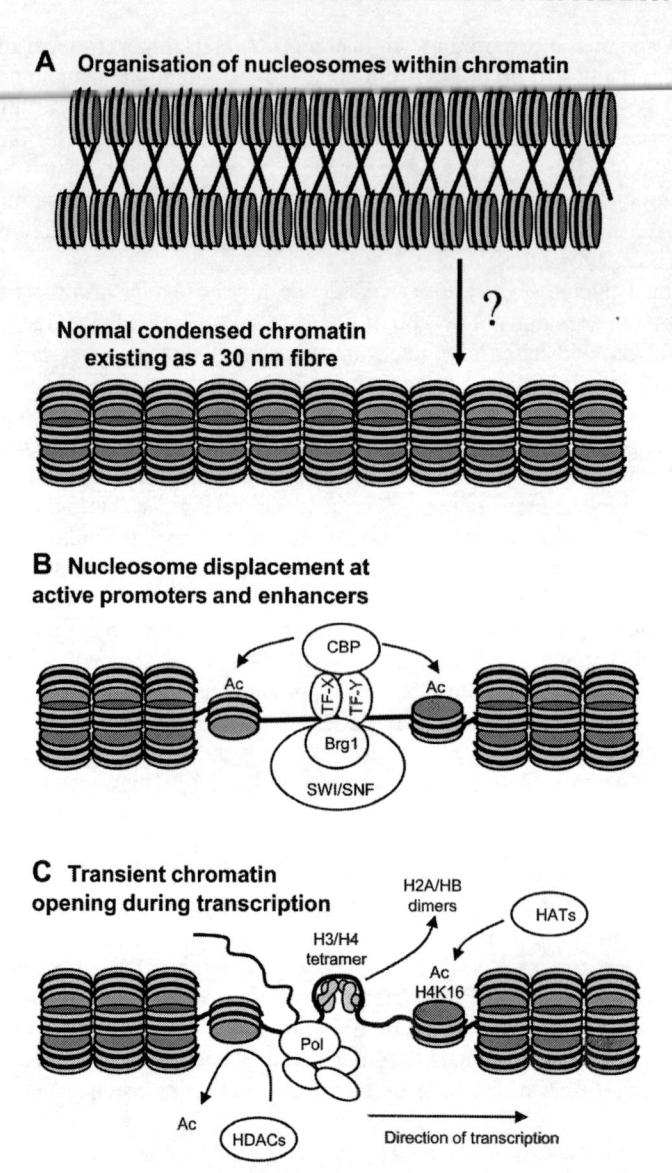

Figure 2. Hypothetical view of the organization and remodeling of the chromatin fiber. A) At the simplest level, nucleosomes are thought to zig-zag backwards and forward within chromatin. The precise details of chromatin fiber structure remain to be determined, but under physiological salt conditions, chromatin can be observed in vitro as a 30 nm diameter fiber. Chromatin is believed to be assembled into much more complex higher-order structures in vivo; B) At active promoters and enhancers it is thought that nucleosomes are either displaced by transcription factor (TF) complexes, or are so extensively modified that much of the nucleosomal DNA is rendered accessible. TFs recruits HATs such as CBP that create a more open chromatin structure and chromatin remodelers such as SWI/SNF that can directly disrupt and/or relocate nucleosomes; C) Elongating polymerases carry a variety of modifications and factors that act directly on chromatin. It is likely that these include HATs that can acetylate histone H4 K16, a modification sufficient to decondense chromatin and other factors such as HMTs that subsequently trigger the recruitment of HDACs such as Rpd3S that return chromatin to the deacetylated once the polymerase has passed.[14]

interact with reduced affinity and thus form less stable nucleosomes This facilitates the displacement of nucleosomes at promoters by the basal transcription machinery.[18]

THE ROLE OF EPIGENETIC MECHANISMS IN CELL DIFFERENTIATION

Research investigating the basis of cell differentiation in the hematopoietic system was instrumental in the development of the concept that stem cells and multipotent precursor cells activate extended sets of genes at low level prior to differentiation.[19] In this context it is important to note that lineage specification and the restriction of developmental potential involve not only the upregulation of genes important for the development of specific blood cell lineages, but that it is just as important to selectively silence lineage inappropriate genes that exist in an activated state in stem cells. This is a general principle of pattern formation that is common to all multicellular organisms and it implies that a regulatory machinery exists which maintains genes in their respective active and silent states and thus maintains cellular identity. It also follows that during the proliferative phases of cell differentiation, such "epigenetic" states have to be faithfully copied during cell division.[20] Another important principle of epigenetics is that such regulatory states can be maintained in the absence of the original initiator.[21] In the last years, significant progress has been made to identify and characterize the components of the epigenetic regulatory machinery. It is beyond the scope of this chapter to review its full complexity but the next chapters will review the general principles and discuss the role of the main players: DNA-methylation and histone modifications.

DNA METHYLATION

DNA methylation represents one of the most stable epigenetic modifications and plays a major role during development in maintaining specific patterns of gene expression.[22-25] In mammals, DNA methylation most commonly involves a symmetrical conversion to 5-methylcytosine on both DNA strands at CpG sequences. This modification is introduced by DNA methyltransferases (DNMTs) that include DNMT3a and DNMT3b which methylate cytosines de novo and DNMT1 which requires a methylated cytosine at one strand of newly replicated DNA and functions to maintain previously installed methylation states during replication.[22,26] DNMT3a contacts chromatin in cooperation with DNMT3L and the activating histone H3 K4 methylation modification blocks binding of DNMT3L, and thereby suppresses DNA methylation in active regions.[25,27,28]

Most of the CpG elements in the genome are, by default, maintained in the methylated state if they exist outside of active regions. A side effect of DNA methylation is that CG sequences are relatively rare in the genome, due to the propensity of 5-methylcytosine to mutate to thymidine. The genome also includes many promoter regions that are highly enriched in CpG sequences, termed CpG islands, that are resistant to DNA methylation. However, these CG islands are themselves significant targets for dysregulation in blood cell diseases and cancer.[29] For example, it is common to find aberrant DNA methylation within the promoter CpG islands of tumor suppressor genes in myelodysplastic disorders,[30] which are now sometimes treated with the "epigenetic" drug 5-Azacytidine to reduce genome-wide levels of DNA methylation.[31]

Active CG island

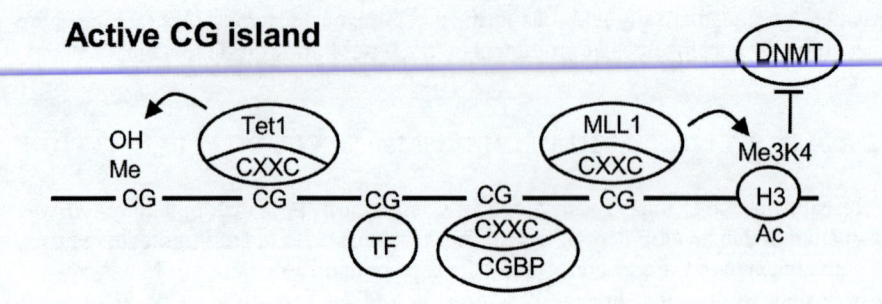

Repressed CG island

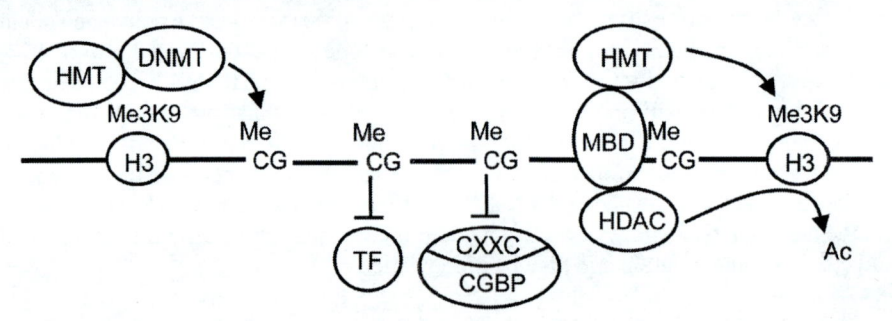

Figure 3. Mechanisms that regulate CpG island activation and repression. CG islands are normally maintained in an active state by specific transcription factors (TFs) and a wide variety of CXXC domain proteins that bind to non-acetylated CpG elements. The balance can be shifted from the activated state (top) to the repressed state (bottom) by the self-reinforcing modifications of DNA methylation and H3K9 methylation.

A recent unbiased genome-wide analysis of sequence patterns characterizing DNA methylation states identified specific transcription factor motifs at those CG islands that were resistant to de novo methylation. Furthermore, this resistance correlated with the fact that these sites were indeed occupied by these specific transcription factors,[32] strongly suggesting that the same factors are responsible for the protection of these sequences from DNA methylation (Fig. 3). How methyl groups are removed from DNA during normal mammalian cell differentiation is still not completely understood and various mechanisms have been proposed.[33]

It was recently shown that the balance between the methylated and nonmethylated DNA state at CpG islands is controlled in part by proteins containing CXXC motifs that bind to nonmethylated CG sequences (Fig. 3). CXXC domain proteins include the H3K4 HMT Set1 and Cfp1 (also known as CGBP or CXXC1) which associates with the H3K4 HMTs Set1 and MLL1.[34-37] CXXC proteins also include Tet1 which a member of the Tet family proteins that hydroxylate 5-methylcytosine.[38,39]

As modeled in Figure 3, the CXXC and HMT proteins provide potential mechanisms for maintaining regions of high CpG content in an unmethylated state. After Tet1 becomes recruited to nonmethylated CpG sequences it can presumably modify and eliminate any adjacent methylation of CpG sequences. Either MLL1 or the Cfp1/Set1 complex can also bind to nonmethylated CpG sequences[34,40] and introduce the H3K4 trimethylation mark (H3K4me3) which suppresses recruitment of the DNMT3a/DNMT3L complex.[25] The Me3H3K4 mark is normally associated specifically with transcribed regions,[37] but CXXC domains provide a mechanism to introduce this modification even in the absence of transcription. Cfp1 was recently shown to play a major genome-wide role in maintaining CpG islands in an active state, being required to introduce the H3K4me3 modification at CpG islands, and it was demonstrated that introduction of an artificial CpG island was sufficient to recruit Cfp1 and establish an active H3K4me3 domain.[34]

Conversely, CpG islands can also be repressed and maintained in a repressed state if they undergo DNA methylation and H3K9 methylation (Fig. 3). These modifications cooperate to maintain the repressed state by promoting recruitment of the H3K9 HMT G9a and DNMTs.[23-25] Once methylated, CpG islands bind proteins containing methylated methyl-CpG binding domains (MBDs) which recruit H3K9 HMTs and HDACs. However, mechanisms controlling the balance of methylation are highly complex with the same proteins in some cases involved in both activation and repression. Hence, Cfp1 can also recruit DNMT1 and loss of Cfp1 leads to a decrease, not an increase, in levels of DNA methylation within both repeat elements and single copy genes.[41] This may indicate that the net balance of Cfp1 function is different at CpG islands, where it is required to introduce H3K4me3, as opposed to interspersed CpG elements where it may promote DNA methylation. MBD1 and DNMT1 also each have both CXXC domains and methylated CpG binding domains meaning that they can drive repression of CpG islands if there is an absence of activating factors.[40]

Tet family proteins are also targets for mutations in blood cell diseases[42] and this could account for the aberrant methylation of CpG island promoters in myeloid malignancies.[30] The Tet2 gene is frequently mutated in Chronic Myelomonocytic Leukemia (CMML)[43,44] and the Tet1 gene (previously termed LCX) is involved in chromosomal translocations in Acute Myeloid Leukemia (AML).[45] Interestingly, Tet2 lacks a CXXC domain, meaning that another class of factor is required to direct Tet2 to CpG elements and this represents another potential point for epigenetic dysregulation.

HISTONE MODIFICATIONS MARKING THE INACTIVE TRANSCRIPTIONAL STATE

In the absence of transcriptional activators, the chromatin of genes adopts a heritable silent state by default, or even a heterochromatic state with distinct biochemical features. DNA of heterochromatic genes is highly methylated and compacted, and harbor inactive histone marks such as methylated histone H3 K9 or K27 which are deposited by the HMTs Su(var)3.9 and EZH2 respectively, the latter being a component of the polycomb family of epigenetic regulators. An important principle is that these DNA and histone modifications serve as binding sites for "readers" of the epigenetic code.[46] The best-characterized examples for such interactions are the recognition of methylated CGs by MBD proteins[47] and the binding of heterochromatin protein 1 (HP1) family members to trimethylated histone H3 lysine 9.[48,49] All of these proteins associate with highly cooperative macromolecular complexes that include histone and DNA modification enzymes which either re-install the inactive mark, or remove active marks and thus sustain an inactive chromatin structure.

This is exemplified by the findings that (i) DNMT1 and the methyl-binding protein MeCP2 both associate with histone deacetylases (HDACs), (ii) DNMT1 interacts with the H3 K9 HMT G9a[50] and (iii) HP1 interacts with both HDACs and DNMTs.[51,52]

Similar to DNA methylation, the aberrant deposition of inactive histone marks is a hallmark of disease processes. Since these modifications are normally highly dynamic and get rewritten depending on the transcription cycle and the presence and absence of extracellular signals,[53] the deposition of an inactive histone mark per se does not lead to permanent gene silencing. However, as described above, one of the hallmarks of cancer cells is the permanent silencing of CpG island promoters of important tumour suppressor genes by aberrant DNA-methylation. It has recently been shown that the binding of such sequences by polycomb complexes and the concomitant deposition of methylated H3 K27 predisposes associated genes to DNA methylation where they are finally inactivated,[54,55] again indicating that the gene silencing machinery operates in a highly cooperative fashion. These experiments also demonstrate that DNA-methylation is the final modification that locks genes into a permanently inactive state.[22]

CHROMATIN MODIFICATIONS ACCOMPANYING GENE ACTIVATION

Recent genome-wide analyses confirmed that histone modifications are deposited in a combinatorial fashion at the cis-regulatory elements of specific genes, reflecting their differential activities.[56,57] The fact that such patterns are not random, and change in response to extracellular stimuli,[58] already hints at the fact that the epigenetic regulatory machinery is directed to specific DNA sequences by sequence specific DNA binding proteins, and their cell type specific combinatorial action directs the differential deposition of histone modifications.

The architecture of the chromatin fiber is modified in many fundamental ways during the process of gene activation. In the first instance, the regulatory machinery gains entry to the ~1% of the genome that comprises the regulatory elements active in any one cell type by creating highly accessible nucleosome-free regions that exist as DHSs.[13] In most cases this involves the cooperative action of different transcription factors, but in some cases the creation of these DHSs is initiated by specialized pioneer factors that have the intrinsic ability to bind to chromatin compacted by histone H1.[59] Other specific factors, such as the transcription factors NFAT and NF-κB, are intimately associated with the induction of DHSs within promoter and enhancer elements in response to activation by immune and pro-inflammatory stimuli.[60,61] NFAT is a key mediator of T cell receptor (TCR) signaling, whereas NF-κB is a key mediator of pro-inflammatory signals such as bacterial lipopolysaccharide (LPS). These types of factors play a key role in creating access for and assisting the recruitment of other factors and represent a pivotal point at which the normal tight control over gene expression can be overridden in a disease context.

Once bound to DNA, transcription factors recruit a host of chromatin modifying activities. Besides the histone modification machinery described above, they also recruit ATP dependent nucleosome remodeling complexes such as SWI/SNF and ISWI that either disrupt or reposition nucleosomes and mobilize arrays of nucleosomes.[62-65] Remodelers can serve both to create nucleosome-free sites for regulatory factors and polymerases and to render nucleosome organization highly dynamic. Remodeling activities play essential roles in mediating inducible responses within the immune system and we have observed that NFAT-dependent enhancers function in part by mediating long-range mobilization of nucleosomes, creating a highly disorganized and dynamic nucleosome array.[66,67] In addition, we showed that transcription factors induced by inflammatory stimuli can activate promoters driving the expression of noncoding RNAs which alter the nucleosomal architecture of cis-regulatory elements by the process of transcription itself.[68] Many inducible transcription factors, including for example AP-1 and CREB, which mediate responses within the immune system, have the ability to recruit HATs such as CBP and p300. This typically leads to the creation of a hyperacetylated and more open state at promoters and enhancers.[62-65]

Similar to mechanisms maintaining the inactive state, histone modifications characteristic for active genes reinforce the active state by providing interaction modules for the transcription machinery. For example, HATs such as GCN5 and subunits of chromatin remodelers such as Brg1 possess bromodomains that recognize H3 K9 acetylation.[69,70] Similarly, H3 K4 trimethylation is recognized by PHD-finger domains as exemplified by that of TFIID which is part of the basal transcription machinery.[71] Moreover, it has recently been shown that this histone modification is required for the maintenance of an active transcriptional state during cell division.[72] However, for normal development it is of vital importance that complexes reinforcing the activated state are tightly regulated. One of the major causes of leukemia is the generation of aberrant epigenetic regulatory proteins as a result of chromosomal translocations. Fusing heterologous domains can lead to the aberrant targeting of activating complexes, as exemplified by a recent study investigating the fusion of the PHD finger of the histone demethylase JARID1A and Nup98.[73] The expression of such a dominant-negative fusion protein leads to a targeting of a nonfunctional complex to H3 lysine di/trimethylated sites where it blocks the demethylation of histones. This causes the maintenance of the active state and eventually, a block in cell differentiation and leukemia.

EPIGENETICS MEETS CHRONIC INFLAMMATION IN LEUKEMIA

One of the hallmarks of many cancers is their aberrant growth, which is based on the fact that many tightly regulated growth-controlling signaling processes are dysregulated and constitutively active in these cells. This is achieved by either autocrine/paracrine stimulation of growth factor receptors or the mutation of other molecules involved in transmitting such signals into the nucleus. In blood cells, this involves signaling molecules such as cytokines, cytokine receptors and kinases, as well as transcription factors integrating immune responses. For example, the direct activation of Ras pathways and/or the suppression or mutation of negative regulators of cytokine signaling pathways can lead to activation of genes such as GM-CSF and hypersensitivity to GM-CSF in myeloid malignancies.[74-78]

The consequence of the chronic activation of inflammatory signals is that transcription factors linking such signals to gene expression control are constitutively active, with the most important factor being NF-κB.[79] In human Hodgkin's lymphoma (HL), the constitutive activation of this transcription factor is required for the survival of leukemic cells.[80] In the majority of cases, HL cells originate from germinal center B cells, but have lost much of their B cell specific gene expression program.[81,82] Interestingly, these cells also express lineage inappropriate genes, including the receptor for colony-stimulating-factor 1 (CSF1R or c-FMS) which is the main growth factor receptor for the macrophage lineage.[82,83] Moreover, it was recently shown that these cells also express CSF-1 itself and this autocrine/paracrine stimulation is required for HL cell survival.[84] However, the most intriguing result from the same study was that aberrant expression of the *CSF1R* gene was not driven by its normal promoter, but originated from an aberrantly activated long terminal repeat (LTR) promoter of the THE1B family of repeats located 6.5 kb upstream of the normal transcription start site. LTRs are remnants of retroviral insertions that have remained in the germline. These elements are normally efficiently epigenetically silenced during embryonic development and this silencing is strictly maintained by DNA methylation and the action of corepressors recruiting HDACs that maintain the presence of inactive histone marks. Moreover, the activation of *THE1B* elements in HL cells was not restricted to one genomic location, but was a widespread phenomenon. As it turned out, HL cells have lost expression of the corepressor MTG8/CBFA2T3 (otherwise known as ETO2). In addition, *THE1B* elements contain functional binding sites for inducible transcription factors, including NF-κB, which are required to activate LTR-driven promoter activity. The artificial recreation of this situation in non HL cells is sufficient to activate LTR-driven expression, indicating that the loss of epigenetic control combined with constitutive activation of otherwise inducible transcription factors is sufficient to override the safeguards that normally protect cells from the activation of LTR promoters. The consequences of these events are cells of B cell origin that have hijacked myeloid-specific survival signals.

THE ROLE OF EPIGENETIC MECHANISMS IN AUTOIMMUNITY

The role of this chapter has up until now been to introduce basic concepts of chromatin structure and the epigenetic mechanisms that control the function of the genome in normal cells and in disease. However, we also need to at least touch on the role of epigenetics in autoimmunity, as this is the main theme of this volume, and many specific examples will be discussed in the following chapters. There is now abundant evidence that disturbance of epigenetic mechanisms in the immune system can lead to autoimmune disease, with perhaps the best example being Systemic Lupus Erythematosus (SLE),[85-87] which will be discussed in depth in this volume in Chapter 9. This is a disease where there is a prevalence of global DNA hypomethylation and demethylation of the regulatory elements of pro-inflammatory genes such as IL-4 and IL-6 in T cells.[85,88] Furthermore, DNA demethylating agents are able to induce lupus-like symptoms.[86] Abnormal patterns of histone acetylation are also found in T cells from lupus patients. Atopy is another condition where DNA demethylation of genes such as interferon gamma can contribute to autoimmunity.[85]

CONCLUSION

The few examples described in this chapter graphically demonstrate that the interplay of transcription factors with the epigenetic regulatory machinery is at the heart of many disease processes. They also demonstrate that the defects of this interplay are specific for each individual disease. The major challenge for the future will be to delineate the mechanisms common to aberrant gene regulation involved in individual disease processes and identify targets for their correction. A tall order.

ACKNOWLEDGEMENTS

Our laboratories are supported by Leukaemia and Lymphoma Research, Cancer Research UK, Yorkshire Cancer Research and the BBSRC.

REFERENCES

1. de Laat W, Klous P, Kooren J et al. Three-dimensional organization of gene expression in erythroid cells. Curr Top Dev Biol 2008; 82:117-139.
2. Gialitakis M, Arampatzi P, Makatounakis T et al. Interferon gamma dependent transcriptional memory via relocalization of a gene locus to PML nuclear bodies. Mol Cell Biol 2010; 30(8):2046-2056.
3. Mirabella F, Baxter EW, Boissinot M et al. The Human IL-3/Granulocyte-Macrophage Colony-Stimulating Factor Locus Is Epigenetically Silent in Immature Thymocytes and Is Progressively Activated during T-Cell Development. J Immunol 2010; 184(6):3043-3054.
4. Chen MJ, Yokomizo T, Zeigler BM et al. Runx1 is required for the endothelial to haematopoietic cell transition but not thereafter. Nature 2009; 457(7231):887-891.
5. Hoogenkamp M, Lichtinger M, Krysinska H et al. Early chromatin unfolding by RUNX1: a molecular explanation for differential requirements during specification versus maintenance of the hematopoietic gene expression program. Blood 2009; 114(2):299-309.
6. Zlatanova J, Leuba SH, van Holde K. Chromatin structure revisited. Crit Rev Eukaryot Gene Expr 1999; 9(3-4):245-255.
7. Luger K, Mader AW, Richmond RK et al. Crystal structure of the nucleosome core particle at 2.8 A resolution. Nature 1997; 389(6648):251-260.
8. Robinson PJ, Fairall L, Huynh VA et al. EM measurements define the dimensions of the "30-nm" chromatin fiber: evidence for a compact, interdigitated structure. Proc Natl Acad Sci USA 2006; 103(17):6506-6511.
9. Schalch T, Duda S, Sargent DF et al. X-ray structure of a tetranucleosome and its implications for the chromatin fibre. Nature 2005; 436(7047):138-141.
10. Williams SP, Athey BD, Muglia LJ et al. Chromatin fibers are left-handed double helices with diameter and mass per unit length that depend on linker length. Biophys J 1986; 49(1):233-248.
11. Woodcock CL, Frado LL, Rattner JB. The higher-order structure of chromatin: evidence for a helical ribbon arrangement. J Cell Biol 1984; 99(1 Pt 1):42-52.
12. Hu Y, Kireev I, Plutz M et al. Large-scale chromatin structure of inducible genes: transcription on a condensed, linear template. J Cell Biol 2009; 185(1):87-100.
13. Gross DS, Garrard WT. Nuclease hypersensitive sites in chromatin. Annu Rev Biochem 1988; 57:159-197.
14. Carrozza MJ, Li B, Florens L et al. Histone H3 methylation by Set2 directs deacetylation of coding regions by Rpd3S to suppress spurious intragenic transcription. Cell 2005; 123(4):581-592.
15. Zippo A, Serafini R, Rocchigiani M et al. Histone crosstalk between H3S10ph and H4K16ac generates a histone code that mediates transcription elongation. Cell 2009; 138(6):1122-1136.
16. Kouzarides T. Chromatin modifications and their function. Cell 2007; 128(4):693-705.
17. Shogren-Knaak M, Ishii H, Sun JM et al. Histone H4-K16 acetylation controls chromatin structure and protein interactions. Science 2006; 311(5762):844-847.
18. Jin C, Felsenfeld G. Nucleosome stability mediated by histone variants H3.3 and H2A.Z. Genes Dev 2007; 21(12):1519-1529.
19. Enver T, Greaves M. Loops, lineage and leukemia. Cell 1998; 94(1):9-12.
20. Probst AV, Dunleavy E, Almouzni G. Epigenetic inheritance during the cell cycle. Nat Rev Mol Cell Biol 2009; 10(3):192-206.
21. Berger SL, Kouzarides T, Shiekhattar R et al. An operational definition of epigenetics. Genes Dev 2009; 23(7):781-783.
22. Bird A. DNA methylation patterns and epigenetic memory. Genes Dev 2002; 16(1):6-21.
23. Berger J, Bird A. Role of MBD2 in gene regulation and tumorigenesis. Biochem Soc Trans 2005; 33(Pt 6):1537-1540.
24. Bird A. The methyl-CpG-binding protein MeCP2 and neurological disease. Biochem Soc Trans 2008; 36(Pt 4):575-583.
25. Cedar H, Bergman Y. Linking DNA methylation and histone modification: patterns and paradigms. Nat Rev Genet 2009; 10(5):295-304.
26. Chen T, Li E. Establishment and maintenance of DNA methylation patterns in mammals. Curr Top Microbiol Immunol 2006; 301:179-201.

27. Ooi SK, Qiu C, Bernstein E et al. DNMT3L connects unmethylated lysine 4 of histone H3 to de novo methylation of DNA. Nature 2007; 448(7154):714-717.
28. Jia D, Jurkowska RZ, Zhang X et al. Structure of Dnmt3a bound to Dnmt3L suggests a model for de novo DNA methylation. Nature 2007; 449(7159):248-251.
29. Sharma S, Kelly TK, Jones PA. Epigenetics in cancer. Carcinogenesis 2010; 31(1):27-36.
30. Boultwood J, Wainscoat JS. Gene silencing by DNA methylation in haematological malignancies. Br J Haematol 2007; 138(1):3-11.
31. Fandy TE. Development of DNA methyltransferase inhibitors for the treatment of neoplastic diseases. Curr Med Chem 2009; 16(17):2075-2085.
32. Gebhard C, Benner C, Ehrich M et al. General transcription factor binding at CpG islands in normal cells correlates with resistance to de novo DNA methylation in cancer cells. Cancer Res 70(4):1398-1407.
33. Zhu JK. Active DNA demethylation mediated by DNA glycosylases. Annu Rev Genet 2009; 43:143-166.
34. Thomson JP, Skene PJ, Selfridge J et al. CpG islands influence chromatin structure via the CpG-binding protein Cfp1. Nature 2010; 464(7291):1082-1086.
35. Ansari KI, Mishra BP, Mandal SS. Human CpG binding protein interacts with MLL1, MLL2 and hSet1 and regulates Hox gene expression. Biochim Biophys Acta 2008; 1779(1):66-73.
36. Tate CM, Lee JH, Skalnik DG. CXXC finger protein 1 restricts the Setd1A histone H3K4 methyltransferase complex to euchromatin. FEBS J 2010; 277(1):210-223.
37. Shilatifard A. Molecular implementation and physiological roles for histone H3 lysine 4 (H3K4) methylation. Curr Opin Cell Biol 2008; 20(3):341-348.
38. Tahiliani M, Koh KP, Shen Y et al. Conversion of 5-methylcytosine to 5-hydroxymethylcytosine in mammalian DNA by MLL partner TET1. Science 2009; 324(5929):930-935.
39. Loenarz C, Schofield CJ. Oxygenase catalyzed 5-methylcytosine hydroxylation. Chem Biol 2009; 16(6):580-583.
40. Allen MD, Grummitt CG, Hilcenko C et al. Solution structure of the nonmethyl-CpG-binding CXXC domain of the leukaemia-associated MLL histone methyltransferase. EMBO J 2006; 25(19):4503-4512.
41. Carlone DL, Lee JH, Young SR et al. Reduced genomic cytosine methylation and defective cellular differentiation in embryonic stem cells lacking CpG binding protein. Mol Cell Biol 2005; 25(12):4881-4891.
42. Mullighan CG. TET2 mutations in myelodysplasia and myeloid malignancies. Nat Genet 2009; 41(7):766-767.
43. Abdel-Wahab O, Mullally A, Hedvat C et al. Genetic characterization of TET1, TET2 and TET3 alterations in myeloid malignancies. Blood 2009; 114(1):144-147.
44. Jankowska AM, Szpurka H, Tiu RV et al. Loss of heterozygosity 4q24 and TET2 mutations associated with myelodysplastic/myeloproliferative neoplasms. Blood 2009; 113(25):6403-6410.
45. Ono R, Taki T, Taketani T et al. LCX, leukemia-associated protein with a CXXC domain, is fused to MLL in acute myeloid leukemia with trilineage dysplasia having t(10;11)(q22;q23). Cancer Res 2002; 62(14):4075-4080.
46. Jenuwein T, Allis CD. Translating the histone code. Science 2001; 293(5532):1074-1080.
47. Klose RJ, Bird AP. Genomic DNA methylation: the mark and its mediators. Trends Biochem Sci 2006; 31(2):89-97.
48. Lachner M, O'Carroll D, Rea S et al. Methylation of histone H3 lysine 9 creates a binding site for HP1 proteins. Nature 2001; 410(6824):116-120.
49. Bannister AJ, Zegerman P, Partridge JF et al. Selective recognition of methylated lysine 9 on histone H3 by the HP1 chromo domain. Nature 2001; 410(6824):120-124.
50. Esteve PO, Chin HG, Smallwood A et al. Direct interaction between DNMT1 and G9a coordinates DNA and histone methylation during replication. Genes Dev 2006; 20(22):3089-3103.
51. Smallwood A, Esteve PO, Pradhan S et al. Functional cooperation between HP1 and DNMT1 mediates gene silencing. Genes Dev 2007; 21(10):1169-1178.
52. Nan X, Ng HH, Johnson CA et al. Transcriptional repression by the methyl-CpG-binding protein MeCP2 involves a histone deacetylase complex. Nature 1998; 393(6683):386-389.
53. Metivier R, Penot G, Hubner MR et al. Estrogen receptor-alpha directs ordered, cyclical and combinatorial recruitment of cofactors on a natural target promoter. Cell 2003; 115(6):751-763.
54. Schlesinger Y, Straussman R, Keshet I et al. Polycomb-mediated methylation on Lys27 of histone H3 premarks genes for de novo methylation in cancer. Nat Genet 2007; 39(2):232-236.
55. Ohm JE, McGarvey KM, Yu X et al. A stem cell-like chromatin pattern may predispose tumor suppressor genes to DNA hypermethylation and heritable silencing. Nat Genet 2007; 39(2):237-242.
56. Wang Z, Zang C, Rosenfeld JA et al. Combinatorial patterns of histone acetylations and methylations in the human genome. Nat Genet 2008; 40(7):897-903.
57. Wang Z, Zang C, Cui K et al. Genome-wide mapping of HATs and HDACs reveals distinct functions in active and inactive genes. Cell 2009; 138(5):1019-1031.

58. Ghisletti S, Barozzi I, Mietton F et al. Identification and characterization of enhancers controlling the inflammatory gene expression program in macrophages. Immunity.
59. Cirillo LA, Lin FR, Cuesta I et al. Opening of compacted chromatin by early developmental transcription factors HNF3 (FoxA) and GATA-4. Molecular Cell 2002; 9(2):279-289.
60. Cockerill PN. NFAT is well placed to direct both enhancer looping and domain-wide models of enhancer function. Sci Signal 2008; 1(13):pe15.
61. Hogan PG, Chen L, Nardone J et al. Transcriptional regulation by calcium, calcineurin and NFAT. Genes Dev 2003; 17(18):2205-2232.
62. Mellor J. Dynamic nucleosomes and gene transcription. Trends Genet 2006; 22(6):320-329.
63. Shahbazian MD, Grunstein M. Functions of site-specific histone acetylation and deacetylation. Annu Rev Biochem 2007; 76:75-100.
64. Berger SL. The complex language of chromatin regulation during transcription. Nature 2007; 447(7143):407-412.
65. Li B, Carey M, Workman JL. The role of chromatin during transcription. Cell 2007; 128(4):707-719.
66. Johnson BV, Bert AG, Ryan GR et al. GM-CSF enhancer activation requires cooperation between NFAT and AP-1 elements and is associated with extensive nucleosome reorganization. Mol Cell Biol 2004; 24(18):7914-7930.
67. Bert AG, Johnson BV, Baxter EW et al. A modular enhancer is differentially regulated by GATA and NFAT elements that direct different tissue-specific patterns of nucleosome positioning and inducible chromatin remodeling. Mol Cell Biol 2007; 27(8):2870-2885.
68. Lefevre P, Witham J, Lacroix CE et al. The LPS-induced transcriptional upregulation of the chicken lysozyme locus involves CTCF eviction and noncoding RNA transcription. Mol Cell 2008; 32(1):129-139.
69. Hassan AH, Prochasson P, Neely KE et al. Function and selectivity of bromodomains in anchoring chromatin-modifying complexes to promoter nucleosomes. Cell 2002; 111(3):369-379.
70. Marmorstein R, Berger SL. Structure and function of bromodomains in chromatin-regulating complexes. Gene 2001; 272(1-2):1-9.
71. Vermeulen M, Mulder KW, Denissov S et al. Selective anchoring of TFIID to nucleosomes by trimethylation of histone H3 lysine 4. Cell 2007; 131(1):58-69.
72. Muramoto T, Muller I, Thomas G et al. Methylation of H3K4 Is Required for Inheritance of Active Transcriptional States. Curr Biol 20(5):397-406.
73. Wang GG, Song J, Wang Z et al. Haematopoietic malignancies caused by dysregulation of a chromatin-binding PHD finger. Nature 2009; 459(7248):847-851.
74. Bowen DT. Chronic myelomonocytic leukemia: lost in classification? Hematol Oncol 2005; 23(1):26-33.
75. Russell NH. Autocrine growth factors and leukaemic haemopoiesis. Blood Rev 1992; 6(3):149-156.
76. Birnbaum RA, O'Marcaigh A, Wardak Z et al. Nf1 and Gmcsf interact in myeloid leukemogenesis. Mol Cell 2000; 5(1):189-195.
77. Parikh C, Subrahmanyam R, Ren R. Oncogenic NRAS rapidly and efficiently induces CMML- and AML-like diseases in mice. Blood 2006; 108(7):2349-2357.
78. Ramshaw HS, Bardy PG, Lee MA et al. Chronic myelomonocytic leukemia requires granulocyte-macrophage colony-stimulating factor for growth in vitro and in vivo. Exp Hematol 2002; 30(10):1124-1131.
79. Van Waes C. Nuclear factor-kappaB in development, prevention and therapy of cancer. Clin Cancer Res 2007; 13(4):1076-1082.
80. Bargou RC, Emmerich F, Krappmann D et al. Constitutive nuclear factor-kappaB-RelA activation is required for proliferation and survival of Hodgkin's disease tumor cells. J Clin Invest 1997; 100(12):2961-2969.
81. Kuppers R. The biology of Hodgkin's lymphoma. Nat Rev Cancer 2009; 9(1):15-27.
82. Mathas S, Janz M, Hummel F et al. Intrinsic inhibition of transcription factor E2A by HLH proteins ABF-1 and Id2 mediates reprogramming of neoplastic B cells in Hodgkin lymphoma. Nat Immunol 2006; 7(2):207-215.
83. Bonifer C, Hume DA. The transcriptional regulation of the Colony-Stimulating Factor 1 Receptor (csf1r) gene during hematopoiesis. Front Biosci 2008; 13:549-560.
84. Lamprecht B, Walter K, Kreher S et al. De–repression of an endogenous long terminal repeat activates the CSF1R proto–oncogene in human lymphoma. Nature Medicine 2010; 16(5):571-579.
85. Szyf M. Epigenetic therapeutics in autoimmune disease. Clin Rev Allergy Immunol 2009.
86. Zhou Y, Lu Q. DNA methylation in T-cells from idiopathic lupus and drug-induced lupus patients. Autoimmun Rev 2008; 7(5):376-383.
87. Richardson B. DNA methylation and autoimmune disease. Clin Immunol 2003; 109(1):72-79.
88. Mi XB, Zeng FQ. Hypomethylation of interleukin-4 and -6 promoters in T-cells from systemic lupus erythematosus patients. Acta Pharmacol Sin 2008; 29(1):105-112.

CHAPTER 3

EPIGENETIC CONTROL OF LYMPHOCYTE DIFFERENTIATION

Eduardo Lopez-Granados

Clinical Immunology Department University Hospital La Paz, Paseo de la Castellana, Madrid
Email: elopezg.hulp@salud.madrid.org

Abstract: Lymphocyte differentiation from haematopoietic stem cells (HSCs) is a multi-step process in which lineage fate choices are made at crucial branch points. Plasticity of common precursors is evidenced by presence of transcriptionally favourable chromatin structures at several lineage-specific loci, making them poised for further priming and regulation. Down the differentiation tree, the interplay between lineage-specific networks of transcription factors and epigenetic modifications gradually decreases the multipotency ability of precursors and increases the compromise of cells within a particular lineage. The maintenance of a cell-specific phenotype is the result of sustained gene expression programs resulting from activation of lineage-specific and repression of lineage-discrepant loci. The peripheral functional specialisation of lymphocytes requires further plasticity, to allow differentiation onto short term effectors cells, or long term memory circulating and resident cells. Impaired differentiation of lymphocytes or deregulated or unbalanced production of certain lymphocytes subsets underlies the pathogenesis of lymphoproliferation, autoimmunity and possibly immunodeficiency. Understanding epigenetic mechanisms governing lymphocyte differentiation would allow future therapeutic interventions to prevent aberrant deviations or promote beneficial cell populations.

INTRODUCTION

Epigenetic marks modulate gene expression without variations in DNA sequence. The epigenetic profile defines the trancriptome and is particular of each cell type, determining cell identity and functional capacity. The two major epigenetic modifications are DNA methylation and histone modifications. DNA methylation occurs primarily at the 5′ position of CpG dinucleotides, a proportion of which cluster in CpG islands located in the promoter

Epigenetic Contributions in Autoimmune Disease, edited by Esteban Ballestar.
©2011 Landes Bioscience and Springer Science+Business Media.

of coding genes and are mostly unmethylated, whereas methylation leads to repression of gene transcription.[1] Increasing evidences demonstrate a role of epigenetic alterations in the aetiology of human diseases, like cancer and more recently autoimmunity.[2,3]

DIFFERENTIATION OF COMMON LYMPHOCYTE PRECURSORS

In adults, lymphocytes, like other blood cell types, are derived from haematopoietic stem cells (HSCs) resident in the bone marrow.[4,5] Moving down the haematopoietic differentiation tree, HSCs gradually lose self-renewing potential, as indicated reconstitution experiments of myeloablated recipients that allowed the identification of long-term and short-term capacity for multilineage reconstitution in different HSCs subpopulations.[6] Self-renewing is completely abrogated in multipotent precursors (MPPs) that can differentiate however into separate lymphoid and myeloid lineages by the initiation of differentiation programs in which gradually the capacity of generating different cells types is lost and the compromise with a given cell type increases.[7] In the classical model of haematopoietic differentiation, a common lymphoid progenitor (CLP) and a common myeloid progenitor (CMP) derived from MPPs were ascribed differentiation potential for each of the separate branches.[8] A fundamental role for the IL7 signalling in mouse lymphocyte development pointed to the expression of the IL-7Rα chain as a main marker differentiating the CLP and the MLP.[9,10] Interestingly, IL-7Rα[-/-] mice lack peripheral T and B lymphocytes whereas human with null mutations in this gene present T cell severe combined immune deficiency but circulating B lymphocytes. This constitutes an example of how, being an excellent tool for understanding of the immune system, conclusions extracted from mouse studies need further confirmation in human cells. CLPs are capable of forming all T, B and NK lymphocytes, whereas MLPs further subdivided in bipotent megakaryocyte/erythroid or macrophage/granulocyte progenitors.[11] In recent years, this model has been revised as several evidences from different research groups indicate that commitment to the lymphoid lineage is dependent on step-wise lost of pluripotency for other cells types. Before committing to the lymphoid lineage, MPPs lose myeloid differentiation potential. The first fundamental crossroad appears to be the loss of potential for megakaryocyte/erithroid differentiation and a first restriction step made by MPPs towards a progenitor with lymphoid and granulocyte/monocyte potential, the lymphoid-primed multipotent progenitors (LMPPs).[4] This population are precursors of early thymic progenitors (ETPs) that migrate to the thymus to start the T-cell differentiation and CLPs that lose macrophage/granulocyte differentiation potential and will further develop to B and NK lymphocytes (Fig. 1).

Specific haematopoietic differentiation programs appear to be determined within certain bone marrow microenviroments or niches, in which a complex interplay of progenitors, endothelial cells and the cytokine milieu promote each particular differentiation path. Location of HSCs and specific progenitors in niches is well orchestrated by chemokyne signalling.[4] The mechanisms that govern cell differentiation at molecular level consist in site specific interactions of networks of activating and repressing transcription factors, chromatin structure and epigenetic modifications. This complexity is far from being well characterised.

Gene expression analyses have revealed that HSCs and lymphoid and myeloid progenitors show certain promiscuity,[12,13] expressing both typical lymphoid and myeloid genes at a low level. This "lineage priming" appears to be a critical step for further

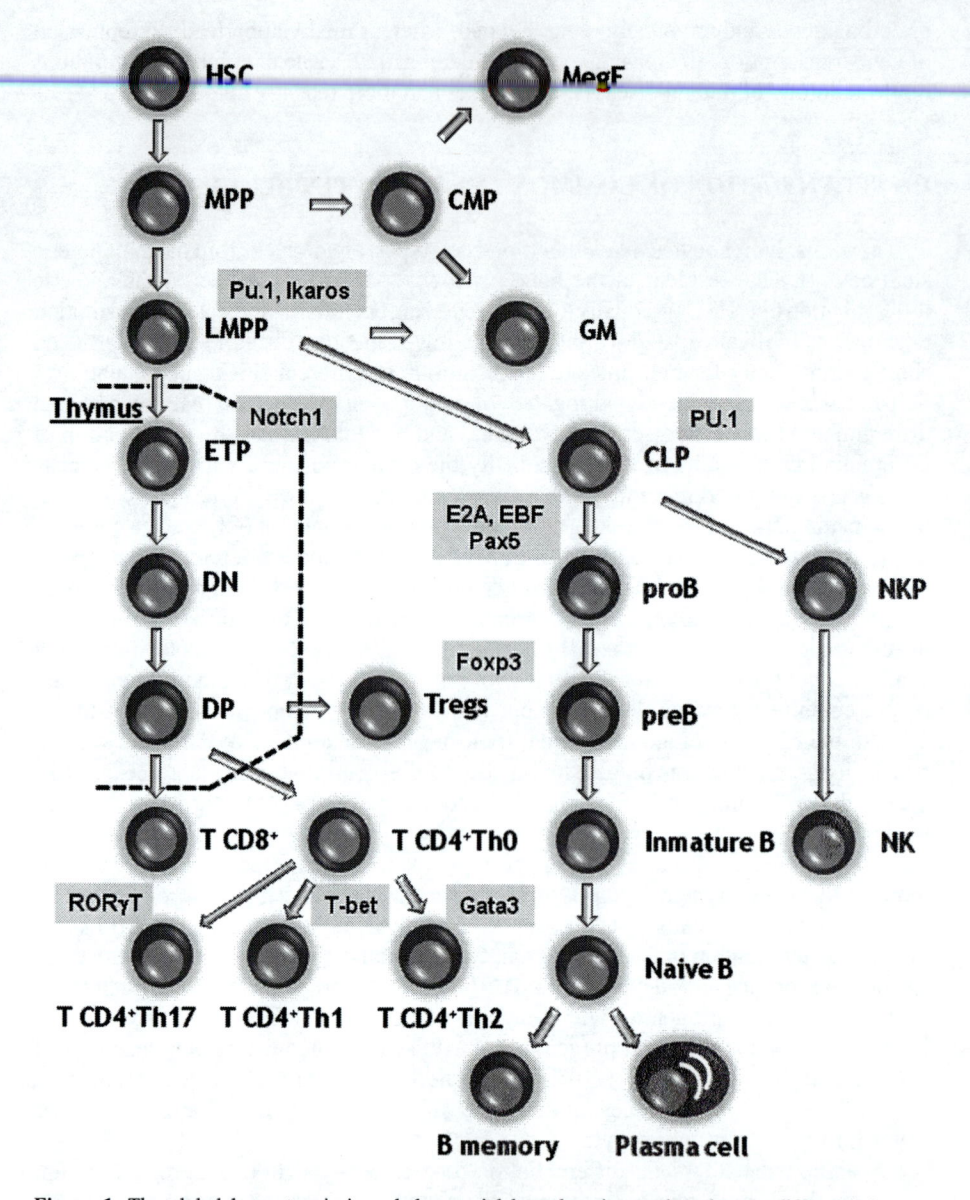

Figure 1. The global haematopoiesis and the crucial branch points at lymphocyte differentiation are depicted. Key transcription factors mediating cell fate commitments are highlighted in grey.

commitment, leaving lineage-associated genes exposed for recruitment of transcription factors and further modulation of chromatin in subsequent lineage differentiation steps.[12,14] Lineage commitment requires the activation of specific differentiation programs, in which both, activation of lineage-specific genes (lineage specification) and repression of genes associated with different other lineages (lineage commitment) are needed for the differentiation of a certain progeny.[12]

Gene expression programs are activated by recruitment of lineage-specific transcription factors and remodelling of chromatin structure mediated by epigenetic changes. Using chromatin immunoprecipitation (ChIP) assays and bisulfite sequencing (BS) analysis (see Chapter 1), changes in histone modifications and DNA methylation associated with transcriptional activity have been evidenced at lineage specific loci in mouse HSCs and MPPs.[15] Patterns of H3K4me2 are similar in multipotent populations, being more prominent at enhancer regions. This is consisting with a transcriptionally permissive status and promiscuous gene "priming" for expression. H3K4me3, a marker of transcriptionally active genes, was identified at the promoter or transcriptional start site (TSS) of cells with the highest gene expression of lineage specific loci and in their closest precursors. In contrast, H3K27me3 which has been associated with silent genes was prominent at the promoter of genes in the cells most distant to those expressing the genes.[15] Similar results have been obtained on multipotent human progenitors from cord blood,[16] in which many lymphoid and myeloid-associated genes are associated with acetylated H4 and H3 and H3K4me2 but not repressive H3K9me3 or H3K27me3 modifications. Progression in the differentiation path of multipotent cells towards the lymphoid or the myeloid lines is associated with loss of H3 and H4 acetylation and the presence of repressive H3K9 and H3K27 modifications at lineage non-associated genes. These results indicate that pluripotency is associated with permissive structures for gene transcription at multiple gene loci suitable for further modifications.[15,16] Decisions on the direction of the development are then linked to more stable modifications that will determine active and inactive genes.

EARLY T- AND B-CELL COMMITMENT

At LMPPs, the action of two key transcription factors, Ikaros and PU.1, tags cells towards lymphoid differentiation by differentiation of early thymic progenitors (ETPs) and common lymphoid progenitors (CLPs) that will differentiate to T, B and NKs cells respectively.[14] At the molecular level, both can act as repressors or activators of gene transcription albeit the epigenetic mechanism behind this activity is not well defined. The initiation of a B-cell progeny is driven by cooperation of the transcription factors EBF1 and E2A, which promote differentiation to the pro-B cell but are not sufficient for fully commitment to the B-cell path.[14] Pax5 is the essential transcription factor for full definition and maintenance of the B-cell phenotype, even in the periphery.[17] Conditional deletion of Pax5 in mature B cells induces de differentiation, plasticity and even T-cell generation.[18] The T-cell potential relies on the Notch signalling pathway, prevented by the transcriptional repressor LRF.[19] B-cell fate is rescued by inhibition of Notch signalling and Pax5 promotes the commitment to B cell partially by the inhibition of Notch.[17] The most consensuated opinion is that CLPs are LMPPs in the process of being committed to the B-cell fate.[14] Although is clear that T and B cells share a common progenitor, the precise point of divergence of the two lines is debated. CLPs can sustain T-cell production when injected in the thymus, but LMPPs already express chemokine receptors for trafficking to the thymus and sustained even higher T-cell production in vivo.[14] ETPs retain myeloid potential, indicating that are not derived from CLPs but more multipotent progenitors.[20,21] ETPs cease their B-cell differentiation potential upon Notch signalling, most likely by repression of B cell specific factors and also induced expression of key

T-cell transcription factors like Gata3 and TCF1.[22] Notch signalling has revealed a clue repressor of non-T cell programs.

REARRANGEMENT OF ANTIGEN RECEPTORS

The hallmark of T and B cells is the expression of extremely diversified antigen T cell and B-cell receptors (TCR and BCR respectively).[23] This requires a sophisticated process of site-specific creation of double-strand DNA breaks, recombination of VDJ genes by recombinant activating genes (RAG)-1 and 2 proteins that bind appropriate recombination signal sequences (RSS) and repair of the DNA breaks by the ubiquitous repairing machinery. The impairment of the recombination process leads to absence of T and B cells and severe immunodeficiency, or chromosomal aberrations and malignant lymphoproliferation, therefore the recombination process must be tightly regulated.[23] One level of regulation is the strict control of RAG gene expression at differentiation steps in which recombination occurs.[24] Other mechanisms must account for lineage and locus-specific accessibility to the recombinases. A chromatin opening model has been proposed, in which RSS are in closed non accessible chromatin until proper signals are received.[25,26] This is consistent with germline transcription of the heavy chain locus, a phenomenon largely known to be associated with recombination.

In early B-cell progenitors and before D_H to J_H recombination, H3 acetylation is abundant in a region extended from D_H to $C\mu$, extending later on to the V_H region. This is probably related with accessibility of the recombinases to the DNA. Additional modifications like H3K4me2 directly correlate with VDJ recombination in T and B cells, whereas H3K9methylation correlates inversely.[27-29]

Hypermethylation blocks recombination as has been shown with recombination substrates methylated in vitro.[30,31] In vivo, methylation could prevent recombination by regulating chromatin accessibility or masking RSS signals. In mouse, IL-7 signalling is crucial for lymphocyte development and IL7R$^{-/-}$ mice present severe immunodeficiency and absent $\gamma\delta$ T cells, due to lack of recombination at the $\gamma\delta$ locus.[32,33] This locus is methylated in the absence of IL-7R signalling and this could contribute to the recruitment of deacetylases, as suggested by the induction of recombination by the histone deacetylase inhibitor trichostatin A (TSA) in the absence of IL-7 signalling.[34,35] On the other hand, different evidences indicate that hypomethylation is necessary but not sufficient for recombination.[23]

Genomic methylation impacts not only on recombination. In vivo experiments of lineage specific demethylation targeting lymphoid-specific helicase Lsh revealed a role for methylation in lymphocyte development and immune response.[36] Lsh is a chromatin remodeler that links remodelling and DNA methylation. Lsh is mostly detected in precursors and activated lymphocytes.[23] Rag$^{-/-}$ mice reconstituted with Lsh$^{-/-}$ lymphocyte precursors showed circulating but reduced numbers of T and B lymphocytes in thymus, spleen and lymph nodes. Proliferative responses to polyclonal mitogens were reduced and T cells showed increased apoptosis upon stimulation.[36] Thus global hypomethylation does not prevent maturation and differentiation of lymphocytes, but impacts on their global production and survival.[23] Another important phenomenon associated with methylation in developing lymphocytes is allelic exclusion. This is a mechanism by which only one of the two alleles for the antigen receptor undergoes recombination.[37] Monoallelic expression ensures a single specificity for the antigen at the variable region of the antigen receptor, a fundamental principle for the antigen driven clonal expansion of lymphocytes.

GENERATION OF B CELLS

The combined activity of E2A, EBF and Pax5 promotes transcription of key B cell genes like mb-1 (Igα), B29 (Igβ), λ5 and VpreB (subrogate light chain) and cd19.[14] Proteins codified by those genes contribute, together with the rearranged μ heavy chain, to the generation of the B-cell receptor (BCR).[38,39] The mb-1 gene promoter is methylated at CpG dinucleotides in HSCs and EBF and E2A promote demethylation and accessibility to Pax5.[40] Chromatin remodelling also participate in this regulation, as recently demonstrated in culture B cells. Knockdown of different components of the SWI/SNF and Mi-2/NuRD complexes result respectively in inhibition or enhancement of Mb-1 transcription promoted by Pax5.[41] Epigenetic control of early B-cell development occurs also at the Cd19 locus.[39] An upstream enhancer is first remodelled in MPPs, facilitating binding of E2A and EBF and Pax5 in pro-B cells.[42] The expression of a functional pre-BCR is a crucial step in B-cell development.[38,43] Once the μ heavy chain has been rearranged it is tested by surface expression in conjunction with subrogate light chain (λ5 and VpreB). The μ heavy chain lacks signalling capacity that is provided by the cytoplasm motifs of Igα and Igβ to complete the pre-BCR. Signalling by this receptor is a fundamental checkpoint in early B maturation, by promoting proliferation and expansion of B precursors that have successfully rearranged the heavy chain gene and subsequent conversion to pre-B cells. Mutations in components of the pre-BCR (μ heavy chain, λ5, Igα and Igβ) or molecules that participate in pre-BCR signalling (BTK and BLNK) are associated in humans to block of B-cell differentiation at the pro-B stage, lack of mature B cells in the periphery and agammaglobulinaemia.[38,43] Efficient signalling through the pre-BCR in needed for the rearrangement of the immunoglobulin κ light chain locus and germ line transcription and histone modifications at the J kappa locus are induced by pre-BCR signalling.[44] Successful rearrangement of light chain will allow the expression of the BCR in the immature B cell that will leave the bone marrow and circulate in the periphery as a mature B cell.

Sustained expression of Pax5 is fundamental to maintain the B-cell commitment in the periphery. Pax5[-/-] KO mice express EBF and E2A, whereas in EBF[-/-] and E2A[-/-] mice Pax5 expression is repressed, indicating that Pax5 acts downstream EBF and E2A.[14] Pax5 has two promoters, a TATA-containing upstream promoter used by B cells and that is inactivated by dense CpG hypermethylation and a TATA-less promoter downstream used by other Pax-5 expressing cells that is repressed by histone deacetylation.[45] Additionally a potent enhancer in intron 5 that is methylated in stem cells becomes active in MPPs.[46] The promoter region is repressed by the Polycomb group in non-B cells and activated at the pro-B cell trough chromatin remodelling induced by EBF.[46] Both promoters and enhancer are fully active in mature lymphocytes. Pax5 maintains B-cell identity by activating B-cell specific and repressing non-B cell genes. ChIP-on-chip experiments in pro-B cells have revealed that Pax5-activated genes contain epigenetic activating marks, such H3 acetylation and H3K4me2 and H3K4me3. In Pax5[-/-] cells these modifications are very reduced or lost.[47-51]

PERIPHERAL B AND PLASMATIC CELL DIFFERENTIATION

Terminal B-cell differentiation and activation are dependent on antigen recognition by the BCR and co stimulatory pathways. Once a naive mature B cells is activated a further specialization decision is taken.[52] At this point some level of plasticity in B cells is present, as suggested by relatively low levels of histone methylation and high levels of histone acetylation.[53] Activated B cells can enter the germinal centre reaction for further modification of the antigen receptor; through somatic hypermutation (SHM) and immunoglobulin class switch recombination (CSR). This path is governed by the Bcl6 transcriptional repressor, expressed at low levels in mature naive B cells but rapidly up-regulated in some B cells after antigen stimulation. Alternatively the B cell can differentiate to plasma cells, producers of low affinity immunoglobulins. This occurs under the action of plasma cell master regulator Blimp-1. These processes are mutually exclusive. By repressing Blimp-1, Bcl6 prevents plasma cell differentiation. Plasma cell formation implies a tremendous change in B-cell phenotype and morphology. For this the complete B-cell expression program has to be repressed, including Pax5 and Bcl6 expression, VDJ recombination to prevent changes in antigen specificity and c-myc to ensure a resting state.[39,54] Expression of XBP-1, a transcriptional factor that regulates antibody secretion is induced by removal of its repressor Pax5.

The mechanisms of gene repression used by Bcl6 and Blimp-1 are varied. Bcl-6 interacts with MTA-3, a subunit of the repressor Mi-2/NuRD complex expressed in germinal centre B cells.[55] The function of this complex requires deacetylation of the central core of Bcl6 itself and of locus-associated histones to repress Blimp-1 expression. Once the germinal centre reaction is completed, if antigen persists plasma cells producing high affinity IgG, IgA or IgE are developed. Antigen stimulation induces MAP kinase-mediated Bcl6 phosphorylation and ubiquitinylation, targeting Bcl6 for proteosomal degradation.[54] This releases Blimp-1 repression and permits plasma cell differentiation. The repressive mechanisms used by Blimp-1 have only been defined by indirect studies. PRD1-BF1, a human ortholog of mouse Blimp-1 acts on fibroblasts and represses INFβ production in response to virus. Several mechanisms contributing to the repression have been identified: competition for promoter biding with activators, association with corepressors that use histone deacetylases or H3K9 methyltransferases.[54] The latest is likely to be the core of sustained gene expression pattern in plasma cells.

DEFECTS IN B-CELL DIFFERENTIATION: IMMUNODEFICIENCIES

Primary immunodeficiencies (PIDs) are an enormous and heterogeneous group of rare diseases affecting the immune system. Most syndromes are monogenic disorders that follow a mendelian inheritance. The syndromes arise as consequence of the role of the mutated gene in the immune cell differentiation. Examples are recombinant activating genes (RAG-1 and RAG-2) mutations in T- B- Severe Combined Immunodeficiency (SCID), or μ heavy chain in autosomal recessive agammaglobulinaemia with absence of mature B cells.[38] Others impair the expression or function of surface or intracellular proteins that are necessary for lymphocyte activation or regulated function and the redundancy or exclusivity of that function defines the severity of the clinical phenotype.

Candidate genes and genomic strategies have identified a causative gene for many of the PID syndromes (over 150 different genes identified to date), but in quite a few traditional genetics has not proved to be very successful identifying the missing gene function. Additionally, although a genetic cause had been identified in a syndrome an a primary constrain to the immune system is well defined, clinical immunologists frequently observe many different course and severities in patients with similar mutations, even within a family.[43]

A possible pathogenic relation between altered epigenetic control of gene transcriptional activity and immunodeficiency is exemplified on the rare immunodeficiency, centromeric instability and facial anomalies (ICF) syndrome. ICF syndrome is a rare autosomal recessive entity and the only human disease associated with mutations in a DNA methyltransferase. Specifically, ICF patients harbour mutations in the DNA methyltransferase 3B (DNMT3B) gene and present a primary immunodeficiency with hypogammaglubulinaemia, leading to recurrent respiratory and intestinal infections, impaired B-cell terminal differentiation and occasional T-cell defects, that can predispose to opportunistic infections.[56] Most ICF patients carry mutations in the catalytic domain of the DNA methyltransferase 3B (*DNMT3B*) gene. Marked hypomethylation of satellite centromere-adjacent heterochromatin is associated with decondensation and chromosomal elongations with formation of multiradials.[56] ICF patients present normal numbers of peripheral B cells, but these are only a naive phenotype, as no memory B cells or plasma cells are present in peripheral blood or the gut. Furthermore, this B cell pool is enriched in potentially self-reactive cells indicating that negative selection and clonal deletion mechanisms are impaired. ICF patients do not typically develop autoimmunity, suggesting that cells are anergic or silenced in vivo.[57] DNMT3B mutations cause deregulation of lymphogenesis associated genes expression. Upregulated genes are associated with low-level DNA methylation in normal cells that is lost in ICF cells concomitant with loss of repressive histone modifications, particularly H3K27m3 and gain of H3K9 acetylation and H3K4me3.[58] The advance in the understanding of the fine epigenetic events that govern lymphocyte differentiation and the analysis of those events in cells from ICF and PID syndromes could shed some light in those syndromes that do not seem to follow a mendelian inheritance or for which substantial heterogeneity in the phenotype is well observed.

CONCLUSION

A better definition of the epigenetic changes driving lymphocyte differentiation will clarify our understanding of the molecular bases of several immune related diseases. Contribution of epigenetic alterations to lymphoid malignancies is well established. Evidences for a similar importance in autoimmune conditions are also being unravelled. Research on immunodeficiency should follow the lead. Although evidences are still scarce, the conceptual frame for a role of epigenetic deregulation in primary immunodeficiency is already in place.

ACKNOWLEDGMENTS

Eduardo Lopez Granados is supported by the SAF2009-09899 research grant from the Spanish Ministry of Science and Innovation.

REFERENCES

1. Delcuve GP, Rastegar M, Davie JR. Epigenetic control. J Cell Physiol 2009; 219(2):243-250.
2. Hatchwell E, Greally JM. The potential role of epigenomic dysregulation in complex human disease. Trends Genet 2007; 23(11):588-595.
3. Javierre BM, Esteller M, Ballestar E. Epigenetic connections between autoimmune disorders and haematological malignancies. Trends Immunol 2008; 29(12):616-623.
4. Lai AY, Kondo M. T and B lymphocyte differentiation from hematopoietic stem cell. Semin Immunol 2008; 20(4):207-212.
5. Kondo M, Weissman IL, Akashi K. Identification of clonogenic common lymphoid progenitors in mouse bone marrow. Cell 1997; 91(5):661-672.
6. Christensen JL, Weissman IL. Flk-2 is a marker in hematopoietic stem cell differentiation: a simple method to isolate long-term stem cells. Proc Natl Acad Sci USA 2001; 98(25):14541-14546.
7. Morrison SJ, Wandycz AM, Hemmati HD et al. Identification of a lineage of multipotent hematopoietic progenitors. Development 1997; 124(10):1929-1939.
8. Akashi K, Traver D, Miyamoto T et al. A clonogenic common myeloid progenitor that gives rise to all myeloid lineages. Nature 2000; 404(6774):193-197.
9. Peschon JJ, Morrissey PJ, Grabstein KH et al. Early lymphocyte expansion is severely impaired in interleukin 7 receptor-deficient mice. J Exp Med 1994; 180(5):1955-1960.
10. von Freeden-Jeffry U, Vieira P, Lucian LA et al. Lymphopenia in interleukin (IL)-7 gene-deleted mice identifies IL-7 as a nonredundant cytokine. J Exp Med 1995; 181(4):1519-1526.
11. Lai AY, Kondo M. Asymmetrical lymphoid and myeloid lineage commitment in multipotent hematopoietic progenitors. J Exp Med 2006; 203(8):1867-1873.
12. Kioussis D, Georgopoulos K. Epigenetic flexibility underlying lineage choices in the adaptive immune system. Science 2007; 317(5838):620-622.
13. Buza-Vidas N, Luc S, Jacobsen SE. Delineation of the earliest lineage commitment steps of haematopoietic stem cells: new developments, controversies and major challenges. Curr Opin Hematol 2007; 14(4):315-321.
14. Dias S, Xu W, McGregor S et al. Transcriptional regulation of lymphocyte development. Curr Opin Genet Dev 2008; 18(5):441-448.
15. Attema JL, Papathanasiou P, Forsberg EC et al. Epigenetic characterization of hematopoietic stem cell differentiation using miniChIP and bisulfite sequencing analysis. Proc Natl Acad Sci USA 2007; 104(30):12371-12376.
16. Maes J, Maleszewska M, Guillemin C et al. Lymphoid-affiliated genes are associated with active histone modifications in human hematopoietic stem cells. Blood 2008; 112(7):2722-2729.
17. Souabni A, Cobaleda C, Schebesta M et al. Pax5 promotes B lymphopoiesis and blocks T-cell development by repressing Notch1. Immunity 2002; 17(6):781-793.
18. Cobaleda C, Jochum W, Busslinger M. Conversion of mature B-cells into T-cells by dedifferentiation to uncommitted progenitors. Nature 2007; 449(7161):473-477.
19. Maeda T, Merghoub T, Hobbs RM et al. Regulation of B versus T lymphoid lineage fate decision by the proto-oncogene LRF. Science 2007; 316(5826):860-866.
20. Wada H, Masuda K, Satoh R et al. Adult T-cell progenitors retain myeloid potential. Nature 2008; 452(7188):768-772.
21. Bell JJ, Bhandoola A. The earliest thymic progenitors for T-cells possess myeloid lineage potential. Nature 2008; 452(7188):764-767.
22. Franco CB, Scripture-Adams DD, Proekt I et al. Notch/Delta signaling constrains reengineering of pro-T cells by PU.1. Proc Natl Acad Sci USA 2006; 103(32):11993-11998.
23. Muegge K, Young H, Ruscetti F et al. Epigenetic control during lymphoid development and immune responses: aberrant regulation, viruses and cancer. Ann NY Acad Sci 2003; 983:55-70.
24. Nagaoka H, Yu W, Nussenzweig MC. Regulation of RAG expression in developing lymphocytes. Curr Opin Immunol 2000; 12(2):187-190.
25. Yancopoulos GD, Alt FW. Developmentally controlled and tissue-specific expression of unrearranged VH gene segments. Cell 1985; 40(2):271-281.
26. Stanhope-Baker P, Hudson KM, Shaffer AL et al. Cell type-specific chromatin structure determines the targeting of V(D)J recombinase activity in vitro. Cell 1996; 85(6):887-897.
27. Schlissel MS. Regulating antigen-receptor gene assembly. Nat Rev Immunol 2003; 3(11):890-899.
28. Bergman Y, Fisher A, Cedar H. Epigenetic mechanisms that regulate antigen receptor gene expression. Curr Opin Immunol 2003; 15(2):176-181.
29. Chowdhury D, Sen R. Stepwise activation of the immunoglobulin mu heavy chain gene locus. EMBO J 2001; 20(22):6394-6403.

30. Cherry SR, Baltimore D. Chromatin remodeling directly activates V(D)J recombination. Proc Natl Acad Sci USA 1999; 96(19):10788-10793.
31. Hsieh CL, Gauss G, Lieber MR. Replication, transcription, CpG methylation and DNA topology in V(D)J recombination. Curr Top Microbiol Immunol 1992; 182:125-135.
32. Hofmeister R, Khaled AR, Benbernou N et al. Interleukin-7: physiological roles and mechanisms of action. Cytokine Growth Factor Rev 1999; 10(1):41-60.
33. Huang J, Muegge K. Control of chromatin accessibility for V(D)J recombination by interleukin-7. J Leukoc Biol 2001; 69(6):907-911.
34. Maki K, Sunaga S, Ikuta K. The V-J recombination of T-cell receptor-gamma genes is blocked in interleukin-7 receptor-deficient mice. J Exp Med 1996; 184(6):2423-2427.
35. Durum SK, Candeias S, Nakajima H et al. Interleukin 7 receptor control of T-cell receptor gamma gene rearrangement: role of receptor-associated chains and locus accessibility. J Exp Med 1998; 188(12):2233-2241.
36. Geiman TM, Muegge K. Lsh, an SNF2/helicase family member, is required for proliferation of mature Tlymphocytes. Proc Natl Acad Sci USA 2000; 97(9):4772-4777.
37. Mostoslavsky R, Kirillov A, Ji YH et al. Demethylation and the establishment of kappa allelic exclusion. Cold Spring Harb Symp Quant Biol 1999; 64:197-206.
38. Lopez Granados E, Porpiglia AS, Hogan MB et al. Clinical and molecular analysis of patients with defects in micro heavy chain gene. J Clin Invest 2002; 110(7):1029-1035.
39. Parra M. Epigenetic events during B lymphocyte development. Epigenetics 2009; 4(7):462-468.
40. Maier H, Ostraat R, Gao H et al. Early B-cell factor cooperates with Runx1 and mediates epigenetic changes associated with mb-1 transcription. Nat Immunol 2004; 5(10):1069-1077.
41. Gao H, Lukin K, Ramirez J et al. Opposing effects of SWI/SNF and Mi-2/NuRD chromatin remodeling complexes on epigenetic reprogramming by EBF and Pax5. Proc Natl Acad Sci USA 2009; 106(27):11258-11263.
42. Walter K, Bonifer C, Tagoh H. Stem cell-specific epigenetic priming and B-cell-specific transcriptional activation at the mouse Cd19 locus. Blood 2008; 112(5):1673-1682.
43. Lopez-Granados E, Perez de Diego R, Ferreira Cerdan A et al. A genotype-phenotype correlation study in a group of 54 patients with X-linked agammaglobulinemia. J Allergy Clin Immunol 2005; 116(3):690-697.
44. Geier JK, Schlissel MS. PreBCR signals and the control of Ig gene rearrangements. Semin Immunol 2006; 18(1):31-39.
45. Danbara M, Kameyama K, Higashihara M et al. DNA methylation dominates transcriptional silencing of Pax5 in terminally differentiated B-cell lines. Mol Immunol 2002; 38(15):1161-1166.
46. Decker T, Pasca di Magliano M, McManus S et al. Stepwise activation of enhancer and promoter regions of the B-cell commitment gene Pax5 in early lymphopoiesis. Immunity 2009; 30(4):508-520.
47. Schebesta A, McManus S, Salvagiotto G et al. Transcription factor Pax5 activates the chromatin of key genes involved in B-cell signaling, adhesion, migration and immune function. Immunity 2007; 27(1):49-63.
48. Cobaleda C, Schebesta A, Delogu A et al. Pax5: the guardian of B-cell identity and function. Nat Immunol 2007; 8(5):463-470.
49. Delogu A, Schebesta A, Sun Q et al. Gene repression by Pax5 in B-cells is essential for blood cell homeostasis and is reversed in plasma cells. Immunity 2006; 24(3):269-281.
50. Pridans C, Holmes ML, Polli M et al. Identification of Pax5 target genes in early B-cell differentiation. J Immunol 2008; 180(3):1719-1728.
51. Holmes ML, Pridans C, Nutt SL. The regulation of the B-cell gene expression programme by Pax5. Immunol Cell Biol 2008; 86(1):47-53.
52. Calame KL, Lin KI, Tunyaplin C. Regulatory mechanisms that determine the development and function of plasma cells. Annu Rev Immunol 2003; 21:205-230.
53. Baxter J, Sauer S, Peters A et al. Histone hypomethylation is an indicator of epigenetic plasticity in quiescent lymphocytes. EMBO J 2004; 23(22):4462-4472.
54. Su IH, Tarakhovsky A. Epigenetic control of B-cell differentiation. Semin Immunol 2005; 17(2):167-172.
55. Fujita N, Jaye DL, Geigerman C et al. MTA3 and the Mi-2/NuRD complex regulate cell fate during B lymphocyte differentiation. Cell 2004; 119(1):75-86.
56. Ehrlich M, Buchanan KL, Tsien F et al. DNA methyltransferase 3B mutations linked to the ICF syndrome cause dysregulation of lymphogenesis genes. Hum Mol Genet 2001; 10(25):2917-2931.
57. BlancoBetancourt CE, Moncla A, Milili M et al. Defective B-cell-negative selection and terminal differentiation in the ICF syndrome. Blood 2004; 103(7):2683-2690.
58. Jin B, Tao Q, Peng J et al. DNA methyltransferase 3B (DNMT3B) mutations in ICF syndrome lead to altered epigenetic modifications and aberrant expression of genes regulating development, neurogenesis and immune function. Hum Mol Genet 2008; 17(5):690-709.

CHAPTER 4

EPIGENETIC CONTROL IN IMMUNE FUNCTION

Peter J. van den Elsen,*[1,2] Marja C.J.A. van Eggermond[1]
and Rutger J. Wierda[1]

[1]Department of Immunohematology and Blood Transfusion, Leiden University Medical Center, Leiden, The Netherlands; [2]Department of Pathology, VU University Medical Center, Amsterdam, The Netherlands
*Corresponding Author: Peter J. van den Elsen—Email: pjvdelsen@lumc.nl

Abstract: This chapter describes recent advances in our understanding how epigenetic events control immune functions with emphasis on transcriptional regulation of *major histocompatibility complex Class I (MHC-I)* and *Class II (MHC-II)* genes. MHC-I and MHC-II molecules play an essential role in the adaptive immune response by virtue of their ability to present peptides, respectively to CD8[+] and CD4[+] T cells. Central to the onset of an adequate immune response to pathogens is the presentation of pathogen-derived peptides in the context of MHC-II molecules by antigen presenting cells (APCs) to CD4[+] T cells of the immune system. In particular dendritic cells are highly specialized APCs that are capable to activate naïve T cells. Given their central role in adaptive immunity, *MHC-I* and *MHC-II* genes are regulated in a tight fashion at the transcriptional level to meet with local requirements of an effective antigen-specific immune response. In these regulatory processes the *MHC2TA* encoded Class II transactivator (CIITA) plays a crucial role. CIITA is essential for transcriptional activation of all *MHC-II* genes, whereas it plays an ancillary function in the transcriptional control of *MHC-I* genes. The focus of this chapter therefore will be on the transcription factors that interact with conserved cis-acting promoter elements and epigenetic mechanisms that modulate cell type-specific regulation of *MHC-I, MHC-II* and *MHC2TA* genes. Furthermore, we will also briefly discuss how genetic and epigenetic mechanisms contribute to T helper cell differentiation.

Epigenetic Contributions in Autoimmune Disease, edited by Esteban Ballestar.
©2011 Landes Bioscience and Springer Science+Business Media.

INTRODUCTION

The products of the *MHC Class I (MHC-I)* and *MHC Class II (MHC-II)* genes encode cell-surface glycoproteins involved in the binding and presentation of antigenic peptides to the T-cell receptors (TCRs) of T-lymphocytes. MHC-I proteins present peptides from endogenous sources, such as those derived from viruses, to CD8[+] T cells, whereas MHC-II molecules mainly present peptides from exogenous sources, such as those derived from extracellular pathogens, to CD4[+] T cells. These tri-molecular interactions of MHC, peptide and TCR are central to the generation of antigen-specific immune responses.

The *MHC-I* gene cluster encodes the highly polymorphic classical MHC-I molecules (Human Leukocyte Antigen (HLA)-A, -B and -C) and the less polymorphic nonclassical MHC-Ib molecules (HLA-E, -F and -G). Whereas the classical MHC-I molecules play essential roles in the detection and elimination of virus-infected cells, tumor cells and transplanted allogeneic cells, the MHC-Ib molecules have specialized immune regulatory functions (reviewed in 1). All cell surface expressed MHC-I and MHC-Ib molecules are associated with the nonpolymorphic β2-microglobulin. The MHC-II genes encode the polymorphic HLA-DR, -DQ and -DP molecules, which are expressed as α- and β-chain heterodimers on the cell surface. MHC-II molecules are central in the initiation of cellular and humoral immune responses, but they have also been implicated as contributing factors for a variety of autoimmune disorders. In contrast to MHC-I molecules, which are expressed in a constitutive fashion on almost all nucleated cells, the constitutive expression of MHC-II molecules is tissue-specific and is restricted to professional antigen presenting cells (APCs) of the immune system (reviewed in ref. 1). These APCs include dendritic cells, macrophages and B cells. All other cell types lack constitutive expression of MHC-II molecules, but their expression can be induced in an environment rich in inflammatory cytokines of which IFNγ is the most potent, or upon activation, such as in human T cells.[2] Because of their crucial role in the adaptive immune response, the genes encoding MHC-I and MHC-II molecules are tightly regulated by genetic and epigenetic mechanisms at the transcriptional level to provide an effective immune response against pathogens.

In its natural state, DNA is packaged into chromatin, a highly organized and dynamic protein-DNA complex, which consists of DNA, histones and nonhistone proteins. The fundamental subunit of chromatin, the nucleosome, is composed of an octamer of four core histones: two each of H2A, H2B, H3 and H4 surrounded by 146 bp of DNA.[3] Epigenetic changes are modifications in the architecture of chromatin without a change in the DNA sequence and determine the accessibility of chromatin. In this way, global gene activation and local control of gene-specific transcription is exerted by components of the epigenetic machinery. Methylation of DNA at CpG dinucleotides and modification or rearrangement of nucleosomes, which include covalent posttranslational modifications of histone tails, are key epigenetic chromatin marks.[4-6] Epigenetic modifications of histone tails include amongst others acetylation and methylation of lysine residues, phosphorylation of serine residues and methylation of arginine residues. The various histone modifications form a code which is read by nonhistone proteins and have varying effects on chromatin structure and gene accessibility.[4] As a rule of thumb, conformationally relaxed chromatin (euchromatin) is a hallmark of potentially active genes and is associated with hypomethylation of CpG dinucleotides in DNA and acetylated histones. Compact chromatin (heterochromatin) is associated with transcriptionally silent genes and is associated with DNA hypermethylation at CpG dinucleotides and nonacetylated histones. The influence of histone methylation on gene expression depends on the exact lysine residue methylated and the number of added methyl groups.[7-11]

These chromatin modifications are exerted by epigenetic regulators such as DNA methyltransferases (DNMTs) and lysine acetyltransferases (KATs) and lysine methyltransferases (KMTs), which are increasingly being implicated as direct or indirect components in the regulation of expression of immune and other (tissue)-specific genes. Methylation and acetylation histone modifications are reversible. Lysine deacetylases (KDACs) and sirtuins (Sirt) remove acetylation modifications, whereas lysine demethylases (KDMs) remove methylation modifications.[12-15] In this way these enzymes promote a return to respectively repressive or active chromatin structure. In addition to this, histone and DNA modification activities are intimately linked. This is exemplified by the finding that triple methylated lysine 9 in histone H3 (H3K9me3) creates a binding platform for the various Heterochromatin Protein-1 (HP1) isoforms, which associate with Dnmt-1, Dnmt3a and Dnmt3b.[7,16-19] In addition, the KMTase Enhancer of Zeste Homologue-2 (EZH2 or KMT6), which trimethylates lysine 27 in histone H3 (H3K27me3), interacts with Dnmt's and in this way EZH2 recruits Dnmt activities to target promoters for CpG methylation.[20] As a result, these reversible epigenetic processes fine-tune gene expression patterns required for fundamental processes in the immune system such as cell activation, proliferation and differentiation. Moreover, it has also become apparent in recent years that many inflammatory disorders, including atherosclerosis, have an epigenetic component contributing to the disease.[21]

In the next paragraphs we will discuss the genetic and epigenetic mechanisms that direct transcriptional regulation of genes devoted to antigen presentation and to differentiation of T helper cells.

TRANSCRIPTIONAL REGULATION OF *MHC* GENES

Activation of *MHC-I* genes, with the exception of *HLA-G*, is mediated by several conserved regulatory elements within the various promoters: enhancer A, IFN-stimulated response element (ISRE) and the SXY-module (comprising the S, X1, X2 and Y-boxes). These conserved regulatory elements play an important role in the inducible and constitutive expression of *MHC-I* genes (reviewed in ref. 1). Of these regulatory elements, the SXY-module is also present is the promoters of *MHC-II* genes (Fig. 1). The sequence and stereo-specific alignment of the various boxes in the SXY-module is highly conserved and critical for its functioning in constitutive and inducible-transcriptional activation of *MHC-I* and *MHC-II* genes.[22,23] The SXY-module is cooperatively bound by a multi-protein complex containing regulatory factor X (RFX; consisting of RFX5, RFXB/ANK and RFXAP),[24-27] cyclic-AMP response element binding protein (CREB)/activating transcription factor (ATF)[22,28] and nuclear factor Y (NFY).[29,30] This complex acts as an enhanceosome driving transactivation of these genes.[22,31] In addition to these factors that assemble directly to the X1/X2 and Y box sequences, the co-activator CIITA (Class II transactivator) is also required. CIITA is essential for *MHC-II* transcription,[32] whilst it contributes to the activation of MHC-I promoters.[33] Given the essential role of CIITA in *MHC-II* transcription, constitutive expression of CIITA coincides with constitutive MHC-II molecule expression in APCs of which dendritic cells are the most efficient APCs. In all other types of cells

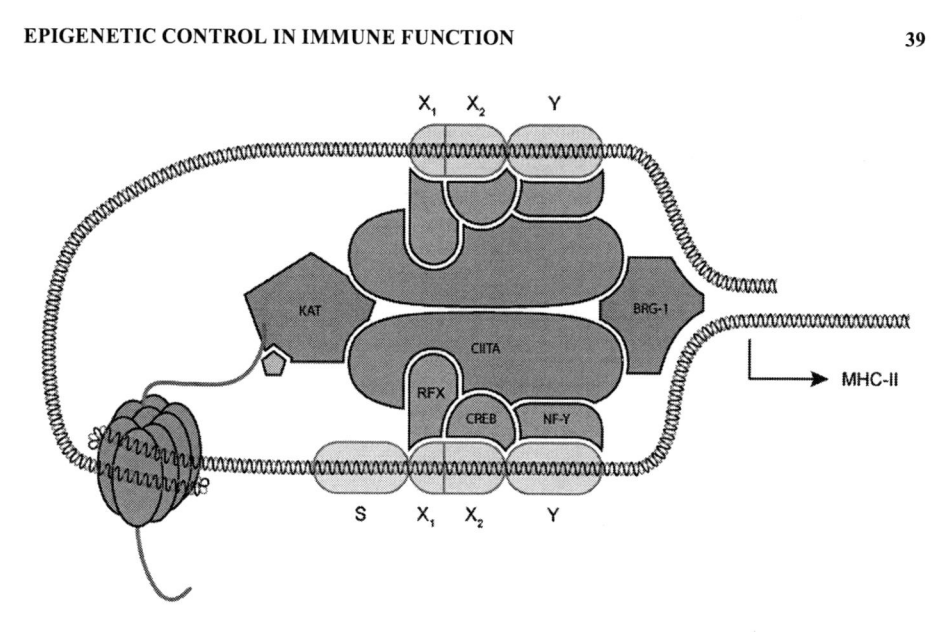

Figure 1. Schematic view of the factors and epigenetic events governing *MHC-II* transcription. Shown are the proximal SXY module and a distal XY element. The proximal SXY module is cooperatively bound by a multiprotein complex consisting of RFX (comprising RFXB/ANK, RFX5 and RFXAP), CREB/ATF and NFY. A similar binding pattern is observed for the more distal XY elements. CIITA interacts with the components of the multiprotein complex to positively regulate *MHC-II* transcription. CIITA recruits histone modification enzymes as detailed in the text, such as KATs and the general chromatin remodeler BRG1. CIITA has the capacity to self associate and this self association may allow bridging of the factors bound to the distal XY elements with the factors bound to the proximal SXY module to form a chromatin loop.

expression of CIITA can be induced by IFNγ resulting in inducible MHC-II expression at the cell surface. Thus CIITA acts as a molecular switch for MHC-II expression. Expression of *MHC-II* genes involves covalent modifications of histones and chromatin remodeling at the *MHC-II* genes. This is illustrated by the notion that IFNγ-induced MHC-II expression results in an increase in histone H3 and H4 acetylation in addition to an increase in the H4K4me3 modification at the MHC-II promoter, while a decrease in H3K9me3 was noted.[34]

LYSINE ACETYLTRANSFERASE/DEACETYLASE ACTIVITIES AND CIITA

CIITA exerts its transactivating function through protein-protein interactions with the components of the MHC-enhanceosome bound to the proximal SXY regulatory module in MHC promoters.[31,35,36] This interaction of CIITA with the MHC-enhanceosome allows for the subsequent association of CIITA with the KATs p300 (KAT3b)/CREB binding protein (CBP or KAT3a) and p300/CBP-associated factor (PCAF or KAT2b), which promote transcription of *MHC-I* and *MHC-II* genes by providing a more open chromatin structure.[22,23,37-39] Furthermore, CIITA also recruits the coactivator-associated arginine methyltransfease-1/protein arginine N-methyltransferase 4 (CARM1/PRMT4).[40,41] Besides acting as a platform for recruitment of KAT activities for transcriptional control of *MHC-I* and *MHC-II* genes, CIITA itself contains intrinsic KAT activity.[42] CIITA-mediated transactivation of MHC promoters was found to rely on this intrinsic KAT activity, which maps to a region in its N-terminus.[42] This KAT activity of CIITA is regulated by its C-terminal GTP-binding domain and is stimulated by GTP.[42] Interestingly, the CIITA KAT activity was found to bypass TATA Box Binding Protein (TBP)-associated factor 250kD ($TAF_{II}250$) in MHC-I promoter activation.[42] Moreover, acetylation of CIITA itself by CBP and/or PCAF at specific lysine residues within the bipartite nuclear localization signal in the amino-terminal region of CIITA governs its nuclear accumulation.[39] As such these KATs control indirectly transcription of *MHC-I* and *MHC-II* genes.

In addition to KATs, CIITA also associates with lysine deacetylases (KDACs), which were found to interfere with CIITA function. KATs and KDACs thereby act as molecular switches for CIITA-mediated transcriptional activation/silencing of *MHC* genes. In this respect, it was found that KDAC1 and KDAC2 interfere in the transcriptional transactivation function of CIITA following IFNγ induction.[43,44] It has been shown in mice that the KDAC1/KDAC2-associated repressor SIN3 homolog A (mSin3A) amplifies this inhibition in CIITA function.[43] Endogenous CIITA and KDAC2 interact and KDAC2 has the potential to deacetylate CIITA in cultured cells.[44] As a result, CIITA is targeted to proteosomal degradation, which leads to a decreased interaction of CIITA with the RFX component RFX5 in a deacetylation dependent manner.[44] Together, these observations reveal that these KDAC activities affect CIITA function on the one hand by disrupting assembly of the MHC-enhanceosome, while on the other hand they interfere in CIITA interactions with the MHC-enhanceosome. The Switch/Sucrose NonFermentable (SWI/SNF) ATPase Brahma-related gene 1 (BRG-1) also associates with CIITA and is required for the CIITA-mediated induction of *MHC-II* genes.[45] The association of CIITA and BRG-1 suggest that the ATP-dependent chromatin remodeling SWI/SNF complex is recruited by CIITA to MHC-II promoters to control transcription of *MHC-II* genes.

Besides the crucial role of the proximal SXY-module in MHC-II promoters in the transcriptional regulation of *MHC-II* genes, the appropriate temporal and spacial expression of *MHC-II* genes in vivo also requires the involvement of additional, long-range regulatory elements. In these processes X-Y or X-box like sequences in the *MHC-II* region play an important role.[46] It has been found that interactions between the proximal elements and more distal X-Y or X-box like sequences (2.3 kb upstream of the HLA-DRA promoter) result in epigenetic changes at the MHC-II promoter.[47,48] In one model, RFX and CIITA can interact with the proximal SXY-module and with distal X-Y or X-box like sequences to form a chromatin loop.[47] Binding of CIITA to the distal X-box like sequences has been demonstrated by a chromatin looping technique.[47] This chromatin loop results in enhanced histone acetylation.[49] Likewise, the transcriptional insulator CCCTC binding factor (CTCF) was found to control *MHC-II* gene expression through long-distance chromatin interactions.[50] The intergenic DNA of the *HLA-DRB1* and *HLA-DQA1* genes hosts a region that was bound by CTCF and acts as a potent enhancer-blocking element.[51] This element and its bound factors was found to interact with *HLA-DRB1* and *HLA-DQA1* genes as determined in a quantitative 3C assay—an assay to detect long-distance chromatin interactions.[50] Subsequently it was demonstrated that CTCF associates with CIITA and RFX5 suggesting that the CTCF bound region and the flanking HLA-DRB1 and HLA-DQA1 proximal promoters may interact.[50]

EPIGENETIC REGULATION OF *MHC2TA* TRANSCRIPTION

As detailed above, CIITA is the 'master regulator' of MHC-II expression.[32] Transcriptional regulation of *MHC2TA*, the gene encoding CIITA, is mediated through the activity of four independent promoter units (CIITA-PI through CIITA-PIV) (Fig. 2A).[52] These promoter units are employed in a cell type- and activation-specific manner. CIITA-PI

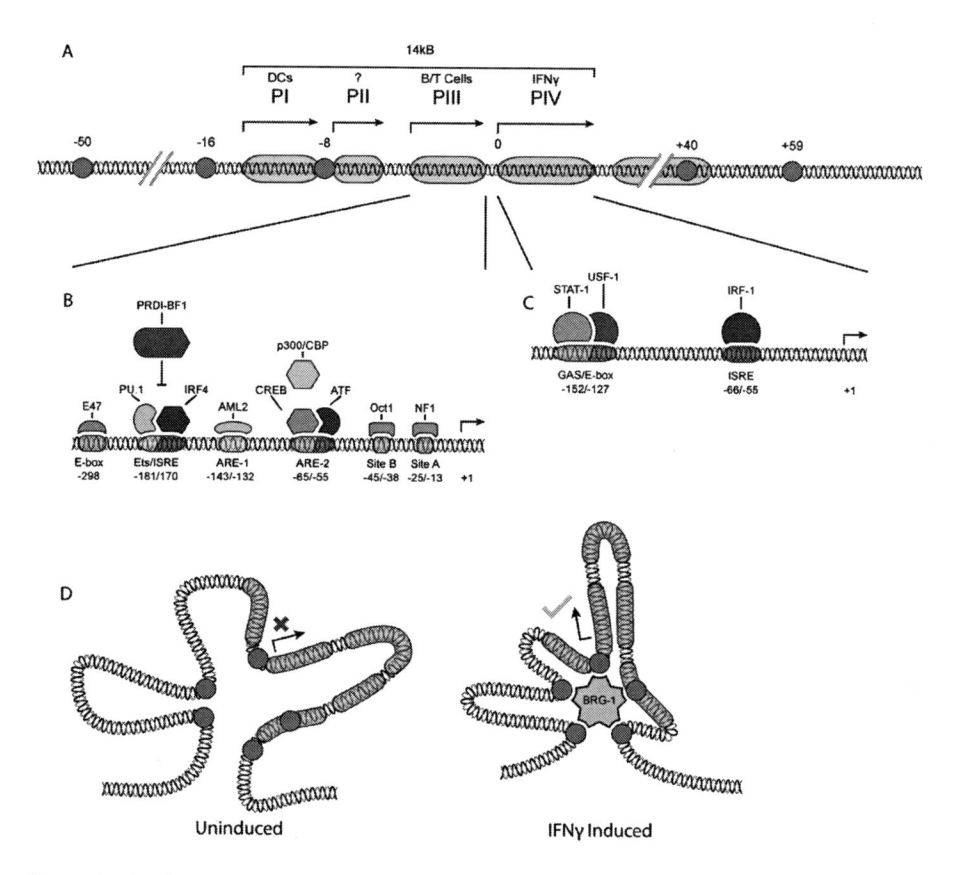

Figure 2. A) Schematic overview of the *MHC2TA* multipromoter region. Shown are the four MHC2TA promoters: CIITA-PI through CIITA-PIV. Grey spheres show BRG-1 binding sites relative to PIV. B) Factors and elements governing CIITA-PIII transactivation in B cells. Shown is the core promoter region of CIITA-PIII and the interacting factors. The localization of the various protein/DNA-binding elements is indicated relative to the transcription start site. Of these factors CREB/ATF has been shown to activate CIITA-PIII and this transactvation can be enhanced by p300/CBP. E47, PU.1 and IRF4 synergize to direct CIITA-PIII expression solely in B cells. C) Factors and elements governing CIITA-PIV transactivation following IFNγ stimulation. The localization of the various protein/DNA binding elements is indicated relative to the transcription start site. After stimulation with IFNγ, the IFNγ activated factor STAT1 binds directly together with USF1 to the GAS/E box motif in CIITA-PIV. Indirectly, STAT1 induces IRF1, which subsequently participates in the activation of CIITA-IV through binding to the ISRE. D) Model for chromatin loop formation of the *MHC2TA* multipromoter region after IFNγ stimulation involving BRG1-dependent distal enhancers (adapted from ref. 107). Grey spheres represent the relative locations of the BRG1-dependent distal enhancers, which interact weakly with each other and CIITA-PIV before IFNγ stimulation. These interactions are stabilized after IFNγ stimulation allowing transcription of the CIITA-PIV isoform.

and CIITA-PIII are used for the constitutive expression in dendritic cells and in B cells, respectively.[52] CIITA-PIV has been shown to be the promoter predominantly involved in IFNγ-inducible expression.[47,55] In addition, in human non-B cells, CIITA-PIII can also be activated by IFNγ through an element located 2 kb upstream of the core CIITA-PIII promoter.[55-57] CIITA-PIII has also been shown to be employed by human T cells upon activation.[2,58] The promoter function of CIITA-PII is still ill-defined. The various MHC2TA promoters each transcribe a unique first exon and are located within a region of approximately 14 kb.[52]

Several regulatory elements in *MHC2TA* promoters and interacting factors that are important for transcriptional activation have been identified. For induction of CIITA-PIV following stimulation with IFNγ, occupation of the GAS-box and the ISRE in CIITA-PIV by signal transducer and activator of transcription (STAT)-1 and the STAT-1 target gene interferon regulatory factor (IRF)-1 is crucial.[53] Furthermore interaction of STAT-1 with upstream stimulatory factor (USF)-1 bound to the E-box adjacent to the GAS is required for stable interaction (Fig. 2C).[53] The IFNγ-mediated activation of CIITA-PIV also results in increased histone H3 and H4 acetylation at CIITA-PIV.[59] This increase in histone acetylation in CIITA-PIV chromatin is already noted prior to recruitment of IRF-1 to the CIITA-PIV promoter.[59] Interestingly, BRG-1 was also found to be an important factor in the IFNγ-mediated transcriptional activation of CIITA-PIV (which will be discussed further in the last paragraph of this section).[60] This notion is derived from studies with cells that lack expression of BRG-1, which failed to induce IFNγ-mediated CIITA expression.[60]

The transcription factor CREB-1 was found to play a key role in the activation of CIITA-PIII through its interaction with CRE-binding sites in the activation response element (ARE)-2 and, depending on the cellular context, in the 5′-UTR of CIITA-PIII.[2,56,58] The KAT CBP was shown to enhance CREB-1 mediated activation of CIITA-PIII in B cells.[56] CIITA-PIII also contains a composite PU.1/IRF-binding element (Site C) and 2 E-box motifs, which plays a crucial role in B-cell-specific transcriptional regulation of CIITA.[61] In B cells the Ets/ISRE-consensus element is bound by PU.1 and IRF-4, whereas the basic helix-loop-helix factor E47 interacts with the E-box motifs. PU.1, IRF-4 and E47 bound to the Ets/ISRE and E-boxes, respectively, synergize to direct B-cell-specific activation of CIITA-PIII (Fig. 2B).[61] This finding is of interest because PU.1, IRF-4 and E47 play an important role in B-cell differentiation and activation. These observations therefore provide a link between MHC-II mediated antigen presentation in B cells and B-cell differentiation and activation events.[61]

During B-cell differentiation to plasma cells, expression of CIITA is extinguished coinciding with loss of MHC-II cell surface expression.[62] This extinction of CIITA and resulting MHC-II molecule expression in plasma cells is mediated by the transcriptional repressor B lymphocyte-induced maturation protein 1 (Blimp-1, also known as Positive Regulatory Domain I-Binding Factor 1, PRDI-BF1).[63,64] The silencing of CIITA expression mediated by CIITA-PIII in plasma cells is most likely resulting from binding of Blimp-1 to the Ets/ISRE-consensus element (Site C) thereby disrupting the interaction of PU.1/IRF-4 to this element.[48,63,64]

Interestingly, besides its repressive activity on CIITA-PIII transactivation, there is also more recent evidence that PRDI-BF1 mediates also repression of CIITA-PIV.[65]

The fact that transcriptional repression by Blimp-1/PRDI-BF1 involves recruitment of KDACs, in particular KDAC1 and KDAC2 and the lysine methyltransferase KMT1C (also known as G9a), which catalyses dimethylation of lysine 9 in histone H3 (H3K9me2), this provides a strong link with epigenetic silencing of *MHC2TA* in plasma cells involving histone acetylation and methylation modifications.[48,66,67] Indeed it was demonstrated by chromatin immunoprecipitation (ChIP) that differences in the levels of activating and repressive histone marks exists involving CIITA-PIII chromatin between B cells and plasma cells.[68] In plasma cells lacking CIITA expression, histone marks associated with gene transcription such as H3 and H4 acetylation and H3K4me2 and H3K4me3 are lost at CIITA-PIII, while the repressive H3K9me2 mark is increased.[68] Interestingly these histone marks were found also to exist at CIITA-PI, CIITA-PII and CIITA-PIV, revealing the involvement of the entire *MHC2TA* multipromoter region. As a consequence of the repressive histone marks and resulting chromatin inaccessibility, the binding of the CIITA-PIII interacting transcription factors (Sp-1, CREB-1, E47, PU.1, IRF-4) was lost in plasma cells.[68]

Chromatin remodeling also plays an important role in *MHC2TA* transcription in dendritic cell maturation.[69,70] Differentiation of monocytes into immature dendritic cells results in the induction of the CIITA-PI isoform, which directs expression of *MHC-II* genes. In immature dendritic cells, MHC-II molecules are largely retained in intracellular compartments. Upon maturation of dendritic cells, the peptide/MHC-II complexes are assembled and transported to the cell surface. During maturation of dendritic cells the increase of transported MHC-II molecules at the cell surface is accompanied by rapid transcriptional silencing of *MHC2TA* transcription.[69] The transcriptional inactivation of the *MHC2TA* multi-promoter locus is mediated by global histone deacetylation involving CIITA-PI, CIITA-PIII and CIITA-PIV[69]. Notably, during differentiation of monocytes into dendritic cells in a mouse model by mGM-CSF, activation of CIITA-PI is accompanied by an increase in histone H3 and H4 acetylation.[70] This increase in histone H3 and H4 acetylation was found to be blocked by IL-10, which resulted in inhibition of *MHC2TA* transcription.[70]

Distal elements and chromatin-remodeling also play an essential role in the transcriptional regulation of *MHC2TA*.[71] As mentioned before, *MHC2TA* has four alternative promoter units each transcribing its first exon (CIITA-PI through CIITA-PIV).[52] Transcriptional activation of the main IFNγ-responsive (CIITA-PIV) promoter was found to be dependent on the interaction with distal elements at -50kb and -8kb, which formed a loop with CIITA-PIV as determined by a chromatin conformation capture assay.[71] Contact was also detected between elements at -50kb and -16 kb. In these long-range interactions, BRG1, the ATPase driving the chromatin remodeling complex SWI-SNF (also called BAF), was constitutively bound to sites at -50kb, -16kb, -8kb and +59kb and also CIITA-IV as detailed above (Fig. 2D).[71] Thus BRG-1 not only is an important factor in the CIITA-mediated activation of MHC-II genes, but also controls the transcriptional activation of *MHC2TA* through long-range chromatin interactions and promoter interactions.

EPIGENETIC *MHC2TA* SILENCING IN CANCER

Downregulation of expression of MHC molecules is frequently noted in tumor cells. The low or lack of cell surface expression of both classes of MHC molecules impairs cellular immune recognition and resulting T-cell-mediated tumor eradication. Several studies have revealed that epigenetic modifications of chromatin play a critical role in the transcriptional silencing of *MHC2TA* and resulting extinction of *MHC-II* genes in cancer. In several cancer cell types, the lack of IFNγ-induced *MHC2TA* transcription is associated with CpG dinucleotide methylation of CIITA-PIV and also of CIITA-PIII DNA.[72-81] Besides CpG dinucleotide methylation, it has been suggested that the lack of

IFN-γ-induced transcription of *MHC2TA* in several cancer types is also associated with histone deacetylase activities.[82-86]

Of interest is the observation made in uveal melanoma tumor cell lines.[87] It was demonstrated that histone methylation played an important role in *MHC2TA* transcriptional silencing. The strongly reduced expression levels of CIITA after IFNγ-induction in an uveal melanoma cell line were found not to correlate with CpG dinucleotide methylation of CIITA-PIV DNA, but with high levels of the H3K27me3 histone modification in CIITA-PIV chromatin as determined by ChIP.[87] Consistent with the transcriptionally silent state of *MHC2TA* was the lack of RNA polymerase II recruitment into CIITA-PIV chromatin after IFNγ-induction in this cell line, while at the same time CIITA-PIV activating transcription factors were recruited.[87] RNA interference-mediated silencing of expression of the KMTase EZH2, resulted in an increment in CIITA mRNA expression levels after IFNγ induction. These observations suggest that EZH2 is involved in the transcriptional downregulation of IFNγ-induced expression of CIITA in uveal melanoma. Notably, the transcriptional silencing of *MHC2TA* by histone methylation in the absence of CpG dinucleotide methylation is in line with the observation that the H3K27me3 modification premarks genes for de novo methylation in cancer.[88] It could therefore be argued that the epigenetic make-up of the CIITA-PIV region in uveal melanoma reflects premarking for de novo methylation of DNA and that this reflects an intermediate epigenetic state of *MHC2TA* in the complete shut down of MHC-II mediated antigen presentation functions.

EPIGENETIC CONTROL OF T HELPER CELL DIFFERENTIATION

All T cells derive from the same precursor: the naïve T cell, which becomes activated after encounter of antigen in the context of MHC-II molecules at the cell surface of APC. After antigenic stimulation in the context of MHC-II, these naïve T cells can be differentiated into diverse T helper cell subsets, which include Th1, Th2, Th17 or T_{reg}. In these differentiation processes specific cytokines and transcription factors, which determine lineage-specificity, play a critical role. In addition, these differentiation events are also regulated by epigenetic processes (for recent reviews see refs. 89-93). These epigenetic mechanisms are necessary to stably maintain gene expression patterns in the differentiated T helper cells and to eliminate the need for feedback loops.

The differentiation of naïve T cells into Th1 or Th2 is determined by the cytokines IL12 and IL4, respectively. In response to these signals, transcription is initiated of lineage specific cytokine genes including *IFNγ* and *IL4*.[92] The *IFNγ* and *IL4* loci are maintained in a 'poised' state in naïve T cells—i.e., they show both repressive and activating epigenetic marks—allowing rapid, early transcription. For instance, the IL4 promoter region exhibits a low basal level of histone H3 acetylation and DNA hypomethylation, but also shows repressive H3K27me3 modifications.[102] In Th1 cells expression of IFNγ is preceded by remodelling of the *IFNγ* locus.[94,95] Whereas in the differentiation to Th2 cells, IL-4 expression is preceded by remodelling of the *IL4* locus, similarly to the *IFNγ* locus remodelling in Th1 cells. Upon initial stimulation of naïve T cells, the lineage determining factors GATA3 and T-bet mediate many of the structural changes to the chromatin.[90,92] These factors will render the *IFNγ* or *IL4* genes, in respectively Th1 and Th2 cells, accessible to regulatory enzymes and other transcription factors.[96-98] This is illustrated by the notion that an increase in the level of expression of IFNγ was found in T cells from *Dnmt* knockout mice and in T cells treated with DNMT inhibitors.[99-101]

When naïve T cells are stimulated under Th1 conditions, transcription activating chromatin marks at the *IL4* locus are replaced with repressive marks, whereas the contrary happens under Th2 stimulating conditions (e.g., at the *IFNγ locus*)(reviewed in 103). Interestingly, differentiated T helper cells display an unconventional association of Polycomp Group (PcG) proteins.[104] Various members of the PcG family of proteins, including EZH2, bound to actively transcribed *IFNγ* and *IL4* genes in differentiating Th1 and Th2 cells.[104] This finding suggests that in addition to suppressing gene transcription, EZH2 might also act as a facilitator of gene transcription in T-lymphocyte differentiation. This might be achieved possibly through long-range interactions with distal regulatory elements.

The transcription factors T-bet and GATA3 are considered to be driving forces in Th1 or Th2 differentiation respectively. The Foxp3 transcription factor is considered the master switch for T_{reg}. The promoter of the Foxp3 transcription factor showed differences in methylation levels between T_{regs} and non-T_{reg} CD4+ cells.[105] Furthermore, this study also showed differences in activating histone marks (H3Ac, H4Ac and H3K4me3) in Foxp3 promoter chromatin. Epigenetic regulation of T cell subtypes has also been shown in vivo. Mice which were treated with the KDAC inhibitor Trichostatin A showed an increase in Foxp3+ CD4+ T_{reg} cells in the lymphoid tissues.[106]

CONCLUSION

CIITA plays a central role in the control of constitutive and induced *MHC-II* gene transcription whereas it plays an ancillary function in constitutive and induced *MHC-I* gene transcription. The CIITA mediated transactivation of *MHC-II* and *MHC-I* genes is achieved through its interaction with the MHC-enhanceosome bound to the conserved SXY-module in MHC-II and MHC-I (with the exception of HLA-G) promoters. When bound to the MHC-enhanceosome, CIITA acts as a platform recruiting various activities involved in histone acetylation and deacetylation in the transcriptional control of *MHC* genes. Furthermore, CIITA is also central to recruitment of more general chromatin remodeling activities and long-range chromatin interactions of MHC-II promoters with distal elements. These activities mediated by CIITA provide tight control of transcription of these genes dedicated to antigen presentation. Moreover, the *MHC2TA* gene itself is tightly regulated at the transcriptional level by both genetic and epigenetic mechanisms. These include methylation of DNA and histone acetylation and methylation modifications. In addition, transcriptional activation of *MHC2TA* is mediated also through long-range chromatin interactions. Because of the involvement of epigenetic mechanisms in the transcriptional control of *MHC2TA* and T helper differentiation, deviations in these tightly regulated epigenetic mechanisms as observed under pathological conditions such as in cancer and autoimmune disease might provide an opportunity for pharmacological interference targeting the enzymes that modify DNA and histones.

ACKNOWLEDGEMENTS

Support of the research of PJvdE was obtained from the Dutch Cancer Society and the Dutch MS Research Foundation.

REFERENCES

1. Van den Elsen PJ, Holling TM, Kuipers HF et al. Transcriptional regulation of antigen presentation. Curr Opin Immunol 2004; 16:67-75.
2. Holling TM, Van der Stoep N, Quinten E et al. Activated human T-cells accomplish MHC class II expression through T-cell-specific occupation of class II transactivator promoter III. J Immunol 2002; 168:763-770.
3. Luger K, Mader AW, Richmond RK et al. Crystal structure of the nucleosome core particle at 2.8 A resolution. Nature 1997; 389:251-260.
4. Jenuwein T, Allis CD. Translating the histone code. Science 2001; 293:1074-1080.
5. Wu C. Chromatin remodeling and the control of gene expression. J Biol Chem 1997; 272:28171-28174.
6. Kuo MH, Allis CD. Roles of histone acetyltransferases and deacetylases in gene regulation. Bioessays 1998; 20:615-626.
7. Stewart MD, Li J, Wong J. Relationship between histone H3 lysine 9 methylation, transcription repression and heterochromatin protein 1 recruitment. Mol Cell Biol 2005; 25:2525-2538.
8. Cao R, Wang L, Wang H et al. Role of histone H3 lysine 27 methylation in Polycomb-group silencing. Science 2002; 298:1039-1043.
9. Ng HH, Ciccone DN, Morshead KB et al. Lysine-79 of histone H3 is hypomethylated at silenced loci in yeast and mammalian cells: a potential mechanism for position-effect variegation. Proc Natl Acad Sci USA 2003; 100:1820-1825.
10. Tachibana M, Sugimoto K, Fukushima T et al. Set domain-containing protein, G9a, is a novel lysine-preferring mammalian histone methyltransferase with hyperactivity and specific selectivity to lysines 9 and 27 of histone H3. J Biol Chem 2001; 276:25309-253.
11. Rice JC, Briggs SD, Ueberheide B et al. Histone methyltransferases direct different degrees of methylation to define distinct chromatin domains. Mol Cell 2003; 12:1591-1598.
12. De Ruijter AJ, Van Gennip AH, Caron HN et al. Histone deacetylases (HDACs): characterization of the classical HDAC family. Biochem J 2003; 370:737-749.
13. Holbert MA, Marmorstein R. Structure and activity of enzymes that remove histone modifications. Curr Opin Struct Biol 2005; 15:673-680.
14. Grozinger CM, Schreiber SL. Deacetylase enzymes: biological functions and the use of small-molecule inhibitors. Chem Biol 2002; 9:3-16.
15. Shi Y, Whetstine JR. Dynamic regulation of histone lysine methylation by demethylases. Mol Cell 2007; 25:1-14.
16. Lachner M, O'Carroll D, Rea S et al. Methylation of histone H3 lysine 9 creates a binding site for HP1 proteins. Nature 2001; 410:116-120.
17. Bannister AJ, Zegerman P, Partridge JF et al. Selective recognition of methylated lysine 9 on histone H3 by the HP1 chromo domain. Nature 2001; 410:120-124.
18. Fuks F, Hurd PJ, Deplus R et al. The DNA methyltransferases associate with HP1 and the SUV39H1 histone methyltransferase. Nucleic Acids Res 2003; 31:2305-2312.
19. Lehnertz B, Ueda Y, Derijck AA et al. Suv39h-mediated histone H3 lysine 9 methylation directs DNA methylation to major satellite repeats at pericentric heterochromatin. Curr Biol 2003; 13:1192-1200.
20. Vire E, Brenner C, Deplus R et al. The Polycomb group protein EZH2 directly controls DNA methylation. Nature 2006; 439:871-874.
21. Wierda RJ, Geutskens SB, Quax PHA et al. Epigenetics in atherosclerosis and inflammation. J Cell Mol Med 2010; in press.
22. Gobin SJP, Van Zutphen M, Westerheide SD et al. The MHC-specific enhanceosome and its role in MHC class I and beta(2)-microglobulin gene transactivation. J Immunol 2001; 167:5175-5184.
23. Ting JP, Trowsdale J. Genetic control of MHC class II expression. Cell 2002; 109:S21-33.
24. Steimle V, Durand B, Barras E et al. A novel DNA-binding regulatory factor is mutated in primary MHC class II deficiency (bare lymphocyte syndrome). Genes Dev 1995; 9:1021-1032.
25. Masternak K, Barras E, Zufferey M et al. A gene encoding a novel RFX-associated transactivator is mutated in the majority of MHC class II deficiency patients. Nat Genet 1998; 20:273-277.
26. Nagarajan UM, Louis-Plence P, DeSandro A et al. RFX-B is the gene responsible for the most common cause of the bare lymphocyte syndrome, an MHC class II immunodeficiency. Immunity 1999; 10:153-162.
27. Durand B, Sperisen P, Emery P et al. RFXAP, a novel subunit of the RFX DNA binding complex is mutated in MHC class II deficiency. EMBO J 1997; 16:1045-1055.
28. Moreno CS, Beresford GW, Louis-Plence P et al. CREB regulates MHC class II expression in a CIITA-dependent manner. Immunity 1999; 10:143-151.
29. Jabrane-Ferrat N, Nekrep N, Tosi G et al. Major histocompatibility complex class II transcriptional platform: assembly of nuclear factor Y and regulatory factor X (RFX) on DNA requires RFX5 dimers. Mol Cell Biol 2002; 22:5616-5625.

30. Louis-Plence P, Moreno CS, Boss JM. Formation of a regulatory factor X/X2 box-binding protein/nuclear factor-Y multiprotein complex on the conserved regulatory regions of HLA class II genes. J Immunol 1997; 159:3899-3909.
31. Masternak K, Muhlethaler-Mottet A, Villard J et al. CIITA is a transcriptional coactivator that is recruited to MHC class II promoters by multiple synergistic interactions with an enhanceosome complex. Genes Dev 2000; 14:1156-1166.
32. Steimle V, Otten LA, Zufferey M et al. Complementation cloning of an MHC class II transactivator mutated in hereditary MHC class II deficiency (or bare lymphocyte syndrome). Cell 1993; 75:135-146.
33. Gobin SJ, Peijnenburg A, Keijsers V et al. Site alpha is crucial for two routes of IFN gamma-induced MHC class I transactivation: the ISRE-mediated route and a novel pathway involving CIITA. Immunity 1997; 6:601-611.
34. Chou SD, Tomasi TB. Spatial distribution of histone methylation during MHC class II expression. Mol Immunol 2008; 45:971-980.
35. Zhu XS, Linhoff MW, Li G et al. Transcriptional scaffold: CIITA interacts with NF-Y, RFX and CREB to cause stereospecific regulation of the class II major histocompatibility complex promoter. Mol Cell Biol 2000; 20:6051-6061.
36. Jabrane-Ferrat N, Nekrep N, Tosi G et al. MHC class II enhanceosome: how is the class II transactivator recruited to DNA-bound activators? Int Immunol 2003; 15:467-475.
37. Kretsovali A, Agalioti T, Spilianakis C et al. Involvement of CREB binding protein in expression of major histocompatibility complex class II genes via interaction with the class II transactivator. Mol Cell Biol 1998; 18:6777-6783.
38. Fontes JD, Kanazawa S, Jean D et al. Interactions between the class II transactivator and CREB binding protein increase transcription of major histocompatibility complex class II genes. Mol Cell Biol 1999; 19: 941-947.
39. Spilianakis C, Papamatheakis J, Kretsovali A. Acetylation by PCAF enhances CIITA nuclear accumulation and transactivation of major histocompatibility complex class II genes. Mol Cell Biol 2000; 20:8489-8498.
40. Zika E, Fauquier L, Vandel L et al. Interplay among coactivator-associated arginine methyltransferase 1, CBP and CIITA in IFN-gamma-inducible MHC-II gene expression. Proc Natl Acad Sci USA 2005; 102:16321-16326.
41. Zika E, Ting JP. Epigenetic control of MHC-II: interplay between CIITA and histone-modifying enzymes. Curr Opin Immunol 2005; 17:58-64.
42. Raval A, Howcroft TK, Weissman JD et al. Transcriptional coactivator, CIITA, is an acetyltransferase that bypasses a promoter requirement for TAF(II)250. Mol Cell 2001; 7:105-115.
43. Zika E, Greer SF, Zhu XS et al. Histone deacetylase 1/mSin3A disrupts gamma interferon-induced CIITA function and major histocompatibility complex class II enhanceosome formation. Mol Cell Biol 2003; 23:3091-3102.
44. Kong X, Fang M, Li P et al. HDAC2 deacetylates class II transactivator and suppresses its activity in macrophages and smooth muscle cells. J Mol Cell Cardiol 2009; 46:292-299.
45. Mudhasani R, Fontes JD. The class II transactivator requires brahma-related gene 1 to activate transcription of major histocompatibility complex class II genes. Mol Cell Biol 2002; 22:5019-5026.
46. Gomez JA, Majumder P, Nagarajan UM et al. X box-like sequences in the MHC class II region maintain regulatory function. J Immunol 2005; 175:1030-1040.
47. Masternak K, Peyraud N, Krawczyk M et al. Chromatin remodeling and extragenic transcription at the MHC class II locus control region. Nat Immunol 2003; 4:132-137.
48. Wright KL, Ting JP. Epigenetic regulation of MHC-II and CIITA genes. Trends Immunol 2006; 27:405-412.
49. Krawczyk M, Peyraud N, Rybtsova N et al. Long distance control of MHC class II expression by multiple distal enhancers regulated by regulatory factor X complex and CIITA. J Immunol 2004; 173:6200-6210.
50. Majumder P, Gomez JA, Chadwick BP et al. The insulator factor CTCF controls MHC class II gene expression and is required for the formation of long-distance chromatin interactions. J Exp Med 2008; 205:785-798.
51. Majumder P, Gomez JA, Boss JM. The human major histocompatibility complex class II HLA-DRB1 and HLA-DQA1 genes are separated by a CTCF-binding enhancer-blocking element. J Biol Chem 2006; 281:18435-18443.
52. Muhlethaler-Mottet A, Otten LA, Steimle V et al. Expression of MHC class II molecules in different cellular and functional compartments is controlled by differential usage of multiple promoters of the transactivator CIITA. EMBO J 1997; 16:2851-2860.
53. Muhlethaler-Mottet A, Di Berardino W, Otten LA et al. Activation of the MHC class II transactivator CIITA by interferon-gamma requires cooperative interaction between Stat1 and USF-1. Immunity 1998; 8:157-166.

54. Piskurich JF, Wang Y, Linhoff MW et al. Identification of distinct regions of 5' flanking DNA that mediate constitutive, IFN-gamma, STAT1 and TGF-beta-regulated expression of the class II transactivator gene. J Immunol 1998; 160:233-240.
55. Piskurich JF, Linhoff MW, Wang Y et al. Two distinct gamma interferon-inducible promoters of the major histocompatibility complex class II transactivator gene are differentially regulated by STAT1, interferon regulatory factor 1 and transforming growth factor beta. Mol Cell Biol 1999; 19:431-440.
56. Van der Stoep N, Quinten E, Van den Elsen PJ. Transcriptional regulation of the MHC class II trans-activator (CIITA) promoter III: identification of a novel regulatory region in the 5'-untranslated region and an important role for cAMP-responsive element binding protein 1 and activating transcription factor-1 in CIITA-promoter III transcriptional activation in B lymphocytes. J Immunol 2002; 169:5061-5071.
57. Van der Stoep N, Quinten E, Alblas G et al. Constitutive and IFNgamma-induced activation of MHC2TA promoter type III in human melanoma cell lines is governed by separate regulatory elements within the PIII upstream regulatory region. Mol Immunol 2007; 44:2036-2046.
58. Wong AW, Ghosh N, McKinnon KP et al. Regulation and specificity of MHC2TA promoter usage in human primary T-lymphocytes and cell line. J Immunol 2002; 169:3112-3119.
59. Morris AC, Beresford GW, Mooney MR et al. Kinetics of a gamma interferon response: expression and assembly of CIITA promoter IV and inhibition by methylation. Mol Cell Biol 2002; 22:4781-4791.
60. Pattenden SG, Klose R, Karaskov E et al. Interferon-gamma-induced chromatin remodeling at the CIITA locus is BRG1 dependent. EMBO J 2002; 21:1978-1986.
61. Van der Stoep N, Quinten E, Marcondes Rezende M et al. E47, IRF-4 and PU.1 synergize to induce B-cell-specific activation of the class II transactivator promoter III (CIITA-PIII). Blood 2004; 104:2849-2857.
62. Silacci P, Mottet A, Steimle V et al. Developmental extinction of major histocompatibility complex class II gene expression in plasmocytes is mediated by silencing of the transactivator gene CIITA. J Exp Med 1994; 180:1329-1336.
63. Piskurich JF, Lin KI, Lin Y et al. BLIMP-I mediates extinction of major histocompatibility class II transactivator expression in plasma cells. Nat Immunol 2000; 1:526-532.
64. Ghosh N, Gyory I, Wright G et al. Positive regulatory domain I binding factor 1 silences class II transactivator expression in multiple myeloma cells. J Biol Chem 2001; 276:15264-15268.
65. Chen H, Gilbert CA, Hudson JA et al. Positive regulatory domain I-binding factor 1 mediates repression of the MHC class II transactivator (CIITA) type IV promoter. Mol Immunol 2007; 44:1461-1470.
66. Yu J, Angelin-Duclos C, Greenwood J et al. Transcriptional repression by blimp-1 (PRDI-BF1) involves recruitment of histone deacetylase. Mol Cell Biol 2000; 20:2592-2603.
67. Gyory I, Wu J, Fejér G et al. PRDI-BF1 recruits the histone H3 methyltransferase G9a in transcriptional silencing. Nat Immunol 2004; 5:299-308.
68. Green MR, Yoon H, Boss JM. Epigenetic regulation during B-cell differentiation controls CIITA promoter accessibility. J Immunol 2006; 177:3865-3873.
69. Landmann S, Muhlethaler-Mottet A, Bernasconi L et al. Maturation of dendritic cells is accompanied by rapid transcriptional silencing of class II transactivator (CIITA) expression. J Exp Med 2001; 194:379-391.
70. Choi YE, Yu HN, Yoon CH et al. Tumor-mediated down-regulation of MHC class II in DC development is attributable to the epigenetic control of the CIITA type I promoter. Eur J Immunol 2009; 39:858-868.
71. Ni Z, Abou El HM, Xu Z et al. The chromatin-remodeling enzyme BRG1 coordinates CIITA induction through many interdependent distal enhancers. Nat Immunol 2008; 9:785-793.
72. Morris AC, Spangler WE, Boss JM. Methylation of class II trans-activator promoter IV: a novel mechanism of MHC class II gene control. J Immunol 2000; 164:4143-4149.
73. Van den Elsen PJ, Van der Stoep N, Viëtor HE et al. Lack of CIITA expression is central to the absence of antigen presentation functions of trophoblast cells and is caused by methylation of the IFN-gamma inducible promoter (PIV) of CIITA. Hum Immunol 2000; 61:850-862.
74. Meissner M, Whiteside TL, Van Kuik-Romein P et al. Loss of interferon-gamma inducibility of the MHC class II antigen processing pathway in head and neck cancer: evidence for posttranscriptional as well as epigenetic regulation. Br J Dermatol 2008; 158:930-940.
75. Holling TM, Van Eggermond MC, Jager MJ et al. Epigenetic silencing of MHC2TA transcription in cancer. Biochem Pharmacol 2006; 72:1570-1576.
76. Van den Elsen PJ, Holling TM, Van der Stoep N et al. DNA methylation and expression of major histocompatibility complex class I and class II transactivator genes in human developmental tumor cells and in T-cell malignancies. Clin Immunol 2003; 109:46-52.
77. Holling TM, Schooten E, Langerak AW et al. Regulation of MHC class II expression in human T-cell malignancies. Blood. 2004; 103:1438-1444.
78. Van der Stoep N, Biesta P, Quinten E et al. Lack of IFN-gamma-mediated induction of the class II transactivator (CIITA) through promoter methylation is predominantly found in developmental tumor cell lines. Int J Cancer 2002; 97:501-507.

79. De Lerma Barbaro A, De Ambrosis A, Banelli B et al. Methylation of CIITA promoter IV causes loss of HLA-II inducibility by IFN-gamma in promyelocytic cells. Int Immunol. 2008; 20:1457-1466.

80. Satoh A, Toyota M, Ikeda H et al. Epigenetic inactivation of class II transactivator (CIITA) is associated with the absence of interferon-gamma-induced HLA-DR expression in colorectal and gastric cancer cells. Oncogene 2004; 23:8876-8886.

81. Morimoto Y, Toyota M, Satoh A et al. Inactivation of class II transactivator by DNA methylation and histone deacetylation associated with absence of HLA-DR induction by interferon-gamma in haematopoietic tumour cells. Br J Cancer 2004;90: 844-852.

82. Chou SD, Khan AN, Magner WJ et al. Histone acetylation regulates the cell type specific CIITA promoters, MHC class II expression and antigen presentation in tumor cells. Int Immunol. 2005; 17:1483-1494.

83. Murphy SP, Holtz R, Lewandowski N et al. DNA alkylating agents alleviate silencing of class II transactivator gene expression in L1210 lymphoma cells. J Immunol 2002; 169:3085-3093.

84. Magner WJ, Kazim AL, Stewart C et al. Activation of MHC class I, II and CD40 gene expression by histone deacetylase inhibitors. J Immunol 2000; 165:7017-7024.

85. Kanaseki T, Ikeda H, Takamura Y et al. Histone deacetylation, but not hypermethylation, modifies class II transactivator and MHC class II gene expression in squamous cell carcinomas. J Immunol 2003; 170:4980-4985.

86. Holtz R, Choi JC, Petroff MG et al. Class II transactivator (CIITA) promoter methylation does not correlate with silencing of CIITA transcription in trophoblasts. Biol Reprod 2003; 69:915-924.

87. Holling TM, Bergevoet MW, Wilson L et al. A role for EZH2 in silencing of IFN-gamma inducible MHC2TA transcription in uveal melanoma. J Immunol 2007; 179:5317-5325.

88. Schlesinger Y, Straussman R, Keshet I et al. Polycomb-mediated methylation on Lys27 of histone H3 premarks genes for de novo methylation in cancer. Nat Genet 2007; 39:232-236.

89. Lee CG, Sahoo A, Im SH. Epigenetic regulation of cytokine gene expression in T-lymphocytes. Yonsei Med J 2009; 50:322-330.

90. Wilson CB, Rowell E, Sekimata M. Epigenetic control of T-helper-cell differentiation. Nat Rev Immunol 2009; 9:91-105.

91. Placek K, Coffre M, Maiella S et al. Genetic and epigenetic networks controlling T helper 1 cell differentiation. Immunology 2009; 127:155-162.

92. Amsen D, Spilianakis CG, Flavell RA. How are T(H)1 and T(H)2 effector cells made? Curr Opin Immunol 2009; 21:153-160.

93. Lee YK, Mukasa R, Hatton RD et al. Developmental plasticity of Th17 and Treg cells. Curr Opin Immunol 2009; 21:274-280.

94. Schoenborn JR, Wilson CB. Regulation of interferon-gamma during innate and adaptive immune responses. Adv Immunol 2007; 96:41-101.

95. Avni O, Lee D, Macian F et al. T(H) cell differentiation is accompanied by dynamic changes in histone acetylation of cytokine genes. Nat Immunol 2002; 3:643-651.

96. Ansel KM, Lee DU, Rao A. An epigenetic view of helper T-cell differentiation. Nat Immunol 2003; 4:616-623.

97. Murphy KM, Reiner SL. The lineage decisions of helper T-cells. Nat Rev Immunol 2002; 2:933-944.

98. Rao A, Avni O. Molecular aspects of T-cell differentiation. Br Med Bull 2000; 56:969-984.

99. Makar KW, Wilson CB. DNA methylation is a nonredundant repressor of the Th2 effector program. J Immunol 2004; 173:4402-4406.

100. Young HA, Dray JF, Farrar WL. Expression of transfected human interferon-gamma DNA: evidence for cell-specific regulation. J Immunol 1986; 136:4700-4703.

101. Young HA, Ghosh P, Ye J et al. Differentiation of the T helper phenotypes by analysis of the methylation state of the IFN-gamma gene. J Immunol 1994; 153:3603-3610.

102. Koyanagi M, Baguet A, Martens J et al. EZH2 and histone 3 trimethyl lysine 27 associated with Il4 and Il13 gene silencing in Th1 cells. J Biol Chem 2005; 280:31470-31477.

103. Ansel KM, Djuretic I, Tanasa B et al. Regulation of Th2 differentiation and Il4 locus accessibility. Annu Rev Immunol 2006; 24:607-656.

104. Jacob E, Hod-Dvorai R, Schif-Zuck S et al. Unconventional association of the polycomb group proteins with cytokine genes in differentiated T helper cells. J Biol Chem 2008; 283:13471-13481.

105. Floess S, Freyer J, Siewert C et al. Epigenetic control of the foxp3 locus in regulatory T-cells. PLoS Biol 2007; 5:e38.

106. Tao R, de Zoeten EF, Ozkaynak E et al. Deacetylase inhibition promotes the generation and function of regulatory T-cells. Nat Med 2007; 13:1299-307.

107. Reith W, Boss JM. New dimensions of CIITA. Nat Immunol 2008; 9:713-714.

CHAPTER 5

DNA METHYLATION AND B-CELL AUTOREACTIVITY

Soizic Garaud,[1] Pierre Youinou[1,2] and Yves Renaudineau*[,1,2]

[1]*Immunologie and Pathology, Université de Brest, Université Européenne de Bretagne, Brest, France;*
[2]*Laboratory of Immunology, CHU Brest, Hôpital Morvan, Brest, France*
Corresponding Author: Yves Renaudineau—Email: yves.renaudineau@univ-brest.fr

Abstract: Although not exclusive, mounting evidence supports the fact that DNA methylation at CpG dinucleotides controls B-cell development and the progressive elimination or inactivation of autoreactive B cell. Indeed, the expression of different B cell specific factors, including Pax5, rearrangement of the B-cell receptor (BCR) and cytokine production are tightly controlled by DNA methylation. Among normal B cells, the autoreactive CD5[+] B cell sub-population presents a reduced capacity to methylate its DNA that leads to the expression of normally repressed genes, such as the human endogenous retrovirus (HERV). In systemic lupus erythematosus (SLE) patients, the archetype of autoimmune disease, autoreactive B cells are characterized by their inability to induce DNA methylation that prolongs their survival. Finally, treating B cells with demethylating drugs increased their autoreactivity. Altogether this suggests that a deeper comprehension of DNA methylation in B cells may offer opportunities to develop new therapeutics to control autoreactive B cells.

INTRODUCTION

Epigenetics is defined as heritable changes in gene expression that did not affect the DNA sequence of the genome. Epigenetic modifications involve either methylation of cytosine in CpG dinucleotides or covalent posttranslational modifications of the histones. In B cells, like in other cells, CpG dinucleotides are globally methylated with the exception of the CpG rich regions called CpG islands. CpG islands are important for control of gene expression and it has been estimated that 50% of human RNA polymerase II-transcribed genes possess CpG islands. Using a high resolution technique to map the entire B-cell CpG methylome, it was observed that 10% of the promoters were repressed by DNA

Epigenetic Contributions in Autoimmune Disease, edited by Esteban Ballestar.
©2011 Landes Bioscience and Springer Science+Business Media.

methylation when analyzing peripheral blood B cells.[1] The CpG methylation process is controlled by DNA methyltransferases (DNMTs), a family that encompasses five members: DNMT1, DNMT3a, DNMT3b, DNMT3L and DNMT2. DNMT1 preferentially methylates hemi-methylated DNA, such as appear during cellular division, whereas DNMT3a and DNMT3b are involved in the de novo introduction of methyl groups on unmethylated DNA. Methylated CpG can limit transcription directly or indirectly via the recruitment of transcriptional repressors, such as the methyl-CpG binding domain proteins (MBD) a group that includes MBD1-4 and MECP. In their turn, MBDs can recruit other repressors like the histone deacetylases (HDAC). HDACs are histone posttranslational modifying enzymes that introduce positive charges in the histone amino terminal protruding tail and permit interactions with the negatively charged DNA, leading to DNA compaction and preventing transcription. Other histone posttranslational modifications have been described, such as methylation (me), ubiquitination, phosphorylation, sumoylation, deimination/citrullinisation, ADP ribosylation and proline isomerisation.[2] Among them, some are repressive (H3K9me2/3, H3K27me3 and H4K20me2/3) while others have been associated with active transcription (H3K4me2, H3K36me2/3 and H3K79me2). As a consequence, DNA methylation and histone modifications control chromatin density which can be divided into dense regions referred to as heterochromatin (increased DNA methylation, histone deacetylation and histone hypermethylation) and into less dense regions referred to as euchromatin (decreased CpG DNA methylation, increased histone acetylation and decreased histone methylation). In lymphocytes, including B cells, epigenetic mechanisms may be reversed and these changes can be rapid, particularly during the cell cycle, in response to a stimulus or after exposure to environmental factors.

B CELLS AND DNA METHYLATION

B-Cell Development

As represented in Figure 1, B-cell development can be divided into three steps. First step, in the bone marrow, B-cell maturation starts from a lymphoid stem cell that differentiates to a progenitor B (pro-B) cell, to a precursor B (pre-B) cell and to an immature B cell. Bone marrow B-cell differentiation is concomitant with the progressive rearrangement of the B-cell receptor (BCR). Second step, immature B cells migrate to the spleen wherein they differentiate through a transitional stage into follicular B cells or marginal zone B cells according to the antigen stimulation if it is T-cell dependant or not, respectively. The transitional B-cell stage is crucial to the acquisition of the B-cell repertoire (positive selection) and to the elimination of autoreactive B cells (negative selection). In humans, circulating transitional B cells have been characterized; they are CD10+, CD24+, CD38++ and CD5+.[3] Third step, follicular B cells proliferate in the germinal center (GC) of lymphoid follicles and differentiate into GC B cells that express high affinity BCR and class-switch isotypes. B cells that leave the GC can develop into memory B cells or plasma cells.

The transcription factor Pax5 plays a crucial role in B-cell development by controlling the commitment of lymphoid progenitors into the B-cell lineage and later by controlling the evolution from pro-B cells to mature B cells at different check points. Pax5 expression is controlled by DNA methylation. Indeed, analysis of the CpG methylation status at the Pax5 locus by Decker et al has revealed that Pax5 regulatory elements are progressively

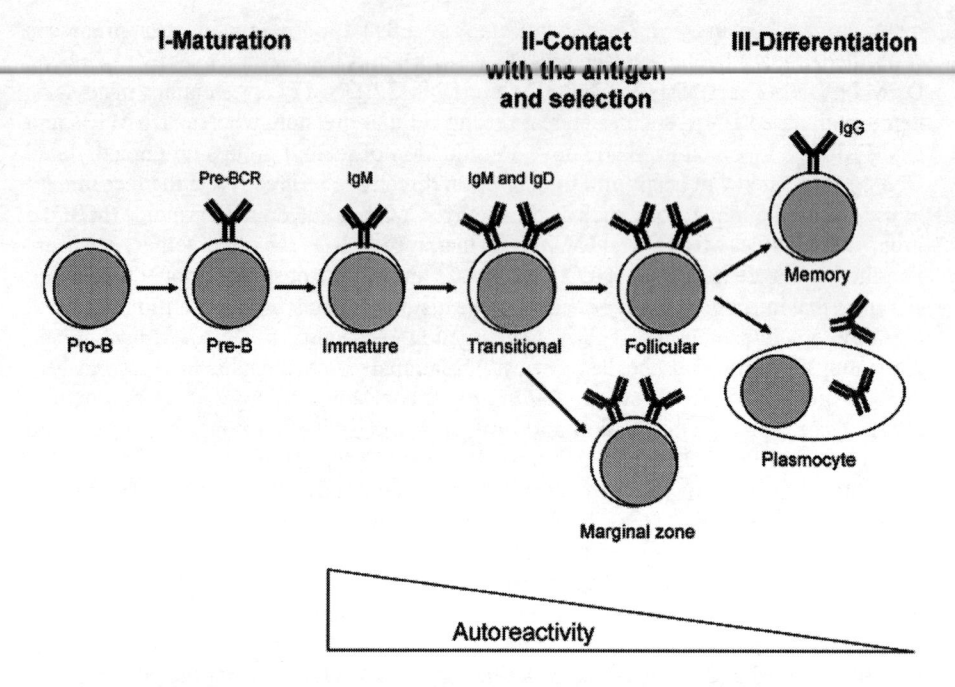

Figure 1. Model of B-cell development. B-cell development occurs in both the bone marrow and peripheral lymphoid tissues such as the spleen and can be divided into three stages. In bone marrow, the first stage, rearrangement of the immunoglobulin locus results in the generation and surface expression of the pre-B cell receptor (pre-BCR) in pre-B cells and finally a mature BCR in immature B cells. In peripheral lymphoid tissues, the second stage, B cells undergo a process of positive and negative selection to eliminate autoreactive cells. Both receptor editing/revision and clonal deletion are important at this stage. Cells completing selection will mature into follicular B cells (or marginal zone B cells). In the germinal center of lymphoid follicles, the third stage and following an immune response, antigen selected B cells develop into either plasmocyte (antibody-secreting B cell) or memory B cells.

demethylated.[4] In lymphoid stem cells, the enhancer but not the promoter starts to be demethylated and from the pro-B cell to the mature B cells both elements are demethylated. At the plasma cell stage, the promoter is remethylated and Pax5 is not expressed. In addition to a direct influence of DNA methylation on Pax5 expression, DNA methylation controls Pax5 binding and transcription factor activity. Thus, explaining that CD79a/ Igα expression starts in pro-B cell, CD19 in preB cell and the human telomerase reverse transcriptase in mature B cell.[5]

B-Cell Receptor

As demonstrated by Sakano et al, sequential rearrangements of the immunoglobulin (Ig) genes are necessary to produce the BCR.[6] In the first step, the rearrangement concerns the D_H to J_H Ig heavy chain in pro-B cells, followed by V_H to D_H-J_H rearrangement at the pre-B cell stage forming the pre-BCR. When Ig_H is completed, the Ig light chain starts its V_L to J_L rearrangement which also proceeds in a stepwise manner since kappa chain rearrangement precedes lambda chain rearrangement. The rearrangement is initiated by two enzymes, Rag1 and Rag2, which form a complex with the well conserved recombination sequence signal (RSS). In GC, the expression of the activation-induced cytidine deaminase (AID) is critical for somatic hypermutation of Ig V-region genes and class-switch recombination of C-region genes.

Since BCR rearrangement may be mutagenic or may produce autoreactive Ig, such a mechanism needs to be hightly regulated. The accessibility hypothesis was proposed to explain that external factors (e.g., IL-7 and IL-4) and/or B cell specific factors (e.g., Pax5) control chromatin accessibility through DNA methylation and histone posttranslational modifications. Several observations support this hypothesis: (1) the Ig locus is highly methylated before V(D)J recombination and undergoes demethylation during gene rearrangement.[7] (2) Demethylation on the Ig light chain occurs after demethylation on the Ig heavy chains.[8] (3) DNA binding and subsequent recombination by Rag1 and Rag2 enzymes is affected when the RSS sequences are methylated.[9] (4) The methylation status of the RSS sequences influences the rearrangement between the frequently and the infrequently rearranged V_H genes.[10] (5) Somatic hypermutations are influenced by DNA methylation since CpG methylation represses AID expression and protects deamination of cytosine to uracil by AID.[11-12]

Cytokine Production

In addition to antibody (Ab) production and antigen presentation, B cells are able to produce cytokines. According to Harris et al and following antigen stimulation, naïve B cells differentiate themselves into effector B cells of Type 1 (Be1) or Type 2 (Be2).[13] On one hand, Be1 cells produce Type 1 cytokines like IFN-γ that provide protection against intracellular pathogens and cancer and, on the other hand, Be2 cells produce Type 2 cytokines like IL-4, IL-5 and IL-13 that are involved in host defense against parasites. In T cells the choice between Type I (IFNγ, IL-2) and Type 2 cytokines (IL-4, IL-5, IL-6 and IL-13) is orchestrated by DNA methylation and histone acetylation.[14] A demonstration that DNA methylation controls cytokine production in B cells has not been provided, but may be suspected.

CD5+ B CELLS

CD5, first described as a T-cell marker, is detected in a subset of B cells referred to as B1 cells as opposed to conventional B2 cells that did not express CD5. B1 cells are further divided into B1a and B1b B cells, the latter sharing all the properties of B1a except the cell surface expression of CD5.[15] Different functions were ascribed for CD5+ B cells: (1) CD5+ B cells produce polyspecific Abs and they are believed to constitute the main source of natural Abs; (2) Repeated BCR stimulation of B cells leads to CD5 expression that controls B-cell activation, maintains transitional and mature B cells in anergy and contributes to the re-expression of Rag1/Rag2 and BCR Ig light chain revision;[3,16-18] (3) CD5+ B cells may also exert their effect through the production of interleukin (IL)-10, which is an immunoregulatory cytokine. Il-10 production is related to the expression of CD5 since transfection of B cells with CD5 is associated with IL-10 production.[19] The role of IL-10 on autoimunity is controversial, on the one hand, IL-10 is exacerbated in SLE patients and, on the other hand, a protective role for IL-10 has been demonstrated in vivo.[20-21]

CD5+ B Cells Are Hypomethylated

The human CD5 gene, which possesses 11 exons, is located on chromosome 11 at position 11q12.2 adjacent to CD6 (Fig. 2). The CD5 and CD6 genes derive from a common ancestor present in fish that has been duplicated after the divergence with birds around 150-200 million years ago, explaining that CD5 and CD6 are highly conserved in avian, bovine, rodent and human. In addition, at the divergence between monkeys from the old world and the new world, around 25 million years ago, a human endogenous retrovirus (HERV) has integrated the 5' portion of the CD5 locus.[22] HERV-CD5 retrovirus is 5,254 bp long and possesses two long terminal repeats (LTR) plus nonfunctional gag-pol and env elements.

In B1a and B1b B cells isolated from humans two transcripts are expressed,[23] a classical one called CD5-E1A and a fusion transcript, called CD5-E1B, that contains the 5' LTR part of the HERV-CD5 element (exon 1B) and the CD5 gene (exons 2-11). Transcription of the fusion transcript CD5-E1B is controlled by DNA methylation and its expression is restricted to B cells.[24] DNA methylation dependence was demonstrated first by testing the activity of the DNMT1 which is reduced in CD5-E1B positive cells (B1a and B1b) in comparison to B2 cells (Fig. 3). In a second instance, it was observed that B cells treated with DNMT inhibitors like procainamide, 5-azacytidine and PD98059 leads to CD5-E1B overexpression. Finally, analysis of the CpG sites in the HERV-CD5 5'LTR using methylation sensitive endonuclease assays followed by PCR and bisulfite sequencing revealed that the methylation status of the U3 promoter present in the 5'LTR is inversely proportional to CD5-E1B expression in B cells (techniques are summarized in Fig. 4).

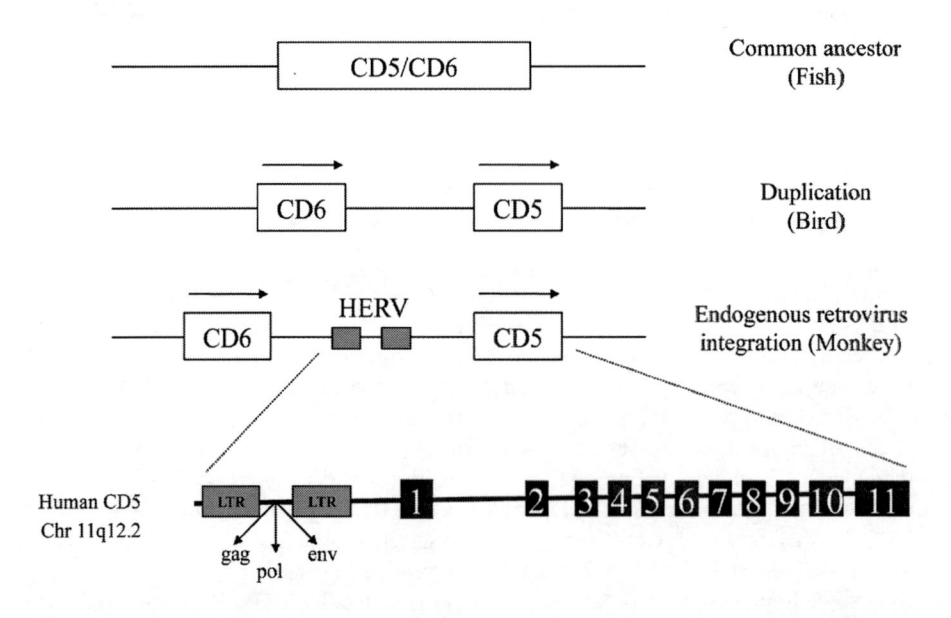

Figure 2. Characterization of CD5 gene. CD5 and CD6 genes have evolved from the duplication of a common ancestral gene. The human CD5 gene maps to the chromosome (Chr) 11q12.2 region, 82kb downstream from the human CD6 gene. A human endogenous retrovirus (HERV) element is integrated in the 5' region of human CD5.

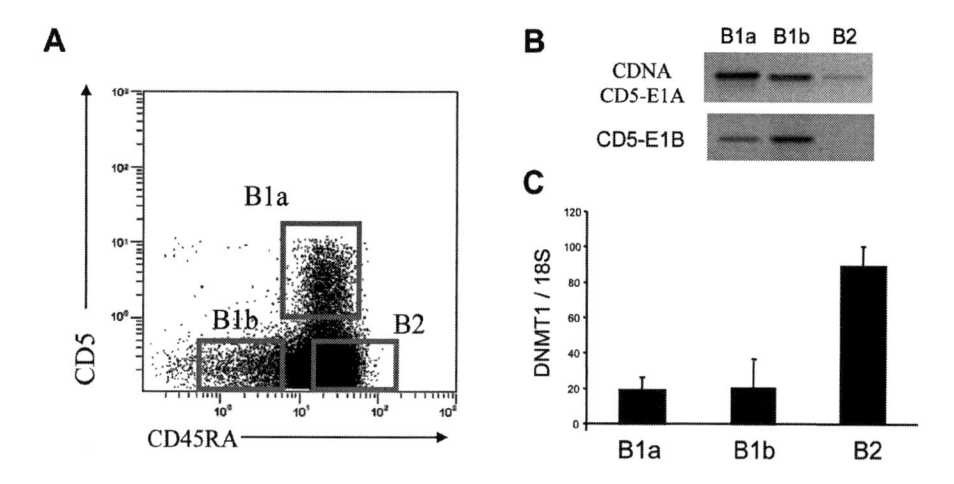

Figure 3. B1 cells are characterized by a reduced capacity to methylate their DNA. A) B1 cells can be discriminated based on their membrane cell surface expression of CD5 and CD45RA.[23] B) The CD5 gene generates two transcripts CD5-E1A and CD5-E1B that are expressed at the cell surface or intracellularly, respectively. CD5-E1A predominates in B1a cells in contrast to CD5-E1B that predominates in B1b B cells. C) Expression of CD5-E1B is controlled by DNA methylation and its expression is inversely proportional to the expression of DNA methyl transferase 1 (DNMT1) as determined by real time PCR.

Endogenous Retrovirus Expression Is Impaired in CD5⁺ B Cells

In addition to CD5-E1B up-regulation, DNA hypomethylation observed in CD5⁺ B cells influences other genes and particularly HERV elements. Such an assertion is based on the observation that HRES-1, another HERV element, is repressed by DNA methylation in B2 cells while the other genes tested (Pax5, CD70, CD19 and Syk) were demethylated.[25] HERVs represent 8% of human chromatin and their contribution to lymphocyte autoreactivity is strongly suspected. Several mechanisms have been proposed to explain how HERV elements contribute to autoreactivity (see review 26 for references). (1) HERV-encoded proteins are considered as foreign antigens that stimulate B cells to produce Abs. Among anti-HERV Abs some of them might cross-react with self proteins by molecular mimicry. For example, Abs against HRES-1 p30gag that cross-react with the nuclear autoantigen U1-snRNP are detected in up to 50% in SLE compared to less than 5% in controls. (2) HERV proteins may act as superantigens which could induce expansion of autoreactive T cells. (3) HERVs may induce immune response dysregulation through their capacity to modulate T-cell activation, cytokine expression and they can activate innate immunity by pattern recognition receptors. (4) HERVs may act as insertional mutagens causing activation, inhibition or alternative splicing of genes involved in immune regulation. One example is the insertion of a HERV element in the CD5 gene that generates the fusion transcript CD5-E1B (see above). CD5-E1B encodes a truncated cytoplasmic protein able to interact with the classical form of CD5, CD5-E1A, forming intracellular aggregates when co-expressed in the same cell.[24] Such an interaction is suspected to contribute to B-cell autoreactivity by downregulating a BCR dampener.[15]

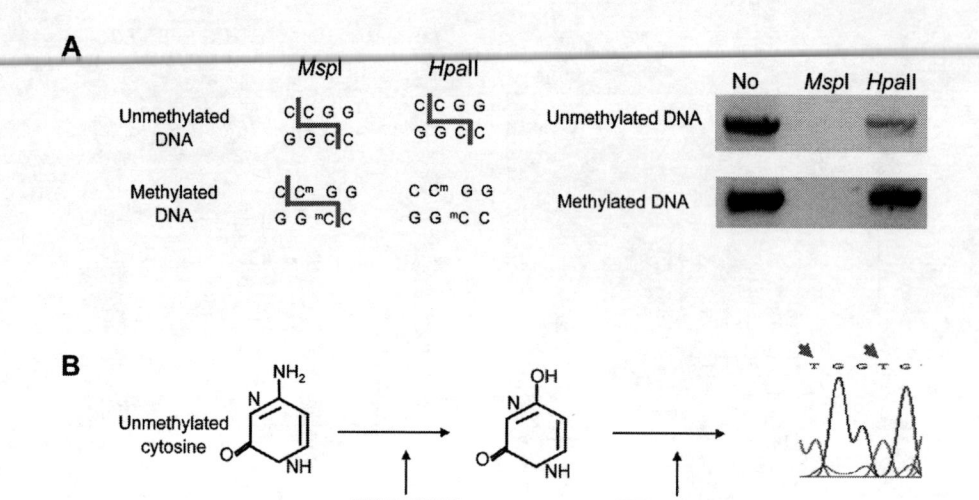

Figure 4. Methods of DNA methylation analysis. A) Methylation-sensitive endonucleases are used to assess the methylation status of CpG sites within a CpG island. This assay is based on the inability of a methylation sensitive restriction enzyme (*Hpa II*) to digest methylated CpG sites, in contrast to a methylation insensitive restriction enzyme (*Msp I*). Digested DNA is analysed by polymerase chain reaction (PCR) showing whether the CpG sequence is preserved, if methylated, or not in the amplified region. B) Bisulfite sequencing is used to determine the pattern of methylation after treatment of DNA with bisulfite that converts unmethylated-cytosine residues to uracil, methylated-cytosine remains unaffected.

AUTOREACTIVE B CELLS

Animal Models

Observing that prolonged treatment with isoniazid, an antituberculous drug, was associated with the development of an SLE-like disease in humans, the influence of long-term oral administration was tested in normal mice.[27] After several weeks murine B cells became autoreactive, antinuclear Abs appeared and the mice developed an SLE-like disease that disappeared after the drug was removed (Fig. 5). Such an effect has been reproduced with procainamide and 5-azacytidine, two other DNA methylation inhibitors and the effects were more pronounced. The direct implication of B cells was confirmed more recently.[28] B cells were purified from mice, treated ex vivo with DNA methylation inhibitors and subsequently reintroduced in syngenic mice by adoptive transfer. This led to the detection of antinuclear Abs in the recipient. Of note, the effect is not restricted to B cells, since Richardson's group has also demonstrated that adoptive transfer of DNA hypomethylated CD4+ T cells, not CD8+ T cells, induced an SLE-like disease with glomerulonephritis and anti-dsDNA Ab deposition in the kidney.[29]

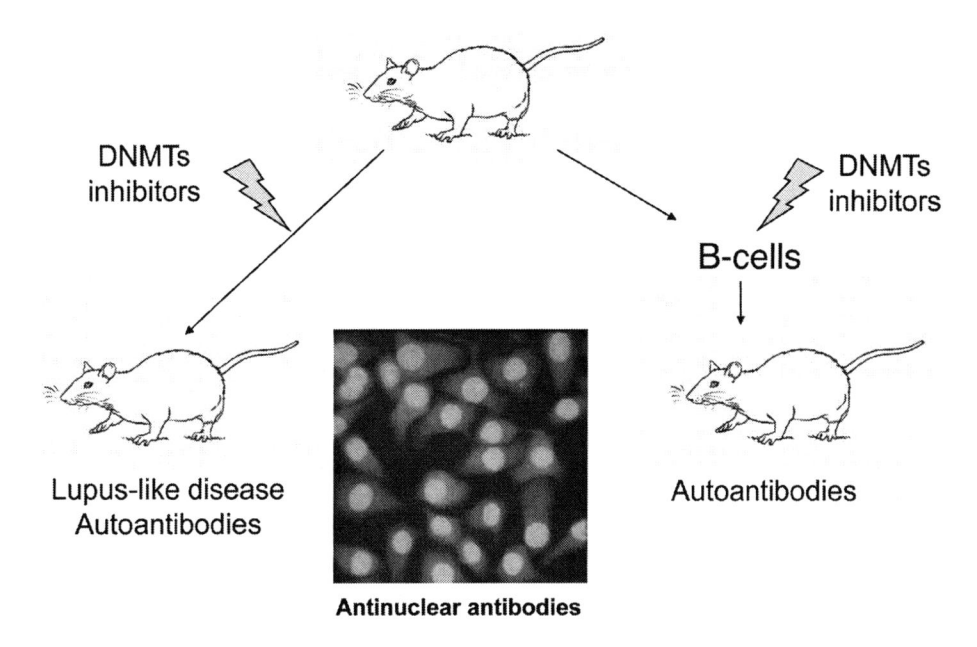

Antinuclear antibodies

Figure 5. Epigenetic alterations in B cells contribute to the pathogenesis of lupus. Both, the long-term oral administration of DNMT inhibitors like hydralazine or isoniazide on one hand (left), or adoptive transfer of bone marrow B cells pretreated with the same drugs to naïve syngeneic mice on the other hand (right), resulted in autoantibody production and a lupus-like disease.

DNA Methylation Is Impaired in SLE B Cells

In SLE, peripheral blood mononuclear cells (PBMC) are characterized by a global DNA hypomethylation status. This was elegantly demonstrated by Javierre and colleagues who compared pairs of monozygotic twins discordant for SLE, rheumatoid arthritis (RA) and dermatomyositis (DM).[30] Indeed, in comparison to the corresponding healthy sibling, PBMC isolated from SLE patients, but neither RA nor DM patients, present a profound DNA methylation defect associated with DNMT1 and DNMT3b reduction and histone acetylation. Among PBMC from SLE patients, CD4+ T cells were first reported to present DNA methylation abnormalities and recently we have also observed that SLE B cells were defective in their capacity to methylate DNA.[25,31] Such a defect has been related to a blockage in the PKC delta/Erk pathway that regulates DNMTs expression.[32] The reason for the initial defect is currently unknown but transgenic mice defective for PKC delta developed an SLE-like disease with B-cell expansion, autoantibody production, IL-6 overexpression and had the constitution of ectopic GC in the absence of stimulation.[33]

IL-6 is a multifunctional cytokine involved in B-cell differentiation/maturation, Ig secretion and T-cell functions. A relation between the IL-6 level detected in the sera and lupus disease activity has been reported, thus providing a clue implicating IL-6 in B-cell autoreactivity.[34] In mice, the treatment of lupus prone mice with an anti-IL-6 mAb prevents the development of an SLE-like disease and the production of anti-dsDNA Abs.[35] The impact of IL-6 in autoreactivity is not completely understood but we have recently proposed that IL-6, by blocking the cell cycle progression at the G0/G1 interface in B cells, controls DNMT1 expression.[25,36,37] Such assertion is based on the observation, in one hand, that addition of IL-6 to normal B cells is associated with a reduction of DNA methylation and DNMT1, while, on the other hand, blocking abnormal IL-6 production with an anti-IL-6-receptor mAb restores DNA methylation in SLE B cells. Interestingly, DNA methylation plays an essential role in IL-6 silencing, suggesting that an amplification loop occurs in SLE B cells.[38,39]

ICF Syndrome and Autoreactivity

The immunodeficiency, centromeric region instability and facial anomalies syndrome (ICF) is a rare genetic disease, less than 50 cases have been reported world wide, that displays DNA hypomethylation.[40] In the majority of cases, ICF is related to mutations in the catalytic domain of the DNMT3b gene. ICF diagnosis is associated with hypogamma-globulinemia or agamma-globulinemia, normal peripheral blood B cell number and cytogenetic abnormalities involving chromosomes 1, 16 and sometimes 9 in mitogen-stimulated lymphocytes. Analysing B cells from ICF patients, BlancoBetancourt, et al have observed that peripheral B cell express autoreactive BCRs, and that terminal differentiation is blocked at the transitional stage.[40] Thus, it could be suspected that DNA methylation controls the negative selection of transitional B cells through an unknown mechanism.

CONCLUSION

Evidence for a role for DNA methylation in the pathogenesis of SLE and common autoimmune diseases has emerged. Patients with SLE have global hypomethylation of DNA with a decrease in the activity of the DNMTs that affects primarily lymphocytes. However and particularly in B cells, the pathways that control DNA methylation and the pathways that are controlled by DNA methylation are poorly understood. Consequently, a better understanding of these pathways may constitutes a revolution in our comprehension of autoreactive B cells.[41]

ACKNOWLEDGMENTS

Authors are grateful to Simone Forest and Geneviève Michel for their secretarial expertise and assistance. Thanks are due also to Dr Wesley H. Brooks (H. Lee Moffitt Cancer Center and Research Institute, Tampa, FL) for editorial assistance. This work was supported by grants from the Conseil Régional de Bretagne, the Conseil Général du Finistère, the College Doctoral International, the Université Européenne de Bretagne and the French Ministry for Education and Research.

REFERENCES

1. Rauch TA, Wu X, Zhong X et al. A human B-cell methylome at 100-base pair resolution. Proc Natl Acad Sci USA 2009; 106:671-8.
2. Dieker J, Muller S. Epigenetic histone code and autoimmunity. Clin Rev Allergy Immunol 2009; DOI: 10-1007/s12016-009-8173-7.
3. Sims GP, Ettinger R, Shirota Y et al. Identification and characterization of circulating human transitional B-cells. Blood 2005; 105:4390-8.
4. Decker T, Pasca di Magliano M, McManus S et al. M. Stepwise activation of enhancer and promoter regions of the B-cell commitment gene Pax5 in early lymphopoiesis. Immunity 2009; 30:508-20.
5. Renaudineau Y, Garaud S, Le Dantec C et al. Autoreactive B-cells and Epigenetics. Clin Rev Allergy Immunol 2009; DOI: 10.1007/s12016-009-8174-6.
6. Sakano H, Maki R, Kurosawa Y et al. Two types of somatic recombination are necessary for the generation of complete immunoglobulin heavy-chain genes. Nature 1980; 286:676-83.
7. Storb U, Arp B. Methylation patterns of immunoglobulin genes in lymphoid cells: correlation of expression and differentiation with undermethylation. Proc Natl Acad Sci USA 1983; 80:6642-6.
8. Xu CR, Feeney AJ. The epigenetic profile of Ig genes is dynamically regulated during B-cell differentiation and is modulated by pre-B-cell receptor signaling. J Immunol 2009; 182:1362-9.
9. Nakase H, Takahama Y, Akamatsu Y. Effect of CpG methylation on RAG1/RAG2 reactivity: implications of direct and indirect mechanisms for controlling V(D)J cleavage. EMBO 2003; 4:774-80.
10. Espinoza CR, Feeney AJ. Chromatin accessibility and epigenetic modifications differ between frequently and infrequently rearranging VH genes. Mol Immunol 2007; 44:2675-85.
11. Fujimura S, Matsui T, Kuwahara K et al. Germinal center B-cell-associated DNA hypomethylation at transcriptional regions of the AID gene. Mol Immunol 2008; 45:1712-9.
12. Larijani M, Frieder D, Sonbuchner TM et al. Methylation protects cytidines from AID-mediated deamination. Mol Immunol 2005; 42:599-604.
13. Harris DP, Haynes L, Sayles PC et al. Reciprocal regulation of polarized cytokine production by effector B and T-cells. Nat Immunol 2000; 1:475-82.
14. Bowen H, Kelly A, Lee T et al. Control of cytokine gene transcription in Th1 and Th2 cells. Clin Exp Allergy 2008; 38:1422-31.
15. Youinou P, Renaudineau Y. The paradox of CD5-expressing B-cells in systemic lupus erythematosus. Autoimmun Rev 2007; 7:149-54.
16. Qian Y, Santiago C, Borrero M et al. Lupus-specific antiribonucleoprotein B-cell tolerance in nonautoimmune mice is maintained by differentiation to B-1 and governed by B-cell receptor signaling thresholds. J Immunol 2001; 166:2412-9.
17. Hippen KL, Tze LE, Behrens TW. CD5 maintains tolerance in anergic B-cells. J Exp Med 2000; 191:883-8.
18. Hillion S, Rochas C, Youinou P et al. Expression and reexpression of recombination activating genes: relevance to the development of autoimmune states. Ann NY Acad Sci 2005; 1050:10-8.
19. Garaud S, Le Dantec C, de Mendoza AR et al. IL-10 production by B-cells expressing CD5 with the alternative exon 1B. Ann NY Acad Sci 2009; 1173:280-5.
20. Gunnarsson I, Nordmark B, Hassan Bakri A et al. Development of lupus-related side-effects in patients with early RA during sulphasalazine treatment-the role of IL-10 and HLA. Rheumatology (Oxford) 2000; 39:886-93.
21. Fillatreau S, Sweenie CH, McGeachy MJ et al. B-cells regulate autoimmunity by provision of IL-10. Nat Immunol 2002; 3:944-50.
22. Renaudineau Y, Vallet S, Le Dantec C et al. Characterization of the human CD5 endogenous retrovirus-E in B lymphocytes. Genes Immun 2005; 6:663-71.
23. Renaudineau Y, Hillion S, Saraux A et al. An alternative exon 1 of the CD5 gene regulates CD5 expression in human B lymphocytes. Blood 2005; 106:2781-9.
24. Garaud S, Le Dantec C, Berthou C et al. Selection of the alternative exon 1 from the CD5 gene down-regulates membrane level of the protein in B lymphocytes. J Immunol 2008; 181:2010-8.
25. Garaud S, Le Dantec C, Jousse-Joulin S et al. IL-6 modulates CD5 expression in B-cells from patients with lupus by regulating DNA methylation. J Immunol 2009; 182:5623-32.
26. Brooks WH, Le Dantec C, Pers JO et al. Epigenetics and autoimmunity. J Autoimmun 2010; 34:J207-19.
27. Cannat A, Seligmann M. Induction by isoniazid and hydrallazine of antinuclear factors in mice. Clin Exp Immunol 1968; 3:99-105.
28. Mazari L, Ouarzane M, Zouali M. Subversion of B lymphocyte tolerance by hydralazine, a potential mechanism for drug-induced lupus. Proc Natl Acad Sci U SA 2007; 104:6317-22.

29. Quddus J, Johnson KJ, Gavalchin J et al. Treating activated CD4+ T-cells with either of two distinct DNA methyltransferase inhibitors, 5-azacytidine or procainamide, is sufficient to cause a lupus-like disease in syngeneic mice. J Clin Invest 1993; 92:38-53.

30. Javierre BM, Fernandez AF, Richter J et al. Changes in the pattern of DNA methylation associate with twin discordance in systemic lupus erythematosus. Genome Res 2010; 20:170-9.

31. Zhao S, Long H, Lu Q. Epigenetic perspectives in systemic lupus erythematosus: Pathogenesis, biomarkers and therapeutic potentials. Clin Rev Allergy Immunol 2009; DOI:10-1007/s12016-009-8165-7.

32. Gorelik G, Fang JY, Wu A et al. Impaired T-cell protein kinase C delta activation decreases ERK pathway signaling in idiopathic and hydralazine-induced lupus. J Immunol 2007; 179:5553-63.

33. Miyamoto A, Nakayama K, Imaki H et al. Increased proliferation of B-cells and auto-immunity in mice lacking protein kinase Cdelta. Nature 2002; 416:865-9.

34. Youinou P, Jamin C. The weight of interleukin-6 in B-cell-related autoimmune disorders. J Autoimmun 2009; 32:206-10.

35. Liang B, Gardner DB, Griswold DE et al. Anti-interleukin-6 monoclonal antibody inhibits autoimmune responses in a murine model of systemic lupus erythematosus. Immunology 2006; 119:296-305.

36. Hillion S, Garaud S, Devauchelle V et al. Interleukin-6 is responsible for aberrant B-cell receptor-mediated regulation of RAG expression in systemic lupus erythematosus. Immunology 2007; 122:371-80.

37. Brown SE, Fraga MF, Weaver IC et al. Variations in DNA methylation patterns during the cell cycle of HeLa cells. Epigenetics 2007; 2:54-65.

38. Dandrea M, Donadelli M, Costanzo C et al. MeCP2/H3meK9 are involved in IL-6 gene silencing in pancreatic adenocarcinoma cell lines. Nucleic Acids Res 2009; 37:6681-90.

39. Mi XB, Zeng FQ. Hypomethylation of interleukin-4 and -6 promoters in T-cells from systemic lupus erythematosus patients. Acta Pharmacol Sin 2008; 29:105-12.

40. BlancoBetancourt CE, Moncla A, Milili M et al. Defective B-cell-negative selection and terminal differentiation in the ICF syndrome. Blood 2004; 103:2683-90.

41. Renaudineau Y. The Revolution of Epigenetics in the Field of Autoimmunity. Clin Rev Allergy Immunol 2009; DOI: 10-1007/s12016-009-8171-9.

CHAPTER 6

ENVIRONMENTAL AGENTS
AND AUTOIMMUNE DISEASES

Frederick W. Miller

National Institute of Environmental Health Sciences, National Institutes of Health, HHS, Bethesda, Maryland, USA
Email: millerf@mail.nih.gov

Abstract: Autoimmune diseases, which comprise over 80 clinically distinct conditions, are characterized by the presence of autoantibodies or autoreactive T cells directed against self structures (autoantigens). While these often incurable disorders appear to be rapidly increasing in recognition throughout the world, their rarity, heterogeneity and complex etiologies have limited our understanding of their pathogeneses. The precise mechanisms for the development of autoimmune diseases are not known, however, evidence from many complementary lines of investigation suggests that autoimmune diseases result from the interactions of both environmental and genetic risk factors. While considerable progress has been made in understanding multiple genetic risk factors for many autoimmune diseases, relatively little information is now available regarding the role of the environment in the development of these illnesses. This chapter examines the limited but growing evidence for the role of the environment in the development and progression of autoimmune diseases, the specific exposures that have been suspected of being involved, the possible mechanisms by which these agents may induce and sustain autoimmune processes and the approaches needed to better understand these issues in the future. Identifying the necessary and sufficient genetic and environmental risk factors for disease holds the promise of allowing for the prevention of some illnesses through avoidance of environmental risk factors by genetically susceptible individuals or via gene or other therapies to correct the effects of deleterious genetic risk factors in the case of unavoidable environmental agents.

Epigenetic Contributions in Autoimmune Disease, edited by Esteban Ballestar.
©2011 Landes Bioscience and Springer Science+Business Media.

INTRODUCTION

Autoimmune diseases are pathologic conditions associated with self-reactive components of the immune system. Most of these illnesses are defined by clinical signs, symptoms and laboratory features that include characteristic autoantibodies or self-directed T-cell responses. Data regarding their incidence and prevalence are limited, but many investigators believe they are increasing for unknown reasons.[1,2] Collectively, over 80 different autoimmune diseases (Table 1) afflict 14-23 million Americans, an estimated 5 to 8 percent of the population.[3] Autoimmune diseases can affect one or more organs in any part of the body and have many clinical manifestations, making them difficult to

Table 1. Diseases with evidence supporting an autoimmune etiology. Source: American Autoimmune Related Diseases Association (http://www.aarda.org/)

- Acute Disseminated Encephalomyelitis (ADEM)
- Acute necrotizing hemorrhagic leukoencephalitis
- Addison's disease
- Agammaglobulinemia
- Allergic asthma
- Allergic rhinitis
- Alopecia areata
- Amyloidosis
- Ankylosing spondylitis
- Anti-GBM/Anti-TBM nephritis
- Antiphospholipid syndrome (APS)
- Autoimmune aplastic anemia
- Autoimmune dysautonomia
- Autoimmune hepatitis
- Autoimmune hyperlipidemia
- Autoimmune immunodeficiency
- Autoimmune inner ear disease (AIED)
- Autoimmune myocarditis
- Autoimmune pancreatitis
- Autoimmune retinopathy
- Autoimmune thrombocytopenic purpura (ATP)
- Autoimmune thyroid disease
- Axonal and neuronal neuropathies
- Balo disease
- Behcet's disease
- Bullous pemphigoid
- Cardiomyopathy
- Castleman disease
- Celiac sprue (nontropical)
- Chagas disease
- Chronic fatigue syndrome
- Chronic inflammatory demyelinating polyneuropathy (CIDP)
- Chronic recurrent multifocal ostomyelitis (CRMO)
- Churg-Strauss syndrome

continued on next page

Table 1. Continued

- Cicatricial pemphigoid/benign mucosal pemphigoid
- Crohn's disease
- Cogans syndrome
- Cold agglutinin disease
- Congenital heart block
- Coxsackie myocarditis
- CREST disease
- Essential mixed cryoglobulinemia
- Demyelinating neuropathies
- Dermatomyositis
- Devic's disease (neuromyelitis optica)
- Discoid lupus
- Dressler's syndrome
- Endometriosis
- Eosinophilic fasciitis
- Erythema nodosum
- Experimental allergic encephalomyelitis
- Evans syndrome
- Fibromyalgia**
- Fibrosing alveolitis
- Giant cell arteritis (temporal arteritis)
- Glomerulonephritis
- Goodpasture's syndrome
- Graves' disease
- Guillain-Barre syndrome
- Hashimoto's encephalitis
- Hashimoto's thyroiditis
- Hemolytic anemia
- Henoch-Schonlein purpura
- Herpes gestationis
- Hypogammaglobulinemia
- Idiopathic thrombocytopenic purpura (ITP)
- IgA nephropathy
- Immunoregulatory lipoproteins
- Inclusion body myositis
- Insulin-dependent diabetes (type1)
- Interstitial cystitis
- Juvenile arthritis
- Juvenile diabetes
- Kawasaki syndrome
- Lambert-Eaton syndrome
- Leukocytoclastic vasculitis
- Lichen planus
- Lichen sclerosus
- Ligneous conjunctivitis
- Linear IgA disease (LAD)
- Lyme disease
- Meniere's disease

continued on next page

Table 1. Continued

- Microscopic polyangiitis
- Mixed connective tissue disease (MCTD)
- Mooren's ulcer
- Mucha-Habermann disease
- Multiple sclerosis
- Myasthenia gravis
- Myositis
- Narcolepsy
- Neuromyelitis optica (see Devic's)
- Neutropenia
- Ocular cicatricial pemphigoid
- Optic neuritis
- Palindromic rheumatism
- PANDAS (Pediatric Autoimmune Neuropsychiatric Disorders Associated with Streptococcus)
- Paraneoplastic cerebellar degeneration
- Paroxysmal nocturnal hemoglobinuria (PNH)
- Parry Romberg syndrome
- Parsonnage-Turner syndrome
- Pars planitis (peripheral uveitis)
- Pemphigus
- Peripheral neuropathy
- Perivenous encephalomyelitis
- Pernicious anemia
- POEMS syndrome
- Polyarteritis nodosa
- Type I, II, and III autoimmune polyglandular syndromes
- Polymyalgia rheumatica
- Polymyositis
- Postmyocardial infarction syndrome
- Postpericardiotomy syndrome
- Progesterone dermatitis
- Primary biliary cirrhosis
- Primary sclerosing cholangitis
- Psoriasis
- Psoriatic arthritis
- Idiopathic pulmonary fibrosis
- Pyoderma gangrenosum
- Pure red cell aplasia
- Raynauds phenomenon
- Reflex sympathetic dystrophy
- Reiter's syndrome
- Relapsing polychondritis
- Restless legs syndrome
- Retroperitoneal Fibrosis
- Rheumatic fever
- Rheumatoid arthritis
- Sarcoidosis

continued on next page

Table 1. Continued

- Schmidt syndrome
- Scleritis
- Scleroderma
- Sjogren's syndrome
- Sperm and testicular autoimmunity
- Stiff person syndrome
- Subacute bacterial endocarditis (SBE)
- Sympathetic ophthalmia
- Systemic Lupus Erythematosus
- Takayasu's arteritis
- Temporal arteritis/Giant cell arteritis
- Thrombocytopenic purpura (TTP)
- Tolosa-Hunt syndrome
- Transverse myelitis
- Ulcerative colitis
- Undifferentiated connective tissue disease (UCTD)
- Uveitis
- Vasculitis
- Vesiculobullous dermatosis
- Vitiligo
- Wegener's granulomatosis

diagnose. Autoimmune diseases also may share many clinical features and risk factors, so that a patient may suffer from more than one autoimmune disorder, or multiple autoimmune diseases may occur in the same family. Since all the autoimmune diseases are mediated by the immune system, the basic treatment is similar and involves the use of immunosuppressive agents and sometimes adjunct or supportive management with occupational or physical therapy. For these and other reasons, the autoimmune diseases should be thought of as a family of related disorders that should be studied collectively as well as individually.[4]

Mechanisms for the development of autoimmune diseases remain obscure despite intense investigation, yet a consensus is emerging that they likely occur as a result of chronic inflammation after selected environmental exposures in genetically susceptible individuals.[5] Despite the great progress that has been made in understanding a number of major histocompatibility complex (MHC) and nonMHC genetic risk factors for autoimmune diseases,[6] relatively little information is now available regarding the role of specific environmental agents in the development of these disorders. This is partly the result of the rarity of these conditions, the lack of easy-to-use and validated exposure biomarkers and environmental assessment tools, difficulties inherent in defining which of many environmental exposures that occur frequently are related to disease, the little formal training in environmental medicine, the few resources dedicated to this area and the lack of consensus approaches for the definition of environmentally associated diseases. As a result, the specific environmental triggers remain unknown for most autoimmune conditions.

It appears that multiple genes need to be present in an individual to induce autoimmune disease[7] and similarly, multiple environmental exposures may also need to occur in a particular sequence, or in tandem, to provoke the chronic immune activation that leads to autoimmunity.[8] Thus, lessons might be learned from studies of similar diseases, such as cancers, which like autoimmune diseases, are complex conditions in which many genetic and environmental risk factors must interact in a correct sequence, before development of disease.[9] For example, a genetic, epigenetic or immune regulatory change induced by one exposure may be necessary before a subsequent exposure can have its effect. Alternatively, mixtures of exposures, including possible combinations of infectious and non-infectious agents, perhaps occurring during critical physiologic windows when persons may be more susceptible to them, may be necessary in order to overcome immune tolerance and induce autoimmunity. Additional general principles from the study of cancer that might be relevant to autoimmunity include: (1) the clinical, pathologic and pathogenetic heterogeneity of different entities as currently defined; (2) the low effect sizes from many environmental exposures requiring large samples for most studies; (3) the possible requirement for inducers, promoters and sustainers of disease at different points in the pathogenetic process; (4) the requirement for interaction with key genetic susceptibility factors; and (5) possible long latencies from exposure to pathogenic agents to the development of immune system alteration and then additional delays to the development of pathology.[10] This latter principle is supported by studies suggesting that cytokine and chemokine elevations, immune activation and autoantibodies precede the development of clinical disease by months to years.[11-13]

In the context of this chapter, environmental exposures will be considered to be all those factors that are not inherited. These are often divided into two general categories, infectious agents—which include viruses, bacteria and parasites—and non-infectious agents—including foods, drugs, devices, occupational exposures, lifestyle patterns, chemical components of air and water, radiation and other incidental exposures.

EVIDENCE SUGGESTING ENVIRONMENTAL AGENTS PLAY A ROLE IN THE DEVELOPMENT OF AUTOIMMUNE DISEASE

The evidence that environmental agents may play a pathogenic role in autoimmune disease comes from many complementary lines of study (Table 2). Although some of these are indirect or anecdotal evidence, taken together, the findings strongly support the notion that most autoimmune diseases do have an important environmental component.[5,14]

An important line of evidence for the role of the environment is that for autoimmune diseases there is generally much less than 50% disease concordance in monozygotic twins.[14,15] Although this may possibly be due to stochastic or other events, this consistent low level of disease concordance in genetically identical persons among all autoimmune disorders studied, as well as the many other lines of evidence implicating environmental factors, argues against this. These findings suggest that even if all the genetic risk factors for a given autoimmune disease were identified, it would not allow for prediction of disease with any greater accuracy than the flip of a coin without the incorporation of environmental, epigenetic or other factors.

The definition of an environmental disease in a person can be achieved by identifying a clinical disorder, which develops soon after a novel exposure (challenge), resolves when the exposure is removed (dechallenge) and then recurs after reintroduction of the same exposure (rechallenge).[16] Classic cases of this type include exposures to defined chemical entities such as drugs, foods, or inhaled toxicants whose effects are short-lived

Table 2. Lines of evidence supporting the role of environmental agents in the development of autoimmune disease

1. Low disease concordance in monozygotic twins
2. Temporal associations with some environmental exposures and later disease onset (challenge)
3. Disease resolution or improvement after removal of the suspect agent (dechallenge)
4. Disease recurrence or worsening after re-exposure to the suspect agent (rechallenge)
5. Seasonality in birth dates in some autoimmune diseases or phenotypes
6. Seasonality in disease onset in some autoimmune diseases or phenotypes
7. Geographic clustering with the onset of disease or disease prevalence
8. Changes in the prevalence or incidence of disease over time
9. Changes in disease frequency when genetically similar cohorts move to different geographic locations
10. Biologic plausibility from animal models that develop disease after specific exposures
11. Genetic risk factors for autoimmune disease regulate immune responses to environmental agents
12. Higher rates of disease in certain occupations
13. Higher rates of disease after higher doses of or more prolonged exposure (a dose-response effect)
14. Epidemiologic associations between particular exposures and certain diseases

Modified from reference 62.

and resolve if the agent is removed. Many xenobiotics (compounds found in an organism but which are not normally produced or expected to be present in it), however, cannot be removed after exposing an organism to them and in these cases this approach is not usually helpful. Exposures in this category include inhaled silica, vaccines, some petrochemicals and medical implants.

The unusual time-space associations of disease onset with some autoimmune illnesses also imply that nongenetic factors play a role in disease development. Examples here are more preliminary and sometimes have not been reproduced, allowing for the possibility that referral or other biases might explain the findings. Nevertheless, investigations have found that certain autoimmune disorders have a seasonal onset[17] or that there is a seasonal association with disease onset in subsets of patients based upon disease-specific autoantibodies.[18,19] Furthermore, studies of Type 1 diabetes have found significant associations with birth dates[20,21] implying that certain exposures at certain times of the year may alter the target tissues or immune systems of fetuses or neonates resulting in later autoimmunity. Infections are often presumed to be the source of seasonal or geographic associations, yet the immune system, like other organ systems, has cyclic patterns[22] that are likely related to light exposure and mediated by melatonin or other neurohormones.[23] Additionally, many non-infectious exposures are seasonal, including exposures to pesticides, chemicals in sunscreens and certain air or water pollutants, so non-infectious agents could account for some of these findings. Geographic clustering or gradients in disease prevalence or incidence have also been found for some autoimmune diseases. These investigations include associations with latitude, suggesting a role of ultraviolet radiation or other associated effects in either inducing disease, as may be the case for dermatomyositis,[24,25] or protecting from disease, as may be the case in multiple sclerosis and Type 1 diabetes.[26]

Changes in the incidence or prevalence of disease over time also suggest a nongenetic etiology given the slow rate of genetic change in a population. Type 1 diabetes, multiple sclerosis, myasthenia gravis, primary biliary cirrhosis Crohn's disease,SLE and myositis all appear to be increasingly prevalent, while rheumatoid arthritis may be decreasing in frequency in some populations.[1,27-31] Studies of genetically similar populations who move to live under different conditions are also interesting. The incidence of both multiple sclerosis and Type 1 diabetes changed as members of a population moved to new regions with higher incidence rates.[32,33]

Unfortunately, the gold standard approach to defining associations of environmental agents with disease—carefully controlled and adequately powered epidemiologic studies—are limited.[5] Large, well-designed, multicenter and sometimes international studies, using appropriate controls and collecting adequate information to minimize confounding, are needed in the future to more fully define the specific environmental risk factors for each disease or phenotype.

DEFINING ENVIRONMENTALLY ASSOCIATED AUTOIMMUNE DISEASES

A general problem in the field of identifying environmental agents that may cause autoimmune disorders is the lack of consensus on the necessary and sufficient evidence needed to define an environmentally associated condition.[2] This is further complicated by medical-legal issues often involved in a number of environmental exposures. To address this problem, a group of experts in the field—members of the American College of Rheumatology Environmentally Associated Rheumatic Disease Study Group—developed consensus on a general structural framework to address this issue and divided the process into four stages.[16]

The first stage is the identification of a single case, or a series of cases, which are clinically suspected of resulting from an exposure (Table 3). The consensus of the group is that such first stage cases need to meet a number of criteria to assure a minimum number of attribution elements are present.[16] A total of at least four of eight possible attribution elements need to be present, including at least three of five primary elements. The five primary elements are: (1) temporal plausibility, taking into account the pharmacokinetics and pharmacodynamics of the agent, the minimum induction time and maximum latency that are thought to be possible; (2) exclusion of other likely causes for the case based on prior experience with the clinical entity and the agent in question; (3) dechallenge if possible (clinical evidence for resolution or improvement in the case after removing the suspect agent); (4) rechallenge if appropriate (clinical evidence for the reinitiation or exacerbation of the case if it is appropriate to give the agent to the patient again) and (5) biologic plausibility based on the known effects of the agent. An additional three secondary elements are: the publication of reports of similar cases (analogy); publication of nearly identical cases (specificity); and evidence that exposure to higher doses or for a more prolonged period is needed for development of disease (a dose-response effect). Also, information regarding the history and clinical examination, laboratory and biopsy results, demographic details, the family history of similar disorders, knowledge of prior infections or physiology-altering exposures, all prior clinical diagnoses and the type/ route/dose/duration/source of the exposure should be detailed in the report.

The second stage involves testing the possible association via epidemiologic studies, using surveillance criteria, to evaluate the relationship between a given exposure

Table 3. Proposed stages for identifying and defining environmentally associated autoimmune diseases

Stage	Description	Proposed Nomenclature for the Syndrome (Example)
Stage 1—Proposing the association	Case reports, defined by adequate criteria, propose a possible association of a specific clinical syndrome with a given exposure	Syndrome following exposure (Rheumatoid Arthritis following Hepatitis B vaccination)
Stage 2—Testing the association	After a number of such cases are reported, surveillance criteria are proposed and epidemiologic and laboratory studies test that hypothesis	Cardinal signs, symptoms and labs but without the putative exposure (Eosinophilia Myalgia syndrome)
Stage 3—Defining criteria for the condition	If studies above support the association, then specific preliminary classification and other criteria are defined for that specific environmental disease	Exposure-associated disorder (L tryptophan-associated Eosinophilia Myalgia syndrome)
Stage 4—Refining criteria for the condition	Criteria are reassessed and refined as necessary as additional data are obtained about the disease to confirm the association	Exposure-induced disorder (Hydralazine-induced Lupus-like disorder)

Modified from reference 16.

and a given syndrome, or by in vitro, in vivo or animal studies as appropriate. Other approaches could be used, such as case-control settings, to determine if the cases that develop after the environmental exposure differ clinically or genetically from those with similar diseases without the exposure or differ from subjects similarly exposed who do not develop disease.

If convincing evidence is obtained that the association is plausible, then the third stage will develop preliminary criteria for that environmentally associated disease. Classification criteria will define, with reasonable sensitivity and specificity, groups of patients with one disorder from closely related diseases. Approaches involving Delphi or Nominal Group Techniques using expert committees and appropriate mathematical algorithms could be used to develop these criteria.[34] Symptom, sign and laboratory criteria should be expressed in clinically sensible and practical formats with precise definitions of constituent elements. The fourth stage repeats the same processes used in the third stage if new information is collected to warrant a redefinition of the disease.

This proposed staging structure has certain limitations, including that the decision as to when to progress from one stage to the next stage remain somewhat subjective, yet it does give an overall framework to plan for future studies and it allows the classification of the environmental agents into groups with levels of evidence for their association with specific syndromes. The current limited information in this field means that most environmental agents suspected of being associated with autoimmune diseases today remain in Stages 1 or 2.

ENVIRONMENTAL AGENTS ASSOCIATED WITH AUTOIMMUNE DISEASES

Infectious Agents

Viruses, bacteria and parasites have all been proposed as possible triggers of autoimmune diseases and yet they also may modulate immune function to possibly prevent the development of autoimmune disease.[35] In fact, the 'hygiene hypothesis' proposes that the recent increases in immune-mediated diseases in developed countries might be related to an early life environment that is relatively deficient in microbial flora.

While many case reports and small case series describe the development of various autoimmune diseases following infections, few epidemiologic investigations have addressed this issue.[36] Controlled studies suggest an increased risk for rheumatoid arthritis and SLE after certain infections by measuring the presence of antibodies to various viral components of Epstein-Barr virus (EBV), Cytomegalovirus (CMV) and Herpes virus in sera or via questionnaires.[5] The evidence that suggests EBV is associated with autoimmune diseases includes an increased presence of antibodies to viral peptides and the ability to amplify EBV genomes by PCR in more autoimmune disease subjects compared to controls, as well as similarities between the products of EBV genes and autoantigens.[37] For further reading on EBV effects on epigenetic control see Chapter 7.

Parvovirus B19 can induce a transient reactive polyarthritis, but several investigations have also suggested parvovirus might be an etiologic agent in autoimmune diseases.[5] In children with an acute onset of arthritis, those with IgM antibodies to B19 developed a chronic arthritis indistinguishable from juvenile rheumatoid arthritis, while those children who lacked IgM antibodies to B19 did not progress to a chronic form of arthritis.[38] In a carefully conducted study in juvenile dermatomyositis, however, investigators failed to find an increase in serum IgG antibodies to parvovirus B19.[39]

New immunologic and molecular screening technologies should allow for the assessment of larger numbers of autoimmune diseases in rapid and efficient ways that could allow for more definitive analyses of the pathogenic role of infections.[40-42]

Drugs

Drugs are some of the best recognized and most often reported agents associated with autoimmunity and autoimmune diseases (Table 4). It is not necessarily the case, however, that drugs are more likely than other chemicals to result in autoimmunity. Rather, it is likely that the widespread use and careful monitoring of drugs by many parties, along with the regulatory oversight and adverse event reporting systems in many countries, has focused more attention on drugs. Also, the rapid metabolism and ease of collection of dechallenge and rechallange evidence has allowed associations in individual patients to be more carefully documented. Hundreds of drugs have been associated in case reports or published case series with a number of immune-mediated or autoimmune illnesses, yet few have met the consensus criteria described above to allow exclusion of confounding factors. Both chemicals and biologic agents used as drugs have been associated with autoimmune disease.

Lupus-like disorders seem to be the most common autoimmune conditions to develop after drug use.[43] These are often characterized by autoantibodies to histones and single-stranded DNA, rather than autoantibodies to double stranded DNA as are found

Table 4. Selected drugs associated in multiple case reports or in case series with autoimmune disorders

Drug	Associated Autoimmune Disorders
α-methyldopa	lupus-like syndrome, hemolytic anemia, thrombocytopenia
allopurinol	lupus-like syndrome, vasculitis
anti-TNFα agents	lupus-like syndrome, hepatitis
bleomycin	scleroderma
captropril	lupus-like syndrome, vasculitis, membranous glomerulopathy
chlorpromazine	lupus-like syndrome, hemolytic anemia
D-penicillamine	lupus-like syndrome, myositis, hypothyroidism, Goodpasture's
estrogens	lupus-like syndrome, myositis
gold salts	lupus-like syndrome, membranous glomerulopathy
hydralazine	lupus-like syndrome, vasculitis
interferon-alpha/beta	lupus-like syndrome, antiphospholipid syndrome, arthritis, hemolytic anemia, thrombocytopenia, hepatitis, myositis, hypothyroidism
interferon-gamma	lupus-like syndrome, myositis, arthritis, hypothyroidism
interleukin-2	scleroderma, antiphospholipid syndrome, arthritis, hypothyroidism
iodine	hypothyroidism
isoniazid	lupus-like syndrome, arthritis, hepatitis, vasculitis, hypothyroidism
L-tryptophan	EMS, scleroderma, myositis, neuropathies
lipid-lowering agents	lupus-like syndrome, myositis, hepatitis
penicillins	hemolytic anemia, lupus-like syndrome
phenytoin	scleroderma, lupus-like syndrome, hepatitis, thrombocytopenia
procainamide	lupus-like syndrome
propylthiouracil	lupus-like syndrome, ANCA+ vasculitis, myositis
quinidine	lupus-like syndrome, arthritis, thrombocytopenia
rifampicin	thrombocytopenia, vasculitis
sulphonamides	lupus-like syndrome, vasculitis
tetracyclines	lupus-like syndrome, arthritis, vasculitis

Reviewed in references 71, 72, 77-80; ANCA: antineutrophil cytoplasmic antibodies; EMS: eosinophilia myalgia syndrome.

more often in idiopathic lupus. Drug related lupus also differs from idiopathic lupus in having more frequent arthritis and less frequent neurologic and renal involvement, as well as having possibly different genetic risk factors. This appears to be a general phenomenon in that many cases of drug-linked disorders often differ from the idiopathic forms in clinical, serologic or genetic features. Nonetheless, the data are very limited in this regard and there are examples where the drug-related cases do not differ from idiopathic ones.

In terms of possible mechanisms for drug-related autoimmunity, there are no common drug structures, binding sites, functions, pathways, metabolites or other features among them that consistently allow prediction of their toxicity. Therefore, a current understanding of the pathogeneses of these syndromes remains incomplete. Collecting adequate numbers of cases in repositories to decipher the genetic and other risk factors that result in drug-induced diseases so that they can someday be predicted and prevented would be a fruitful approach in this area.

Occupational Exposures

Limited but growing epidemiologic and experimental data have linked a number of occupational exposures to autoimmune diseases (Table 5). Silica, solvents, pesticides and ultraviolet radiation are of particular concern.[5,10] Strong associations have been reported in investigations of silica dust and rheumatoid arthritis, lupus, scleroderma and antineutrophil cytoplasmic autoantibody (ANCA) associated glomerulonephritis.[44]

Table 5. Occupational exposures associated with autoimmune diseases in epidemiologic studies

Exposure	Disease	Summary of Results
Crystalline silica	Scleroderma	3-fold increased risk in 4 occupational cohort studies; mixed results in 5 population-based case-control studies
	Rheumatoid arthritis	3-fold (or higher) increased risk in 5 occupational cohort studies
	Lupus	>10 fold increased risk in 3 occupational cohort studies
	ANCA + vasculitis	4-fold increased risk in 3 case-control studies
Ionizing radiation	Autoimmune thyroid disease	~3.5 risk in females among 4299 workers in Pomerania.
Solvents	Scleroderma	Mixed results, but some evidence of 2-3 fold increased risk with specific solvents (e.g., paint thinners and removers, trichloroetheylene) and with "any" solvent
	Undifferentiated connective tissue disease	2-fold increased risk with paint thinners and removers, mineral spirits; 3-fold increased risk with specific solvent-related occupations
	Rheumatoid arthritis	Weak or no association with specific solvents, but 2-fold increased risk among spray painters and lacquer workers
	Multiple sclerosis	2-3 fold increased risk with solvent exposures in most studies
Mercury	Lupus	~3 fold risk in the Carolina Lupus Study
Mineral oil	Rheumatoid arthritis	Slight increased risk in Swedish men
Pesticides	Rheumatoid arthritis	Weak associations (relative risks <2.0 seen with pesticide exposure and in farmers and horticultural workers
	Lupus	~4 fold risk after mixing pesticides
Ultraviolet radiation	Multiple sclerosis	Reduced risk (OR 0.74) of multiple sclerosis and mortality with increased occupational exposure to sunlight

Reviewed in reference 10 and reference 5 with additional information from reference 81. OR: odds ratio; ANCA: antineutrophil cytoplasmic antibodies.

Less strong associations are seen for solvent exposures (in scleroderma, undifferentiated connective tissue disease and multiple sclerosis) and for farming or pesticide exposures (in rheumatoid arthritis).

Assessing the role of occupational exposures in disease presents a number of problems. These include: (1) there are few biomarkers for specific chemical exposures acutely and none that capture lifetime cumulative exposures: (2) few validated and easy to use occupational exposure questionnaires; (3) limited power of relatively small studies resulting in imprecise risk estimates; and (4) possible confounding from multiple exposures in occupations that makes it difficult to ascertain the primary associations.

Non-Occupational Exposures

Many other non-occupational exposures have been studied and have been proposed to be associated with autoimmune diseases (Table 6). Evidence supporting these proposed associations include case reports, case series, in vitro assays, animal model studies and epidemiologic investigations, yet most have not been confirmed by appropriate independent study.[45]

Smoking tobacco has been reported to result in increased risks of rheumatoid arthritis, autoimmune thyroid disease and Crohn's disease in several studies, but inconsistent results were found in studies of smoking and SLE. Of interest, smoking appears to be associated with a reduced risk of ulcerative colitis implying that different compounds in tobacco smoke may alter risk for different diseases in a variety of ways or have different effects in different genetic backgrounds.

Heavy metals, including mercury, cadmium, gold salts and beryllium have been associated with different diseases, some of which have features of autoimmunity. Also, animal models have convincingly demonstrated inflammatory and autoimmune responses to these compounds, which appear to differ in different genetic backgrounds.[46]

Vaccines have raised controversy relating to concerns about their involvement in a number of different diseases. Because they are foreign proteins often injected with adjuvants into muscle to induce immune responses, immune-mediated adverse events would not be unexpected.[47,48] A number of autoimmune diseases have been reported to develop following various vaccinations, yet only a few have been deemed associated with disease by the Advisory Committee on Immunization Practices[49] and are now compensated by the National Vaccine Injury Compensation Program (http://www.hrsa.gov/vaccinecompensation/). These include chronic arthritis after rubella virus vaccines, thrombocytopenic purpura after measles vaccines and brachial neuritis or Guillain-Barre syndrome after certain swine flu or tetanus vaccines. While other illnesses are possibly caused by immunizations, as suggested by case reports or animal models, most epidemiologic studies have not shown significant associations.[50]

Medical devices, particularly silicone breast implants, remain controversial agents that have been proposed to be associated with multiple autoimmune or connective tissue disorders. Studies have been hampered by litigation involved in adverse events following silicone implants and the lack of adequate regulatory review prior to their initial use. Nonetheless, most studies, although underpowered for rare disorders, have not found significant associations with common autoimmune diseases.[51,52] Yet, some investigators believe that rare or atypical autoimmune diseases and fibromyalgia remain inadequately studied.[53,54] An investigation of 37 patients with the rare autoimmune muscle disease called myositis that developed after a variety of silicone implants found significantly different

Table 6. Non-occupational exposures proposed as possible risk factors for autoimmune diseases

Exposure	Disease	Comments and References
Cigarette smoking	Rheumatoid arthritis	Studies suggest relative risks of 1.5-3 with a greater effect in men, seropositive disease and those with the shared RA epitope[82-84]
	Autoimmune thyroid disease	Meta-analyses suggest 2-3 fold increased risks of Grave's and Hashimoto's[85]
	Inflammatory bowel disease	Smoking increases risks for Crohn's disease but decreases risks for ulcerative colitis[86]
	Lupus	Increased risk in current smokers[87]
Dietary gluten	Celiac disease	Gluten-induces disease in genetically susceptible hosts[88]
Dietary meat and protein	Rheumatoid arthritis	Increased risk noted in a European study[89]
Heavy metals	Multiple syndromes	"Pink disease" (acrodynia) and glomerulopathy from mercury toxicity; related syndromes with elements of autoimmunity from cadmium and gold salt toxicity; granulomatous pneumonitis from beryllium exposure; support for genetic risk factors in animal models[90-92]
Hormones	Lupus	Mixed results but larger studies suggest a trend for estrogens[5]
Vaccines	Multiple syndromes	Arthritis after rubella virus vaccines; thrombocytopenia after measles vaccines; Guillain-Barre syndrome after swine flu vaccine and tetanus; controversy remains over others[50]
Collagen implants	Myositis	In one study OR = 5.1; 95% CI, 2.3 to 9.6 for all forms of myositis[56]
Silicone implants	Multiple syndromes	Most studies do not find associations with common autoimmune diseases;[51,52] rare or atypical connective tissue disease and fibromyalgia remain inadequately studied.[53,54]
Stress	Grave's disease	Stressful life events preceding the diagnosis were significantly higher than controls (OR = 6.3, CI = 2.7–14.7.[59]
Ultraviolet radiation	Lupus	Increased risk with >1 severe sunburn in youth[93]
	Dermatomyositis and anti-Mi-2 antibodies	Positive correlation of the proportion of dermatomyositis and anti-Mi-2 antibodies with global surface sunlight intensity on 4 continents [24] and in women in the US.[25]

OR: odds ratio; CI: 95% confidence interval; ANCA: antineutrophil cytoplasmic antibodies; Modified from reference 62.

immunogenetic backgrounds compared to 453 myositis patients without implants.[55] Of interest, collagen implants have also been associated with the development of myositis.[56] And, recent reports of multiple cases of scleroderma following silicone breast implants suggest that additional studies in this area may be warranted.[57]

Stressful life events may boost immune responses through induction of TNF-alpha, IL-1 and IL-8 and by inhibiting TGF-beta production.[58] Therefore, conditions that are associated with significant changes in stress system activity may modulate the neuroendocrine-immune axis and perturb systemic cytokine balances resulting in proinflammatory changes and disease induction. Anecdotal reports suggest that significant stressful life events have preceded the development of many autoimmune diseases. A large population-based, case control study of Grave's disease showed that patients had more negative life events in the 12 months preceding the diagnosis of Grave's and negative life-event scores were also significantly higher.[59] Other diseases have not been adequately studied.

THE IMPORTANCE OF GENE-ENVIRONMENT INTERACTIONS IN AUTOIMMUNE DISEASES

Most common human diseases likely arise from a combination of genetic and environmental risk factors and understanding these interactions is critical to defining risk and focusing preventative measures at the individual level.[14,60] The familial nature of many complex diseases suggests an underlying genetic susceptibility, but environmental or epigenetic factors must be important since in many conditions monozygotic twins are often not concordant for disease.[61] The current scientific view is that virtually all clinical traits will show gene-environment interaction when studied in adequate detail with appropriately powered analyses. Yet, these data are not available in adequate numbers of individuals to allow for these analyses to be performed for most diseases. Evidence of statistical interactions between genetic and environmental risk factors is often used as evidence for the existence of an underlying mechanistic interaction. Gene-environment interactions may be additive or multiplicative or they may be negative (or antagonistic) when protective genes or protective environmental exposures interact. Figure 1 depicts the possible interactions of environmental agents and genetics to result in the development of autoimmune phenotypes and emphasizes the role of possible protective factors.

The complex pattern of inheritance of most human diseases suggests that interactions of multiple unlinked genes and likely multiple environmental factors are needed to produce the phenotype.[8] Genetic hallmarks of complex phenotypes are: (1) that the alleles associated with implicated polymorphic genes are alone neither necessary nor sufficient for the development of disease and (2) that these alleles are not severe, null mutations, but rather are often functional and relatively common in the general population. Data suggest that most of these alleles have arisen because of random mutation and positive selection in past environments, but these same alleles are often disadvantageous in our current environments that include many drugs and other chemical compounds, as well as infectious agents, that were not present during most of human evolution.[62] Thus, the understanding of environmental factors and their effects should always consider the contributing roles of genetic risk and protective factors.[63]

POSSIBLE MECHANISMS BY WHICH ENVIRONMENTAL AGENTS MAY INDUCE AUTOIMMUNE DISEASE

The mechanisms for the role of environmental agents in inducing autoimmune diseases are poorly understood. Yet, a variety of theories have been put forward to explain how

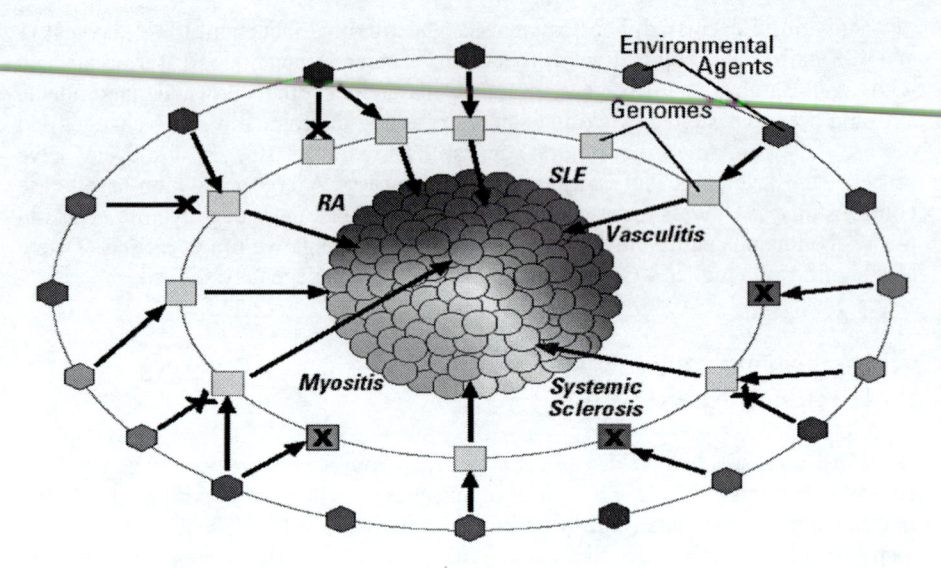

Figure 1. Possible phenotypes of autoimmune diseases resulting from different gene–environment interactions. Each autoimmune disease as currently defined is composed of multiple phenotypes, which in their indivisible form could be called elemental disorders. These are represented here as spheres, each of which would be defined by a unique combination of symptoms, clinical signs and laboratory abnormalities. Each elemental disorder could result from a unique pathogenesis as a result of the interactions between the necessary and sufficient genetic and environmental risk factors. Each box represents an individual's genome and each hexagon a particular environmental exposure. As shown, certain combinations of genotypes and environmental exposures induce specific disease phenotypes, while other combinations have no effect or can even be protective (as indicated by an X). RA, rheumatoid arthritis; SLE, systemic lupus erythematosus. Reproduced with permission from reference 5.

xenobiotics and other exposures may induce disease.[45] The diversity of these theories themselves, however, points to the lack of understanding of even the most carefully-defined environmentally associated diseases. Evidence also implies that different pathogenic mechanisms are likely at work in different syndromes.

One popular theory for how chemicals may induce autoimmunity is their binding to self molecules to induce novel structures, which then overcome immune tolerance. This "hapten hypothesis" is supported by clinical and laboratory evidence in the case of drug-induced hematologic autoimmune disorders.[64] Agents may also alter the cellular level or location of autoantigens or decrease their removal. An example of this would be ultraviolet radiation, which is known to upregulate certain autoantigens, alter their subcellular distribution and induce apoptotic cells, which are cleared at a slower rate in autoimmune individuals.[65-68] Post-translational modification of proteins may also induce an immune attack. This has been postulated to occur when tobacco smoke alters broncho-alveolar cell proteins by inducing citrillination, changing the amino acid arginine to citrulline. Such citrullinated proteins are common targets for autoantibodies in rheumatoid arthritis.[69] Molecular mimicry is defined as an immune response to an environmental agent that cross-reacts with a host antigen and this process is likely responsible for rheumatic fever following β hemolytic streptococcus infection as well as ant-Sm autoantibodies in lupus patients following EBV infection.[5] Other studies have found that over expression of CD70, a T-cell costimulatory molecule encoded by the *TNFSF7* gene, on CD4[+]

lupus T cells, as well as on procainamide- and hydralazine-treated T cells, is due to demethylation of a genetic element that suppresses CD70 expression when methylated.[70] These and other related findings suggest that epigenetic modifications following exposure to drugs, chemicals and other environmental agents may contribute to the induction of autoimmunity. Direct activation of the immune system occurs after the use of a number of therapeutic cytokines, including Type I interferons and interleukins and is the likely mechanism for the development of a number of autoimmune diseases following their use.[71,72] Other agents, including crystalline silica and certain silicones, also likely induce autoimmunity and autoimmune disorders via their direct effects on immune activation.[73]

An overall understanding of mechanisms for environmental effects needs to consider the concept of heterogeneity within the currently defined autoimmune diseases. A hypothesis that addresses this issue has been termed the "elemental disorder hypothesis". This concept posits that each autoimmune disease, as currently recognized, contains many stable and distinct phenotypes, which in their indivisible form are referred to as elemental disorders.[5,74] In this scenario, an elemental disorder is defined as a unique sign-symptom-laboratory complex that results from a distinct pathogenesis as a result of the interaction of the necessary and sufficient genetic and environmental risk factors (Fig. 1). If this concept is true, elemental disorders are likely complicating most studies of disease today via "comparisons of apples and oranges". Identifying elemental disorders should greatly increase the homogeneity of populations under study and significantly decrease the numbers of individuals needed for genetic, environmental, pathogenic and therapeutic studies. In the future, elemental disorder identification could allow for the prevention of some illnesses by avoidance of environmental risk factors or via gene or other therapy to correct deleterious genetic risk factors. The definition of genetic and environmental protective factors is equally important as these could also be harnessed to possibly prevent disease.

As mentioned before, many of the principles of carcinogenesis could be applied to the development of autoimmune diseases. The general concept here is that the pathogenic process could involve multiple sequential stages and that each stage may be dependent on the effects of prior agents. Beginning with genetic susceptibility, the action of one or more initiators of immune dysregulation that induce autoantibodies (autoimmunity) may first be necessary, followed by the subsequent effects of one or more promoters that would result in clinical pathology (autoimmune disease) and finally the effects of one or more sustainers of inflammation that would maintain autoimmune disease over time.[62]

CONCLUSION

Understanding the interactions of those elements that are necessary for autoimmune disease development offers the promise of preventing or treating autoimmune diseases in novel ways. To accomplish this, however, critical questions remain to be answered. Which particular gene-environment interactions lead to which specific clinical syndromes? What are the detailed pathogenic mechanisms involved? Is every autoimmune disease, as currently understood, actually composed of many subsets or "elemental disorders", each of which may be defined by a unique pathogenesis resulting from interactions of the necessary and sufficient risk factors? Can selected autoimmune diseases be better treated, cured, or even prevented through answers to some of the above questions?

Our complex and increasingly artificial environment complicates exposure assessments. Because more than 80,000 chemicals are registered for use in commerce in the United States to be included in our foods, personal care products, drugs, household cleaners and a host of industrial processes, we do not know the full range of environmental agents we are exposed to on a daily basis. Additionally, the long term effects of most of these chemicals on the immune system are unknown.

Parallel to whole genome scans, which have revolutionized our thinking about genetic risk factors for disease, the possibility of whole environmental scans should also be explored. Such global approaches appear daunting today, but new integrated systems biology methods, along with nanotechnology techniques for real-time individual analyte measurements in multiple tissues and worldwide geographic information systems and remote sensing measurements offer promise in this area.[75,76] Additionally, integrating validated exposure questionnaires with biomarkers for exposures from RNA expression signatures, proteomic or metabolomic analyses and antibody microarrays to capture the immune memory of a lifetime of exposures, could revolutionize our capacity to define environmental risk factors in the future.[62]

Many other challenges have prevented further understanding of the environmental risk factors that might trigger autoimmune diseases in genetically susceptible individuals. Nevertheless, a number of coordinated initiatives may be useful in overcoming these obstacles and making more progress in the future. These include: developing more validated exposure assessment tools and bioassays; increased training in the evaluation of environmental exposures; additional data on the incidence, prevalence and demographic information for autoimmune diseases; integrated databases and biorepositories; better coordination between animal model and human studies; increased worldwide integration of environmental exposures with geographic information systems. Critical for all these efforts is increased funding for understanding the environmental exposures that initiate, promote and sustain autoimmune disorders. These investments are likely very cost effective as they would have important clinical and financial implications for improving the public health.

ACKNOWLEDGEMENTS

I thank Drs. Lori Love and John Harley for many useful discussions and concepts. This research was supported by the Intramural Research Program of the National Institute of Environmental Health Sciences at the NIH.

REFERENCES

1. Bach JF. The effect of infections on susceptibility to autoimmune and allergic diseases. N Engl J Med 2002; 347(12):911-920.
2. WHO Task Group on Environmental Health Criteria. Environmental Health Criteria 236. Principles and Methods for Assessing Autoimmunity Associated with Exposure to Chemicals. 236, 1-324. 2006. WHO Report.
3. NIH Autoimmune Diseases Coordinating Committee. NIH Autoimmune Diseases Research Plan. 1-83. 2002. U.S. Department of Health and Human Services Report.
4. National Institutes of Health Autoimmune Diseases Coordinating Committee. Progress in Autoimmune Diseases Research. 1-126. 2005. Bethesda, NIH Report. NIH Publication No. 05-5140.

5. Gourley M, Miller FW. Mechanisms of disease: Environmental factors in the pathogenesis of rheumatic disease. Nat Clin Pract Rheumatol 2007; 3(3):172-180.
6. Gregersen PK, Olsson LM. Recent advances in the genetics of autoimmune disease. Annu Rev Immunol 2009; 27:363-391.
7. Gregersen PK. Modern genetics, ancient defenses and potential therapies. N Engl J Med 2007; 356(12):1263-1266.
8. Hewagama A, Richardson B. The genetics and epigenetics of autoimmune diseases. J Autoimmun 2009.
9. Sarasin A. An overview of the mechanisms of mutagenesis and carcinogenesis. Mutat Res 2003; 544(2-3):99-106.
10. Cooper GS, Miller FW, Germolec DR. Occupational exposures and autoimmune diseases. Int Immunopharmacol 2002; 2(2-3):303-313.
11. Miller FW, Twitty SA, Biswas T et al. Origin and regulation of a disease-specific autoantibody response. Antigenic epitopes, spectrotype stability and isotype restriction of anti-Jo-1 autoantibodies. J Clin Invest 1990; 85(2):468-475.
12. Arbuckle MR, McClain MT, Rubertone MV et al. Development of autoantibodies before the clinical onset of systemic lupus erythematosus. N Engl J Med 2003; 349(16):1526-1533.
13. Kokkonen H, Soderstrom I, Rocklov J et al. Up-regulation of cytokines and chemokines predates the onset of rheumatoid arthritis. Arthritis Rheum 2010; 62(2):383-391.
14. Cooper GS, Miller FW, Pandey JP. The Role of Genetic Factors in Autoimmune Disease: Implications for Environmental Research. Environ Health Perspect 1999; 107(Suppl 5):693-700.
15. Leslie RD, Hawa M. Twin studies in auto-immune disease. Acta Genet Med Gemellol (Roma) 1994; 43:71-81.
16. Miller FW, Hess EV, Clauw DJ et al. Approaches for identifying and defining environmentally associated rheumatic disorders. Arthritis Rheum 2000; 43(2):243-249.
17. Samuelsson U, Carstensen J. Space-time clustering at birth and at diagnosis of type 1 diabetes mellitus in relation to early clinical manifestation. J Pediatr Endocrinol Metab 2003; 16(6):859-867.
18. Leff RL, Burgess SH, Miller FW et al. Distinct seasonal patterns in the onset of adult idiopathic inflammatory myopathy in patients with anti-Jo-1 and anti-signal recognition particle autoantibodies. Arthritis Rheum 1991; 34(11):1391-1396.
19. Sarkar K, Weinberg CR, Oddis CV et al. Seasonal influence on the onset of idiopathic inflammatory myopathies in serologically defined groups. Arthritis Rheum 2005; 52(8):2433-2438.
20. Willis JA, Scott RS, Darlow BA et al. Seasonality of birth and onset of clinical disease in children and adolescents (0-19 years) with type 1 diabetes mellitus in Canterbury, New Zealand. J Pediatr Endocrinol Metab 2002; 15(5):645-647.
21. Ursic-Bratina N, Battelino T, Krzisnik C et al. Seasonality of birth in children (0-14 years) with type 1 diabetes mellitus in Slovenia. J Pediatr Endocrinol Metab 2001; 14(1):47-52.
22. Haus E, Smolensky MH. Biologic rhythms in the immune system. Chronobiol Int 1999; 16(5):581-622.
23. Nelson RJ, Drazen DL. Melatonin mediates seasonal changes in immune function. Ann N Y Acad Sci 2000; 917:404-415.
24. Okada S, Weatherhead E, Targoff IN et al. Global surface ultraviolet radiation intensity may modulate the clinical and immunologic expression of autoimmune muscle disease. Arthritis Rheum 2003; 48(8):2285-2293.
25. Love LA, Weinberg CR, McConnaughey R et al. Ultraviolet radiation intensity predicts the relative distribution of dermatomyositis and anti-Mi-2 autoantibodies in women. arth and rheum. Arthritis Rheum. 2009; 60:2499-504
26. Ponsonby AL, McMichael A, van dM I. Ultraviolet radiation and autoimmune disease: insights from epidemiological research. Toxicology 2002; 181-182:71-78.
27. Oddis CV, Conte CG, Steen VD et al. Incidence of polymyositis-dermatomyositis: a 20-year study of hospital diagnosed cases in Allegheny County, PA 1963-1982. J Rheumatol 1990; 17:1329-1334.
28. Cooper GS, Stroehla BC. The epidemiology of autoimmune diseases. Autoimmun Rev 2003; 2(3):119-125.
29. Onkamo P, Vaananen S, Karvonen M et al. Worldwide increase in incidence of Type I diabetes—the analysis of the data on published incidence trends. Diabetologia 1999; 42(12):1395-1403.
30. Uramoto KM, Michet CJ Jr, Thumboo J et al. Trends in the incidence and mortality of systemic lupus erythematosus, 1950-1992. Arthritis Rheum 1999; 42(1):46-50.
31. Jacobson DL, Gange SJ, Rose NR et al. Epidemiology and estimated population burden of selected autoimmune diseases in the United States. Clin Immunol Immunopathol 1997; 84(3):223-243.
32. Noseworthy JH, Lucchinetti C, Rodriguez M et al. Multiple sclerosis. N Engl J Med 2000; 343(13):938-952.
33. Dahlquist G. The aetiology of type 1 diabetes: an epidemiological perspective. Acta Paediatr Suppl 1998; 425:5-10.

34. Philen RM, Posada dlP, Hill RH et al. Epidemiology of the toxic oil syndrome. Arch Toxicol Suppl 1997; 19:41-52.
35. Striso P, Ghlrardellu A, Dotaioa C et al. Infections and autoimmunity: the multifaceted relationship. J Leukoc Biol 2009.
36. Ercolini AM, Miller SD. The role of infections in autoimmune disease. Clin Exp Immunol 2009; 155(1):1-15.
37. Poole BD, Templeton AK, Guthridge JM et al. Aberrant Epstein-Barr viral infection in systemic lupus erythematosus. Autoimmun Rev 2009; 8(4):337-342.
38. Oguz F, Akdeniz C, Unuvar E et al. Parvovirus B19 in the acute arthropathies and juvenile rheumatoid arthritis. J Paediatr Child Health 2002; 38(4):358-362.
39. Mamyrova G, Rider LG, Haagenson L et al. Parvovirus B19 and onset of juvenile dermatomyositis. JAMA 2005; 294(17):2170-2171.
40. Feng Y, Ke X, Ma R et al. Parallel detection of autoantibodies with microarrays in rheumatoid diseases. Clin Chem 2004; 50(2):416-422.
41. Palacios G, Druce J, Du L et al. A new arenavirus in a cluster of fatal transplant-associated diseases. N Engl J Med 2008; 358(10):991-998.
42. Wu W, Tang YW. Emerging molecular assays for detection and characterization of respiratory viruses. Clin Lab Med 2009; 29(4):673-693.
43. Hess EV, Mongey AB. Drug-related lupus. Bull Rheum Dis 1991; 40:1-8.
44. Parks CG, Conrad K, Cooper GS. Occupational exposure to crystalline silica and autoimmune disease. Environ Health Perspect 1999; 107 Suppl 5:793-802.
45. Pollard KM, Hultman P, Kono DH. Toxicology of Autoimmune Diseases. Chem Res Toxicol 2010.
46. Bagenstose LM, Salgame P, Monestier M. Murine mercury-induced autoimmunity: a model of chemically related autoimmunity in humans. Immunol Res 1999; 20(1):67-78.
47. gmon-Levin N, Paz Z, Israeli E et al. Vaccines and autoimmunity. Nat Rev Rheumatol 2009; 5(11):648-652.
48. Israeli E, gmon-Levin N, Blank M et al. Adjuvants and autoimmunity. Lupus 2009; 18(13):1217-1225.
49. Advisory Committee on Immunization Practices. Update: Vaccine Side Effects, Adverse Reactions, Contraindications and Precautions Recommendations of the Advisory Committee on Immunization Practices (ACIP). MMWR Morb Mortal Wkly Rep 1996; 45(RR-12):1-35.
50. Wraith DC, Goldman M, Lambert PH. Vaccination and autoimmune disease: what is the evidence? Lancet 2003; 362(9396):1659-1666.
51. Tugwell P, Wells G, Peterson J et al. Do silicone breast implants cause rheumatologic disorders? A systematic review for a court-appointed national science panel. Arthritis Rheum 2001; 44(11):2477-2484.
52. Janowsky EC, Kupper LL, Hulka BS. Meta-analyses of the relation between silicone breast implants and the risk of connective-tissue diseases. N Engl J Med 2000; 342(11):781-790.
53. Brown SL. Epidemiology of silicone-gel breast implants. Epidemiology 2002; 13(3 Suppl):S34-S39.
54. Brown SL, Langone JJ, Brinton LA. Silicone breast implants and autoimmune disease. J Am Med Womens Assoc 1998; 53(1):21-4, 40.
55. O'Hanlon T, Koneru B, Bayat E et al. Immunogenetic differences between Caucasian women with and those without silicone implants in whom myositis develops. Arthritis Rheum 2004; 50(11):3646-3650.
56. Cukier J, Beauchamp RA, Spindler JS et al. Association between bovine collagen dermal implants and a dermatomyositis or a polymyositis-like syndrome. Ann Int Med 1993; 118:920-928.
57. Levy Y, Rotman-Pikielny P, Ehrenfeld M et al. Silicone breast implantation-induced scleroderma: description of four patients and a critical review of the literature. Lupus 2009; 18(13):1226-1232.
58. Elenkov IJ, Chrousos GP. Stress, cytokine patterns and susceptibility to disease. Baillieres Best Pract Res Clin Endocrinol Metab 1999; 13(4):583-595.
59. Winsa B, Adami HO, Bergstrom R et al. Stressful life events and Graves' disease. Lancet 1991; 338(8781):1475-1479.
60. Luppi P, Rossiello MR, Faas S et al. Genetic background and environment contribute synergistically to the onset of autoimmune diseases. J Mol Med 1995; 73:381-393.
61. Dooley MA, Hogan SL. Environmental epidemiology and risk factors for autoimmune disease. Curr Opin Rheumatol 2003; 15(2):99-103.
62. Miller FW. Non-infectious Environmental Agents and Autoimmunity. In: Rose NR, Mackay IR, eds. The Autoimmune Diseases. 4 ed. New York: Elsevier; 2006:1297-1308.
63. Miller FW. Genetics of environmentally-associated rheumatic disease. In: Kaufman LD, Varga J, eds. Rheumatic Diseases and the Environment. London: Arnold Publishers; 1999:33-45.
64. Mintzer DM, Billet SN, Chmielewski L. Drug-induced hematologic syndromes. Adv Hematol 2009; 2009:495863.
65. Casciola-Rosen LA, Anhalt G, Rosen A. Autoantigens targeted in systemic lupus erythematosus are clustered in two populations of surface structures on apoptotic keratinocytes. J Exp Med 1994; 179(4):1317-1330.

66. Hall JC, Casciola-Rosen L, Rosen A. Altered structure of autoantigens during apoptosis. Rheum Dis Clin North Am 2004; 30(3):455-71, vii. Review.
67. Burd CJ, Kinyamu HK, Miller FW et al. UV radiation regulates Mi-2 through protein translation and stability. J Biol Chem 2008; 283(50):34976-34982.
68. Kuhn A, Beissert S. Photosensitivity in lupus erythematosus. Autoimmunity 2005; 38(7):519-529.
69. Klareskog L, Stolt P, Lundberg K et al. A new model for an etiology of rheumatoid arthritis: smoking may trigger HLA-DR (shared epitope)-restricted immune reactions to autoantigens modified by citrullination. Arthritis Rheum 2006; 54(1):38-46.
70. Strickland FM, Richardson BC. Epigenetics in human autoimmunity. Epigenetics in autoimmunity—DNA methylation in systemic lupus erythematosus and beyond. Autoimmunity 2008; 41(4):278-286.
71. Burdick LM, Somani N, Somani AK. Type I IFNs and their role in the development of autoimmune diseases. Expert Opin Drug Saf 2009; 8(4):459-472.
72. Scherer K, Spoerl D, Bircher AJ. Adverse drug reactions to biological response modifiers. J Dtsch Dermatol Ges 2010.
73. Cooper GS, Miller FW. Environmental influences on autoimmunity and autoimmune diseases. In: Luebke R, editor. Immunotoxicology and Immunopharmacology. Third ed. New York: CRC Press; 2007 p. 437-454.
74. Shamim EA, Miller FW. Familial autoimmunity and the idiopathic inflammatory myopathies. Current Rheumatology Reports 2000; 2(2):201-211.
75. Galloway TS, Brown RJ, Browne MA et al. The ECOMAN project: A novel approach to defining sustainable ecosystem function. Mar Pollut Bull 2006; 53(1-4):186-194.
76. Sloan CD, Duell EJ, Shi X et al. Ecogeographic genetic epidemiology. Genet Epidemiol 2009; 33(4):281-289.
77. Bigazzi PE. Autoimmunity caused by xenobiotics. Toxicology 1997; 119(1):1-21.
78. D'Cruz D. Autoimmune diseases associated with drugs, chemicals and environmental factors. Toxicol Lett 2000; 112-113:421-432.
79. Love LA, Miller FW. Noninfectious environmental agents associated with myopathies. Curr Opin Rheumatol 1993; 5(6):712-718.
80. Hess EV. Environmental chemicals and autoimmune disease: cause and effect. Toxicology 2002; 181-182:65-70.
81. Volzke H, Werner A, Wallaschofski H et al. Occupational exposure to ionizing radiation is associated with autoimmune thyroid disease. J Clin Endocrinol Metab 2005; 90(8):4587-4592.
82. Stolt P, Bengtsson C, Nordmark B et al. Quantification of the influence of cigarette smoking on rheumatoid arthritis: results from a population based case-control study, using incident cases. Ann Rheum Dis 2003; 62(9):835-841.
83. Krishnan E. Smoking, gender and rheumatoid arthritis-epidemiological clues to etiology. Results from the behavioral risk factor surveillance system. Joint Bone Spine 2003; 70(6):496-502.
84. Kallberg H, Padyukov L, Plenge RM et al. Gene-gene and gene-environment interactions involving HLA-DRB1, PTPN22 and smoking in two subsets of rheumatoid arthritis. Am J Hum Genet 2007; 80(5):867-875.
85. Vestergaard P. Smoking and thyroid disorders—a meta-analysis. Eur J Endocrinol 2002; 146(2):153-161.
86. Timmer A. Environmental influences on inflammatory bowel disease manifestations. Lessons from epidemiology. Dig Dis 2003; 21(2):91-104.
87. Costenbader KH, Karlson EW. Cigarette smoking and systemic lupus erythematosus: a smoking gun? Autoimmunity 2005; 38(7):541-547.
88. Alaedini A, Green PH. Narrative review: celiac disease: understanding a complex autoimmune disorder. Ann Intern Med 2005; 142(4):289-298.
89. Pattison DJ, Symmons DP, Lunt M et al. Dietary risk factors for the development of inflammatory polyarthritis: evidence for a role of high level of red meat consumption. Arthritis Rheum 2004; 50(12):3804-3812.
90. Dally A. The rise and fall of pink disease. Soc Hist Med 1997; 10(2):291-304.
91. Bigazzi PE. Autoimmunity and heavy metals. Lupus 1994; 3(6):449-453.
92. Fontenot AP, Kotzin BL. Chronic beryllium disease: immune-mediated destruction with implications for organ-specific autoimmunity. Tissue Antigens 2003; 62(6):449-458.
93. Bengtsson AA, Rylander L, Hagmar L et al. Risk factors for developing systemic lupus erythematosus: a case-control study in southern Sweden. Rheumatology (Oxford) 2002; 41(5):563-571.

CHAPTER 7

EPIGENETIC DYSREGULATION OF EPSTEIN-BARR VIRUS LATENCY AND DEVELOPMENT OF AUTOIMMUNE DISEASE

Hans Helmut Niller,*,[1] Hans Wolf,[1] Eva Ay[2] and Janos Minarovits[2]

[1]Institute for Medical Microbiology and Hygiene of the University of Regensburg, Regensburg, Germany;
[2]Microbiological Research Group of the National Center for Epidemiology, Budapest, Hungary
*Corresponding Author: Hans Helmut Niller—Email: hans-helmut.niller@klinik.uni-regensburg.de

Abstract: Epstein–Barr virus (EBV) is a human herpesvirus that persists in the memory B-cells of the majority of the world population in a latent form. Primary EBV infection is asymptomatic or causes a self-limiting disease, infectious mononucleosis. Virus latency is associated with a wide variety of neoplasms whereof some occur in immune suppressed individuals. Virus production does not occur in strict latency. The expression of latent viral oncoproteins and nontranslated RNAs is under epigenetic control via DNA methylation and histone modifications that results either in a complete silencing of the EBV genome in memory B cells, or in a cell-type dependent usage of a couple of latency promoters in tumor cells, germinal center B cells and lymphoblastoid cells (LCL, transformed by EBV in vitro). Both, latent and lytic EBV proteins elicit a strong immune response. In immune suppressed and infectious mononucleosis patients, an increased viral load can be detected in the blood. Enhanced lytic replication may result in new infection- and transformation-events and thus is a risk factor both for malignant transformation and the development of autoimmune diseases. An increased viral load or a changed presentation of a subset of lytic or latent EBV proteins that cross-react with cellular antigens may trigger pathogenic processes through molecular mimicry that result in multiple sclerosis (MS), systemic lupus erythematosus (SLE) and rheumatoid arthritis (RA).

INTRODUCTION

Epstein-Barr virus (EBV), a ubiquitous human γ-herpesvirus, causes usually asymptomatic infection in children. Upon primary infection of adolescents or adults, however,

---

Epigenetic Contributions in Autoimmune Disease, edited by Esteban Ballestar.
©2011 Landes Bioscience and Springer Science+Business Media.

infectious mononucleosis (IM) may develop. A monoclonal EBV-infection of tumor cells is observed in a wide variety of human lymphomas, like Burkitt's lymphoma (BL), Hodgkin's lymphoma (HL), extranodal natural killer (NK) T cell lymphoma, or lymphoproliferations in severely immune suppressed patients (posttransplant lymphoproliferative disease, PTLD) and epithelial cancers, like undifferentiated nasopharyngeal carcinoma (NPC), gastric carcinoma, or possibly breast carcinoma and leiomyosarcoma, a mesothelial tumor (for review see refs. 1,2). Furthermore, EBV is associated with a panel of common autoimmune diseases, like rheumatoid arthritis (RA), systemic lupus erythematosus (SLE) and multiple sclerosis (MS) (for review see ref. 3).

NATURAL HISTORY

Altogether, about 90% of the world population is infected with EBV. The virus is secreted by the salivary glands and transmitted through direct contact between mother and child. When transmitted, EBV infects either squamous epithelial cells or resting B lymphocytes close to the surface of tonsillar epithelia or other lymphoid organs in Waldeyer's ring. The B cells by themselves are considered necessary and possibly even sufficient, while epithelial cells may be seen as helpful enhancers for virus production, for transfering the virus to other individuals and for establishing latency in B cells.[4]

In industrialized countries, primary infection in up to 50% of cases occurs later than the first decade of life (for review see ref. 5). In this case, virus transmission is mostly through intimate contacts between adolescents, hence, a synonym for IM is kissing disease. After an incubation time of two to four weeks, primary infection may be accompanied by symptoms like tonsillitis, fever, malaise, lymphadenopathy in up to 50% of cases, the more severe courses being diagnosed as IM, sometimes with hepatosplenomegaly and skin rash. Primary infection of B cells in the oropharynx leads to a general infection of the circulating blood B cell pool, normally in the range of 0,1 to 1%, in extreme cases of 10% of all circulating B cells and up to 50% of all circulating memory B cells.[6] EBV infected B cells in lymphoid organs and in the blood proliferate in response to the latent viral proteins and RNAs.[7] Besides, they easily switch to the lytic cycle of virus replication, important for the viral spread between cells. The large number of infected B cells in the peripheral blood expressing numerous highly immunogenic viral antigens elicits a vigorous immune response which clears the infection[8] (for review see ref. 9). Defence cells can amount to 60% of all white blood cells, like in acute leukemia. Clinical symptoms are only relieved with the decline of both the infected B cells and activated T cells.[10]

ESTABLISHMENT OF EBV LATENCY

There are two different models on the natural course of primary B-cell infection and the establishment of EBV latency. One model suggests that EBV infects naive B cells and induces their proliferation via expression of EBV-encoded nuclear antigens (EBNAs) and latent membrane proteins (LMPs) (latency Class III, see below).[11,12] In this model, EBV accompanies the physiological antigen activation of B cells and changes its expression program in dependence of the B-cell differentiation stage. Thus, EBV infected B cells enter the germinal centre (GC) where they stay protected from apoptosis through the expression of several viral latency gene products. Finally, the cells are thought to mature into resting memory B cells that either do not express the EBNAs at all (latency Class 0) or express EBNA 1 only when they divide (latency Class I). Contrary, through laser capture microdissection of IM tonsils, EBV-infected cells were not found to pass through a physiological GC reaction, but GC or memory B cells were directly infected by EBV.[13,14] The directly infected GC cells differentiated into memory B cells without further participation in the GC reaction. Recent data confirm that EBV-infected B cells do mostly not participate in normal GC reactions, because a normal GC reaction would result in clones of hundreds to thousands of infected B cells.[15,16] It is clear that in vitro EBV is equally able to infect both naive and memory B cells.[17] In summary, a small number of EBV-infected cells may regularly undergo abortive GC reactions. The strong constitutive CD40-related signal of LMP1 seems to prohibit the formation of a normal GC.[18] Rarely, EBV may indeed participate in GC reactions, but only under the nonphysiological conditions of antigenic hyperstimulation of the B-cell system, e.g., when the organism is infected by malaria, by other parasites or infectious mononucleosis (HIV), or after organ transplantation.[19-21]

After the acute phase of primary infection is over, the virus persists lifelong in the organism, residing latently in memory B cells. Almost all viral promoters are silenced by epigenetic mechanisms in latency. Therefore, neither lytic replication nor EBV-mediated activation of B-cell proliferation takes place. Due to the viral retreat into surface epithelia and due to the minimal gene expression program in memory B cells, EBV remains nearly invisible for the immune system. Lytic reactivation starts with the overexpression of two viral immediate early (IE) switch genes BRLF1 and BZLF1, coding for transcription factors Rta and Zta which trigger a gene expression cascade that finally leads to virus production.[22,23] The EBV infected plasma cell is usually killed in the process of lytic reactivation.

LATENCY-ASSOCIATED VIRAL GENE PRODUCTS

Latently infected cell lines and tumor cells may be described by their distinct viral gene expression patterns. EBV latency classes are divided into two major groups, based on the activity of the viral C promoter (Cp) linked with the expression of the main transforming protein EBNA2[24] (for review see ref. 2 and references therein; see also below).

The first group (latency Classes 0, I and II, Cp-off latency) exhibits restricted viral gene expression patterns that exclude EBNA2. Class I latency in BL biopsies is the prototype of Cp-off latency. Only two noncoding small RNAs (EBERs), a family of multiply-spliced BamHI A rightward transcripts (BARTs), including its intronic cluster of 22 microRNAs (miRNAs)[25-28] and the nuclear antigen EBNA1 are expressed. In Class II latency, as typically found in HD, two LMPs are expressed, in addition. Resting memory B cells either do not express the EBNAs at all (latency 0) or just EBNA1, when they divide. In the epithelial Class I/II cancers NPC and gastric carcinoma, BARF1 is latently expressed, in addition.

The second group (latency Class III, Cp-on latency) is characterized through the expression of all EBV latency genes including the major immortalizing transcription factor EBNA2. Class III latency cells, as found in lymphoblastoid cell lines (LCLs) and in most cells of the classical PTLDs, express the EBERs, the BARTs, all six EBNAs, including the BHRF1-cluster of 3 miRNAs[25,26] and the LMPs. By and by, all EBV latency genes have been implicated either in cell transformation and immortalization, mostly accompanied with Cp-on latency, or in oncogenesis that is primarily accompanied with Cp-off latency.

CpG METHYLATION OF EBV GENOMES AND LATENCY PROMOTERS

Based on the analysis of dinucleotide frequencies, Honess et al. suggested that after establishing latency EBV genomes are subjected to methylation in their natural host cells.[29] Indeed, although unmethylated double stranded linear EBV genomes are packaged into the virions during lytic replication, high resolution methylation mapping of EBV latency promoters in memory B cells confirmed that EBV genomes were highly methylated in certain regions in normal B lymphocytes present in peripheral blood.[30,31] The viral genomes in latently infected cell lines are subject to extensive epigenetic silencing as well. A systematic study revealed that the latent EBV genomes are highly methylated in BL biopsies and cell lines (latency I) and nude mouse passaged NPC lines (latency II), whereas LCLs (latency III) carried hypomethylated or unmethylated viral episomes.[32] This suggested that de novo methylation of latent EBV genomes by cellular DNA methyltransferases occurs in a cell type specific manner.

The methylation patterns of the currently known viral latency promoters were extensively studied in different EBV latency classes in various cell types. These include the EBER promoters (EBER1p and EBER2p), the alternative promoters for EBNA transcripts (Wp, Cp and Qp), the promoter (BARTp or CSTp) for the complementary strand transcripts, the LMP2A promoter LMP2Ap and the bidirectional promoter for LMP1 and LMP2B (for review see refs. 33,34). With the exception of Qp, the methylation status of latent EBV promoters correlates remarkably well with promoter activity.

Certain regions of the latent EBV genomes are exempt from methylation even in cells carrying highly methylated viral episomes. These include the latent origin of EBV DNA replication (*oriP*) and the EBER 1 and 2 transcription units.[35,36] In addition, switching on of Cp where transcripts for EBNA 1-6 are initiated was accompanied by demethylation of its regulatory region.[37] In addition, histone modifications characteristic of an open chromatin structure also regularly mark the active EBV latency promoters.[3] These data support the idea that functionally important regions carry unique epigenetic marks even in viral episomes characterized by high overall CpG methylation.

THE EBV LATENCY GENE PRODUCTS

EBERs. The EBER genes code for two small nuclear RNAs.[38,39] The abundantly transcribed EBERs are complexed with the La protein that plays a role in systemic lupus erythematosus and ribosomal protein L22.[40,41] They also bind to the double stranded RNA dependent protein kinase PKR[42,43] and thereby block the interferon-α dependent signal transduction pathway that would normally induce apoptosis in a virus infected cell. The EBERs have been shown to exert anti-apoptotic and tumorigenic functions.[44,45] Furthermore, besides blocking PKR, there must be additional ways for the EBERs to block apoptosis.[46,47] A substantial amount of EBER1 was found to be released from EBV-infected cells.[48] This may have important implications for immunopathologic diseases, including autoimmune phenomena, because EBER1 induced signaling from toll-like receptor 3 (TLR3) and maturation of dendritic cells (DCs) in vitro. The EBER1 stimulated DCs produced interferon-β (IFN-β) and interleukin 12 (IL-12). It is important to note that sera from patients with infectious mononucleosis, chronic active EBV infection and EBV-associated haemophagocytic lymphohistiocytosis contained a higher level of EBER1 than sera obtained from healthy individuals.[48]

EBNAs. The Epstein-Barr viral nuclear antigens (EBNAs) are mostly transcription factors that play a critical role in the maintenance of the viral episome, in the immune recognition of infected cells and the process of cellular immortalization and morphological transformation.

EBNA1. EBNA1 is a transcription and replication factor binding to the latent viral replication origin oriP and to Qp (Figs. 1 and 2). EBNA1 messages are also expressed in lytic infection, from the lytic cycle promoter Fp. It is the only viral replication factor required for nuclear maintenance and cell cycle regulated replication of the viral genome via oriP. By binding EBNA1, the FR element of oriP works as a long distance enhancer for several viral promoters and as a nuclear matrix attachment element.[49-53] Almost the entire N-terminal half of the EBNA1 protein is composed of an irregular copolymer of the amino acids glycine and alanine that prevents EBNA1 from being degraded by the proteasome[54] (Fig. 1). Nevertheless, EBNA1 is an immunogenic viral protein that may play an important role in autoimmune diseases[55,56] (see below; Table 1; Figs. 1 and 2).

EBNA2. EBNA2 is the viral protein mainly responsible for transactivating the major latency promoters Cp, LMP1p and LMP2Ap and cellular promoters involved in the

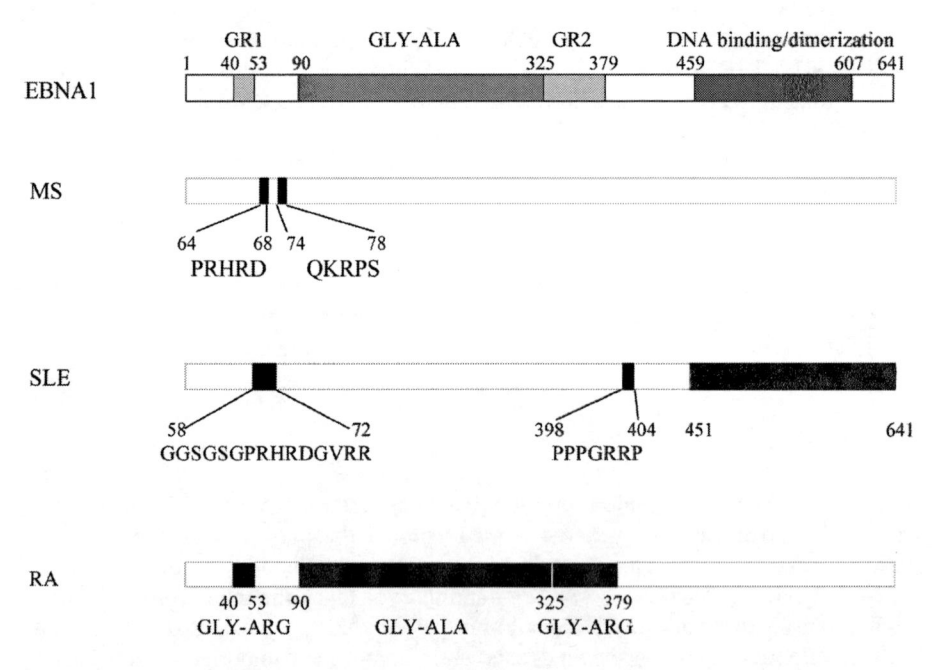

Figure 1. Peptides and domains of EBNA1 associated with autoimmune diseases. On the upper part of the figure GR1 and GR2 designate glycine-arginine-rich linking regions; GLY-ALA stands for a glycine-glycine-alanine-rich region inhibiting proteasome-mediated degradation of EBNA1. Numbers indicate amino acid positions. Black rectangles within the white bars indicate peptides or domains associated with multiple sclerosis (MS), systemic lupus erythematosus (SLE) and rheumatoid arthritis (RA). The peptide PRHRD seems to be involved in the pathogenesis of both MS and SLE.

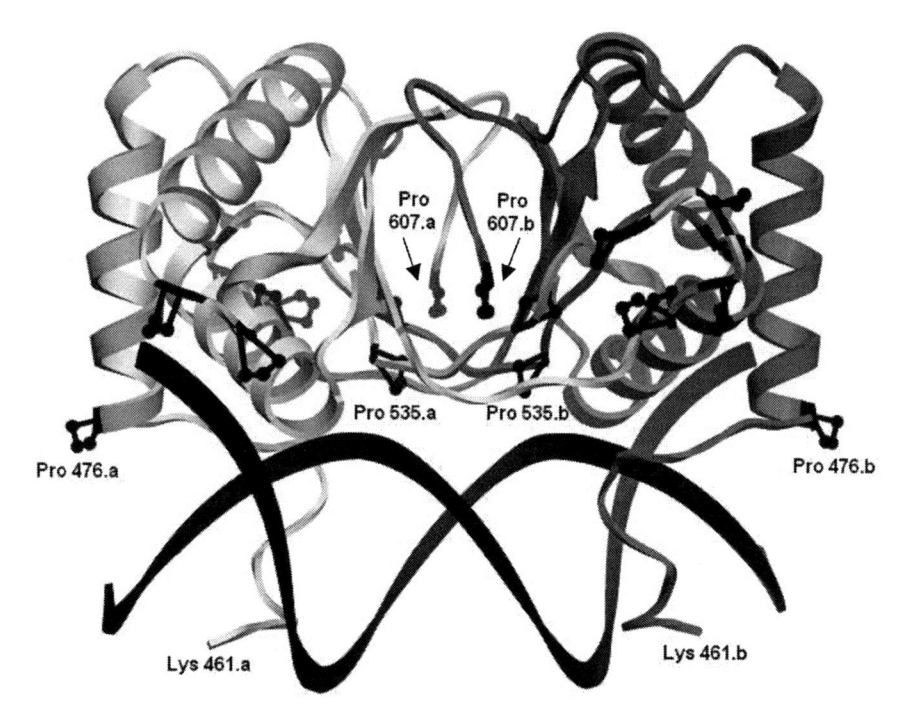

Figure 2. A model of EBNA1 interacting with DNA. The DNA binding and dimerization domain of EBNA1 (residues 461-607, implicated in the pathogenesis of systemic lupus erythematosus) is shown as a dimer, contacting DNA. Numbers indicate amino acid positions in the chains of monomer a and b. The figure was generated using the Chimera program and the Protein Data Bank (model 1B3T).

Table 1. Latent Epstein-Barr virus proteins implicated in the pathogenesis of autoimmune diseases

Protein	Peptide or Domain	Disease	Suggested Mechanism
EBNA1	PRHRD	MS	Cross reaction with myelin basic protein
	QKRPS	MS	Cross reaction with myelin basic protein
	aa 302-641	MS	Cross reaction with myelin basic protein
	GGSGSGPRHRDGVRR	SLE	Cross reaction with the Ro 60 kDa protein
	PPPGRRP	SLE	Antigenic mimicry with Sm B′/B epitopes
	aa 35-58	SLE	Cross reaction with the Sm D1 protein
	aa 451-461	SLE	Cross reaction with Sm proteins
	gly-ala repeat	RA	Cross reaction with collagen and keratin
	gly-arg rich regions	RA	Deamination, citrullination, cross reaction with citrullinated cellular proteins
EBNA2	aa 354-373	SLE	Cross reaction with the Sm D1 protein
	aa 1-116	SLE	Cross reaction with Sm proteins

MS: multiple sclerosis; SLE: systemic lupus erythematosus; RA: rheumatoid arthritis.

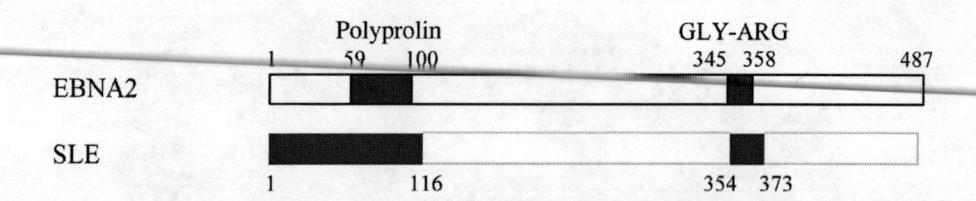

Figure 3. Peptides and domains of EBNA2 associated with autoimmune disease. Polyproline designates a proline rich region; GLY-ARG stands for a glycine-arginine-rich region. Numbers indicate amino acid positions. Black rectangles within the white bar indicate domains associated with systemic lupus erythematosus (SLE).

immortalization and morphological transformation of B cells in vitro (establishment of LCLs). Viruses carrying an EBNA2 deletion are unable to transform B cells.[57,58] Promoter activation by EBNA2 is through indirect binding to promoter DNA via interaction with a cellular protein, CBF1.[59] Specific targets of EBNA2 activation are the cellular genes for the B-cell growth receptor CD23 and the EBV receptor CD21.[60,61] EBNA2 makes the resting B-cell enter the cell cycle and switch from G0 to G1. Similarly to EBNA1, EBNA2 may also contribute to the pathogenesis of autoimmune diseases (Table 1, Fig. 3).

EBNA-LP. EBNA-LP (EBNA5) is the first protein expressed in the B-cell transformation process. Its mRNA is transcribed across the internal W repeat. Viruses with LP mutations do not efficiently transform B cells.[62] LP is a transcriptional coactivator for EBNA2 and greatly increases immortalization efficiency.[63,64]

EBNA3. Among the EBNA3 protein family, EBNA3A and C are required for the morphological transformation of B lymphocytes, just like EBNA2, while EBNA3B mutant viruses are able to immortalize B cells with the same efficiency as wild type viruses.[65,66] Like EBNA2, all three members of the EBNA3 protein family interact with promoter DNA of many genes through binding CBF1 and modulate the transcriptional effects of EBNA2, mostly negatively.[67-69]

BARTs. The BamHI A region transcripts (BARTs), also called complementary strand transcripts (CSTs) are at particularly high levels expressed in NPC cells, at lower levels also in BL, LCL, gastric carcinoma and in HD cells. The CSTs are an mRNA family with complex splicing pattern of partially overlapping exons. Possibly they play a role in tumorigenesis.[70] The expression and function of their open reading frames RPMS1, A73, BARF0 and RK-BARF0 is under investigation.[71] Like the EBNA3 proteins, they seem to modulate EBNA2 transcriptional activation through the CBF1 binding sites of promoter DNA and to modify Notch signaling pathways.[72,73]

LMPs. The LMPs (LMP1, LMP2A, LMP2B) are integral membrane proteins that can modulate signal transduction. LMP2A blocks B-cell receptor (BCR) signalling and induction of lytic EBV infection via BCR cross-linking, while LMP1 affects the CD40 signal transduction pathway. LMP1 also upregulates the B-cell activation molecules, B-cell activating factor (BAFF) and A proliferation inducing ligand (APRIL), both TNF-receptor-like cell surface receptors. BAFF overexpression correlates with systemic lupus erythematosus. Thus, through the overexpression of B-cell activators, EBV might be involved in the development of autoimmune diseases, too.[74] LMP1 and LMP2A allow the EBV infected B cell to survive independently of its contact with the antigen and with the T helper cell. Therefore, both membrane receptors can contribute to the apoptosis resistance of the infected cell in a vulnerable phase of B-cell differentiation. LMP2A is expressed from the LMP2A promoter, whereas in epithelial cells LMP1 is transcribed from the terminal repeat promoter for LMP1.[75,76] Furthermore, a bidirectional promoter used in lymphoid cells for both LMP1 and LMP2B and a shorter splice form of LMP2A, has been described earlier.[75,77] LMP2B is a negative-regulator of LMP2A. Thus LMP2B overexpression increased the magnitude of EBV switching from its latent to its lytic form upon BCR cross-linking.[78,79] Due to an increased apoptosis resistance, LMP2A might promote autoimmune responses through bypassing tolerance checkpoints.[80] In addition, both LMP1 and LMP2A may alter cellular gene expression patterns via up-regulation of DNA methyltransferase 1 (DNMT1) that results in CpG methylation mediated silencing of distinct promoters.[81,82]

miRNAs. These are encoded in two clusters and processed from the BHRF1 and BART transcripts. Their function is unknown in most cases. However, miR-BHRF1-3 downregulates the interferon-inducible T-cell attracting chemokine CXCL11/I-TAC in diverse EBV-positive non-Hodgkin's lymphoma cell lines.[83] miR-BART-22 modulates LMP2A expression in NPC cells.[84] Several BART-cluster 1 miRNAs downregulate LMP1 protein expression.[85] miR-BART-2 downregulates the viral polymerase protein BALF5.[86] miR-BART-5 is abundantly expressed in NPC and gastric carcinoma cells. It modulates the pro-apoptotic protein "p53 upregulated modulator of apoptosis" (PUMA) to facilitate the survival of infected tumor cells.[87] miR-BART2-5p downregulates NK-cell ligand MICB, thereby mediating immune evasion of infected cells.[88]

MOLECULAR MECHANISMS OF EBV ASSOCIATED AUTOIMMUNE DISEASES

A causal role in the generation of malignancies is well established for EBV. EBV-infected tumors are characterized by a high load of genetic and epigenetic alterations of the cellular genomes (for review see ref. 89). In addition to a series of malignancies, the evidence for an involvement of EBV in the generation of autoimmune diseases is condensing, although final proof is still lacking. The possible causal association of frequent autoimmune diseases, like multiple sclerosis (MS), systemic lupus erythematosus (SLE) and rheumatoid arthritis (RA) with EBV-infection has been extensively reviewed.[3,90] The generation of autoreactive T cell clones during infectious mononucleosis, the antigenic cross-reactivity between viral antigens and self antigens, i.e., molecular mimicry, or the immortalization of preexisting autoreactive B cells through infection with EBV, with the consequent enhancement of autoimmunity may be the molecular mechanisms involved in EBV triggering the loss of self tolerance which leads to autoimmunity.[90] While molecular mimicry is conceivable for all viruses, its ability to latently infect and immortalize B cells makes EBV unique in this respect.[91] Autoimmune diseases are complex and multifactorial, as genetic, epigenetic and environmental risk factors are always involved. A familial predisposition may be explained by a common overlapping set of susceptibility genes for autoimmunity in general.[92] Many autoimmune diseases occur with higher frequency in women. Therefore, sex hormones may play a role. Since one of two X chromosomes is silenced in female cells, epigenetic dysregulation on the inactive X may also contribute to more frequent autoimmune disease in women. A multitude of genes involved in immune defects and the development of autoimmunity is located on the X chromosome. Some of them are epigenetic regulatory genes (for review see refs. 93,94).

MULTIPLE SCLEROSIS

MS is a relatively common neurological disease, characterized by chronic inflammation and demyelination within the central nervous system (for review see refs. 95,96). MS seems to be based on a hyperreactive immune system and an increased vulnerability of the blood brain barrier.[97] Autoreactive T cells against myelin basic protein and glia cells are supposed to play a key role in the molecular pathology. Diverse infectious agents, including the reactivation of human endogenous retroviruses (HERVs), have been considered as cofactors.[95,98,99] Transcriptional functions of EBV transactivate human endogenous retroviruses (HERVs) which may be toxic for oligodendrocytes.[100,101]

Metaanalysis showed a clear epidemiological connection between EBV infection and MS. EBV infection by itself is a risk factor, since infection in early childhood leads to an MS risk in the young adult age 10 fold higher than in non-infected individuals. Correspondingly, pediatric MS patients showed far higher EBV seropositivity rates than healthy children.[102,103] Among adults, nearly all MS patients are seropositive to EBV, in contrast to control groups.[104] Besides infection itself, EBV infection that occurs too late in life, namely in the adolescent age, leading to IM constitutes another risk factor, confering a further two- to threefold increase of the risk to develop MS.[95,104,105] Correspondingly, an epidemiological link between the diverse EBV-associated diseases HD, MS and NPC may be measurable in very large population samples.[106]

Several studies showed an altered immune response against EBV in MS patients. Significant increases of EBV antibody titers in serum, mainly IgG against EBNA1, were found years before MS outbreak.[107,108] Contrary to EBNA1, a high antibody titer against VCA seemed to be protective against MS.[109] Antibodies from the CSF of MS patients reacted with EBNA1 at a very high frequency, while antibodies from control CSFs were mostly unreactive. There are protein homologies between EBNA1 and myelin basic protein (MBP) that might explain a potential cross-reactivity of EBNA1 antibodies against MBP[110] (Table 1, Fig. 1). Antibodies in the CSF of MS patients directed against the two EBV antigens, EBNA1 and BRRF2 have been found to represent the most frequent oligoclonal specificities.[111] Furthermore, peptide mimics have been found between myelin basic protein (MBP) and viral peptides that are recognized by the same CD4+T-cell receptor.[112] A strong cross-reactivity was found between peptides from MBP amino acids 85-99 and the viral DNA polymerase BALF5 amino acids 627-641 (Table 2). Both peptides have a different amino acid sequence, but due to structural similarities are recognized by the same T-cell receptor in the context of the two different HLA DR2 haplotypes that remarkably confer the strongest genetic risk for MS. DRB1*1501 presents the MBP peptide and DRB5*0101 the EBV peptide.[113] EBV reactive T cells recognizing EBV infected B-cells were isolated from the CSF of a small panel of MS patients.[114] CD4+ T cells cross-reacting with MBP and EBV BALF5 were also found in the blood or CSF of two MS patients. T cell clones established from the CSF of one patient cross-recognized both peptides.[115]

Furthermore, specific differences in the T cell response between MS patients and the healthy have been found. Th1 specific responses against EBNA1 were increased

Table 2. Lytic Epstein-Barr virus proteins implicated in the pathogenesis of autoimmune diseases

Protein	Peptide or Domain	Disease	Suggested Mechanism
BRRF2	Full length protein; aa 385-537	MS	?
BALF5	TGGVYHFVKKHVHES	MS	Antigenic mimicry
BALF4	QKRAAQRAA	RA	Shared epitope with HLA antigens
BOLF1	TYWQLNQNL and SLTRDDAEYL	JIA	Antigenic mimicry, EBV-self HLA cross-reactive T cells
BALF2	ATEEEEAV	JIA	Antigenic mimicry, EBV-self HLA cross-reactive T cells

MS: multiple sclerosis; RA: rheumatoid arthritis; JIA: juvenile idiopathic arthritis.

and the epitope recognition of EBNA1 by CD4[+] T cells was broader in MS patients.[56] Contrary, the frequency of CD8[+] T cells against EBV did not differ between patients and the healthy.[56,116] Also the EBV genome load in the peripheral blood of MS patients was the same as in the healthy.[56]

Recently, EBV RNA and immunoreactivity for EBV antigens have been found in B cells within white matter lesions and meningeal ectopic follicles in the brains of a high rate of MS patients.[117] (for review see refs. 118-120). These findings are still disputed, as other groups could not reproduce them.[121-123] The discrepancy might be explained by technical differences, e.g., use of frozen versus paraffin embedded autopsy tissue. In any case, it is important to clarify the controversy.

SYSTEMIC LUPUS ERYTHEMATOSUS

SLE is a chronic inflammatory multisystem autoimmune disease, which mostly attacks the skin, joints, kidneys and central nervous system, but can damage any other organ. It is characterized by the regular presence of a set of IgG autoantibodies against nuclear antigens (antinuclear antibody, ANA), like the Ro/La-complex including the viral EBER-RNAs,[40] cellular chromatin including dsDNA, spliceosomal Sm components and spliceosomal nRNP (nuclear ribonucleoprotein) components, or other nuclear antigens. Epitope spreading has been regularly observed with the duration of clinical disease. Deposited immune complexes can lead to organ failure in the long run.

More than 20 genetic loci associated with SLE have been described, with the MHC-II locus playing an important role (for review see ref. 93). Interestingly, the X-linked gene for "Methyl-CpG binding protein 2" (MeCP2) at Xq28 which contributes to chromatin silencing has also been associated with lupus.[124] Impaired DNA methylation in T cells may constitute an important epigenetic mechanism for SLE development. The treatment of CD4[+] T cells with 5-azacytidine or other demethylating drugs led to the recognition of inappropriate antigens and to autoimmunity. This correlated with the demethylation of a set of genes involved in the interaction between T-cell receptor and self Class II MHC antigens. The injection of such demethylated cells into syngeneic mice led to a lupus like disease (for review see ref. 93). A conditional Erk pathway signaling defect in a transgenic mouse model led to the same epigenetic dysregulation of DNMT1 and the overexpression of methylation sensitive genes as in T cells of SLE patients and also to the production of autoantibodies.[125] Therefore, demethylated autoreactive CD4+ cells seem to break self tolerance and activate SLE in the genetically predisposed. For further reading on DNA methylation changes in SLE see Chapter 9.

The miR-17-92 miRNA cluster is frequently amplified in lymphomas and other cancers. Transgenic mice overexpressing miR-17-92 in their lymphocytes developed lymphoproliferations, autoimmunity and SLE-like disease. This miRNA cluster suppressed the tumor suppressor PTEN and the proapoptotic protein Bim.[126] Bim expression was regularly found to be downregulated through epigenetic silencing in EBV-infected B cells, but not in EBV-negative cells.[127] Thus, Bim silencing may provide a connection between SLE and EBV infection.

Among all infectious agents, seroreactivity to EBV is most closely associated with SLE in a significant way. Therefore, EBV has become a leading candidate as a potential SLE trigger. Several case reports describe the beginning of a SLE immediately after IM (for review see refs. 128,129). Several cases of EBV-associated hemophagocytic syndrome in SLE have been reported (for review see ref. 129). 99% of SLE patients have antibodies against EBV, while only 90% of the general population is seropositive.[130] This difference is even more pronounced and highly significant in children and young adults. While 99% of young SLE patients are seropositive, only 70% of the general age cohort react to EBV.[131] Furthermore, SLE onset is frequently preceded by primary EBV infection and seroconversion in a highly significant fashion.[130] Early autoantibodies in a subset of SLE patients against amino acids 169 to 180 TKYKQRNGWSHK of the Ro 60kD protein classically cross-reacted with amino acids 58 to 72 GGSGSGPRHRDGVRR of the EBV protein EBNA1 (Table 1, Fig. 1). Rabbits immunized with either peptide developed antibodies against additional epitopes within Ro 60kD, but also against epitopes within other proteins, like Sm B/B′, nRNP and against dsDNA, just as they are observed in human disease. Furthermore, either peptide led to the rapid appearance of severe SLE symptoms in rabbits, including kidney damage and leukopenia and a regular crossreactivity of antibodies to both peptides.[132] The Sm B/B′ octapeptide PPPGMRPP seems to be a common founder autoantigen in many SLE patients.[133,134] Epitope spreading has been reproduced through immunization with highly conserved Sm B/B′ founder peptides in different animal species.[133,135,136] Rabbits immunized with two Sm B/B′ octapeptides PPPGMRPP and PPPGIRGP developed autoantibodies against those peptides, but also against many other autoantigenic structures typical for SLE and also develop clinical symptoms typical for human SLE.[137] Development of autoantibodies in a cohort of pediatric patients was frequently preceded by anti-EBNA1 antibodies. While EBNA1 antibodies in the healthy are mostly directed against the large glycine-alanine repeat of EBNA1, the EBNA1-antibodies of SLE patients mostly reacted against other epitopes including ones crossreactive to Ro and Sm.[138] Antigenic mimicry was found between the proline-rich repetitive Sm B′/B epitope PPPGMRPP and the EBNA1 motif PPPGRRP (Table 1, Fig. 1). Therefore, it was possible to trigger clinical SLE in rabbits through immunization with the EBV peptide PPPGRRP.[139] Expression of the entire EBNA1 protein in mice led to the appearance of antibodies against Sm B′/B and dsDNA.[140] An additional peptide that was fished with anti-Sm B/B′ antibodies from a phage display library mimicked a peptide sequence from the viral major DNA binding protein of EBV.[141] Another crossreactivity in a subset of SLE patients was found between amino acids 354 to 373 of EBNA2 peptide GRGKGKSRDKQRKPGGPWRP and amino acids 101 to 119 of lupus Sm D1 antigenic peptide GRGRGRGRGRGRGRGGPRR[142]

(Table 1, Fig. 3). Sm D1 peptide 95 to 119 showed cross-reactivity also with EBNA1 peptide 35 to 58.[143] Further antibody specificities against the proline rich epitopes of the Sm proteins were found to cross-react to the poly-proline tracts at the carboxy terminus (amino acids 451 to 641) of EBNA1 (Table 1, Figs. 1 and 2) and the amino terminus (amino acids 1 to 116) of EBNA2 in SLE and other systemic connective tissue diseases[144] (Table 1, Fig. 3). One may speculate, that on the genetic background of SLE patients the production of EBV induced autoantibodies cannot be controlled and they even tend to expand to other specificities over the years.

While antigenic mimicry might explain the initiation of SLE through EBV, there is also a different steady state response of the SLE patients' immune system to latent EBV infection compared with healthy control populations. Significantly more SLE patients than normal controls carried EBV genomes in their blood.[145] The number of EBV infected B cells in the blood of SLE patients was approximately elevated 10 fold comparable to the ranges that are found in the immunosuppressed and the overall viral genome load was up to 40 fold higher in SLE patients, however, even without immunosuppressive medication.[146-148] While their B cells are not intrinsically defective, SLE patients most likely have defects in several subsets of their T cells and are, therefore, unable to control latent EBV infection.[147,149,150] This may indicate that EBV infection is actually not causal for SLE, but that this underlying T-cell immune dysfunction may be the cause of both, an easier infectability through EBV and a tendency to develop autoimmune disease. In addition, one may speculate that the increased portion of EBV infected B cells may contribute to autoantibody production in SLE patients.[146]

How an increased EBV load could initiate or perpetuate SLE remains to be determined. It is noteworthy however, that LMP1 (one of the EBV encoded oncoproteins, see above) induces B cells to express BAFF (B-cell-activating factor belonging to the TNF family).[74] Induction of BAFF by LMP1 appears to be an important link between EBV infection and the genesis of autoimmune diseases, because it connects a latent viral protein to the defects of B-cell tolerance checkpoints described in SLE patients.[151] Thus, BAFF overexpression potentially induced by EBV may subvert B-cell self tolerance.

LMP1, in addition to upregulating BAFF expression, also induced APRIL, a proliferation inducing ligand in B-cells and could trigger T-cell independent Ig heavy chain switch.[74] LMP2A, another EBV encoded transmembrane protein could trigger class switch recombination, too, although to a lesser extent than LMP1.[74] Switching to IgG may lower the sensitivity of B cells to negative regulatory signals mediated by CD22.[152] Both LMP1 and LMP2 expression was detected in 29% and 18% of enriched B-cell samples of SLE patients, respectively.[148] We conclude, therefore, that EBV has the means to initiate and perpetuate key pathological changes related to SLE.

RHEUMATOID ARTHRITIS

RA is an extremely widespread systemic autoimmune disease with a highly disabling impact that affects about 2% of the world population (for review see refs. 93,153). It is characterized by an inflammatory infiltration of CD4+ T cells and NK cells into the synovia of the joints. Secretion of inflammatory cytokines like IL1, IL6 and TNF-α play a pathogenic role (for review see ref. 154). Just as for MS and SLE, both environmental and genetic risk factors play an interconnected role (for review see ref. 155). Epigenetic dysregulation may play a role in the aberrant gene expression pattern and reactivation of LINE1 retrotransposon in synovial fibroblasts.[156] For further reading on epigenetic aspects of RA pathogenesis see Chapter 10. Several genetic loci are associated with RA risk, especially the alleles HLA-DRB1*0401, 0404, 0405, 0408 within the MHC-II complex.[93,157,158] These alleles contain peptide sequence homologies to EBV glycoprotein gp110 (BALF4). BALF4 is normally one of the most abundant EBV proteins in late lytic infection and also serves as a target of antibody dependent cell-mediated cytotoxicity against EBV-infected cells.[159] The so called shared epitope motif QKRAA is the strongest known genetic risk factor for developing RA[160] (Table 2). Antigenic homologies have been observed between EBV proteins BOLF1, a viral tegument protein and BALF2, the major viral DNA binding protein and presumable DNA recombinase[161] and MHC-DRB1 allele epitopes (Table 2). Those crossreactivities seem to play a pathogenic role in juvenile idiopathic arthritis.[162]

Further observations also suggest a role for EBV in the pathogenesis of RA.[163] EBV antibodies against VCA, EBNA and EA antigens are increased, EBV-infected cell number is significantly higher and the viral genome load in the blood of RA patients is elevated about 10 fold.[164,165] Furthermore, the synovia of RA patients is frequently infected with EBV.[164,166] There are occasional reports of antiviral treatment ameliorating RA symptoms in severely ill patients.[154,167] Another possible treatment option besides acyclovir and derivatives may be the use of retinoic acids that are strongly inhibitory for the proliferation of EBV infected lymphoblasts.[168]

Autoantibodies in RA are cross-directed both against the glycine-alanine repeat of EBNA1 and against collagen and keratin filaments in the affected synovia[169-173] (Table 1, Fig. 1). Further autoantibodies are directed against the shared epitope motif QKRAA, both within the EBV glycoprotein gp110 (BALF4) and at amino acid position 70 to 74 of the third hypervariable region of the β-chain of the HLA-DRB1*0401 protein.[160,174] Furthermore, suppressor T-cell function is impaired in RA patients.[175] In RA patients that carry the shared antigen epitope at their DRB1 locus the frequency of T cells recognizing gp110 of EBV is decreased which might lead to a poor T cell control of EBV infection.[176] Further, there is a clonal expansion of a dysfunctional population of CD8+ suppressor T cells specific for EBV peptides.[177] Further, the synovium is infiltrated with CD8+ T cells that recognize EBV antigens including lytic antigens from the immediate early and early class.[178,179] Deiminated proteins like fibrinogen, filaggrin and keratin that carry cyclic citrulline instead of arginine are found in the synovia of RA patients.[180] Also EBNA1 can become deiminated within its glycine-arginine rich sequences (Table 1, Fig. 1). The citrullinated sequence of EBNA1 might induce anticitrullinic antibodies in RA patients.[181] Autoantibodies against those citrullinated proteins play a role in the development of RA and are higly specific for the diagnosis of RA.[182] Furthermore, anticitrulline autoantibodies are found years before disease onset and are, therefore, predictive for later RA development.[183]

CONCLUSION

EBV may trigger autoimmunity through diverse mechanisms (Tables 3 and 4). Another possibility, however, may be that there are host factors predisposing both for autoimmunity and for a dysregulated immune response against EBV. For example, a dysfunction of regulatory T cells might lead both to an increased tendency towards

Table 3. Mechanisms implicated in Epstein-Barr virus-associated autoimmune phenomena

Mechanism	Autoimmune Disease
Generation of autoreactive T-cell clones (in infectious mononucleosis patients?)	MS
Antigenic cross reactivity/mimicry	MS, SLE, RA
Immortalization of preexisting autoreactive B-cells by Epstein-Barr virus infection	MS (?), SLE (?), RA (?)

MS: multiple sclerosis; SLE: systemic lupus erythematosus; RA: rheumatoid arthritis.

Table 4. Potential mechanisms facilitating the development of Epstein-Barr virus-associated pathogenetic and patho-epigenetic changes in major autoimmune diseases

Mechanism	Autoimmune Disease
1. Increased viral load due to the activation of lytic EBV replication and/or insufficient immunological control of latent EBV infection	MS (?), SLE, RA
2. Activation of TLR3 and induction of dendritic cell maturation and IFN-β and IL-12 production by EBER1 RNA released from EBV infected cells	MS, SLE, RA
3. Epigenetic dysregulation of latent EBV gene expression in memory B cells, resulting in 4, 5, 6, 7, 8, 9, 10 and 11	MS, SLE, RA
4. Silencing of cellular gene sets by promoter methylation due to the up-regulation of DNMT1 by LMP1 and LMP2A (e.g., Bim, coding for a proapoptotic protein)	MS, SLE, RA
5. Induction of BAFF by LMP1 resulting in the subversion of B-cell tolerance	MS, SLE, RA
6. Induction of APRIL by LMP1, facilitating B-cell proliferation	MS, SLE, RA
7. Induction of T-cell independent Ig heavy chain switch by LMP1 and LMP2A modulating B-cell sensitivity to regulatory signals	MS, SLE, RA
8. Expression of EBNA2 leading to the expansion of B-cells carrying EBV genomes	MS, SLE, RA
9. miRNAs processed from EBV transcripts may affect B-cell maturation and contribute to the subversion of self-tolerance	MS, SLE, RA
10. EBNA2 and EBV-encoded miRNAs may alter cellular gene expression patterns and direct thereby B-cell migration to atopic sites	MS (?)
11. miR-BART2-5p may down-regulate the NK-cell ligand MICB, resulting in immune evasion	MS, SLE, RA

autoimmunity and to a hyperreactive immune response against EBV. Therefore, a causal relationship between EBV infection and autoimmunity is not proven so far. The ultimate test of causality might be established through the introduction of an EBV vaccination for certain risk groups.[184,185] In addition, a molecular link between the expression of specific EBV-proteins and specific epigenetic alterations in immune cells and of the immune system may also be suitable to establish a causal relationship between EBV-infection and autoimmunity.

REFERENCES

1. Thompson MP, Kurzrock R. Epstein-Barr virus and cancer. Clin Cancer Res 2004; 10:803-821.
2. Niller HH, Wolf H, Minarovits J. Epstein-Barr Virus. In: Minarovits J, Gonczol E, Valyi-Nagy T, eds. Latency Strategies of Herpesviruses. New York: Springer, 2007:154-191.
3. Niller HH, Wolf H, Minarovits J. Regulation and dysregulation of Epstein-Barr virus latency: implications for the development of autoimmune diseases. Autoimmunity 2008; 41:298-328.
4. Hadinoto V, Shapiro M, Sun CC et al. The dynamics of EBV shedding implicate a central role for epithelial cells in amplifying viral output. PLoS Pathog 2009; 5:e1000496.
5. Crawford DH. Biology and disease associations of Epstein-Barr virus. Philos Trans R Soc Lond B Biol Sci 2001; 356:461-473.
6. Hochberg D, Souza T, Catalina M et al. Acute infection with Epstein-Barr virus targets and overwhelms the peripheral memory B-cell compartment with resting, latently infected cells. J Virol 2004; 78:5194-5204.
7. Tierney RJ, Steven N, Young LS et al. Epstein-Barr virus latency in blood mononuclear cells: analysis of viral gene transcription during primary infection and in the carrier state. J Virol 1994; 68:7374-7385.
8. Tosato G, Magrath I, Koski I et al. Activation of suppressor T-cells during Epstein-Barr-virus-induced infectious mononucleosis. N Engl J Med 1979; 301:1133-1137.
9. Moss DJ, Burrows SR, Silins SL et al. The immunology of Epstein-Barr virus infection. Philos Trans R Soc Lond B Biol Sci 2001; 356:475-488.
10. Silins SL, Sherritt MA, Silleri JM et al. Asymptomatic primary Epstein-Barr virus infection occurs in the absence of blood T-cell repertoire perturbations despite high levels of systemic viral load. Blood 2001; 98:3739-3744.
11. Thorley-Lawson DA, Gross A. Persistence of the Epstein-Barr virus and the origins of associated lymphomas. N Engl J Med 2004; 350:1328-1337.
12. Souza TA, Stollar BD, Sullivan JL et al. Peripheral B-cells latently infected with Epstein-Barr virus display molecular hallmarks of classical antigen-selected memory B-cells. Proc Natl Acad Sci USA 2005; 102:18093-18098.
13. Kurth J, Spieker T, Wustrow J et al. EBV-infected B-cells in infectious mononucleosis: viral strategies for spreading in the B-cell compartment and establishing latency. Immunity 2000; 13:485-495.
14. Kurth J, Hansmann ML, Rajewsky K et al. Epstein-Barr virus-infected B-cells expanding in germinal centers of infectious mononucleosis patients do not participate in the germinal center reaction. Proc Natl Acad Sci USA 2003; 100:4730-4735.
15. Roughan JE, Thorley-Lawson DA. The intersection of Epstein-Barr virus with the germinal center. J Virol 2009; 83:3968-3976.
16. Roughan JE, Torgbor C, Thorley-Lawson DA. Germinal center B-cells latently infected with Epstein-Barr virus proliferate extensively but do not increase in number. J Virol 2010; 84:1158-1168.
17. Ehlin-Henriksson B, Gordon J, Klein G. B-lymphocyte subpopulations are equally susceptible to Epstein-Barr virus infection, irrespective of immunoglobulin isotype expression. Immunology 2003; 108:427-430.
18. Uchida J, Yasui T, Takaoka-Shichijo Y et al. Mimicry of CD40 signals by Epstein-Barr virus LMP1 in B lymphocyte responses. Science 1999; 286:300-303.
19. Lenoir GM, Bornkamm G. Burkitt's Lymphoma, a human cancer model for the study of the multistep dvelopment of cancer: proposal for a new scenario. In: Klein G, ed. Advances in Viral Oncology. New York: Raven Press, 1987:173-206.
20. Araujo I, Foss HD, Hummel M et al. Frequent expansion of Epstein-Barr virus (EBV) infected cells in germinal centres of tonsils from an area with a high incidence of EBV-associated lymphoma. J Pathol 1999; 187:326-330.
21. Niller HH, Salamon D, Ilg K et al. EBV-associated neoplasms: alternative pathogenetic pathways. Med Hypotheses 2004; 62:387-391.
22. Marschall M, Leser U, Seibl R et al. Identification of proteins encoded by Epstein-Barr virus trans-activator genes. J Virol 1989; 63:938-942.
23. Sinclair AJ, Brimmell M, Shanahan F et al. Pathways of activation of the Epstein-Barr virus productive cycle. J Virol 1991; 65:2237-2244.
24. Niller HH, Salamon D, Banati F et al. The LCR of EBV makes Burkitt's lymphoma endemic. Trends Microbiol 2004; 12:495-499.

25. Pfeffer S, Zavolan M, Grasser FA et al. Identification of virus-encoded microRNAs. Science 2004; 304:734-736.
26. Cai X, Schafer A, Lu S et al. Epstein-Barr virus microRNAs are evolutionarily conserved and differentially expressed. PLoS Pathog 2006; 2:e23.
27. Grundhoff A, Sullivan CS, Ganem D. A combined computational and microarray-based approach identifies novel microRNAs encoded by human gamma-herpesviruses. RNA 2006; 12:733-750.
28. Zhu JY, Pfuhl T, Motsch N et al. Identification of novel Epstein-Barr virus microRNA genes from nasopharyngeal carcinomas. J Virol 2009; 83:3333-3341.
29. Honess RW, Gompels UA, Barrell BG et al. Deviations from expected frequencies of CpG dinucleotides in herpesvirus DNAs may be diagnostic of differences in the states of their latent genomes. J Gen Virol 1989; 70(Pt 4):837-855.
30. Robertson KD, Ambinder RF. Methylation of the Epstein-Barr virus genome in normal lymphocytes. Blood 1997; 90:4480-4484.
31. Paulson EJ, Speck SH. Differential methylation of Epstein-Barr virus latency promoters facilitates viral persistence in healthy seropositive individuals. J Virol 1999; 73:9959-9968.
32. Minarovits J, Minarovits-Kormuta S, Ehlin-Henriksson B et al. Host cell phenotype-dependent methylation patterns of Epstein-Barr virus DNA. J Gen Virol 1991; 72:1591-1599.
33. Li H, Minarovits J. Host cell-dependent expression of latent Epstein-Barr virus genomes: regulation by DNA methylation. Adv Cancer Res 2003; 89:133-156.
34. Minarovits J. Epigenotypes of latent herpesvirus genomes. Curr Top Microbiol Immunol 2006; 310:61-80.
35. Ernberg I, Falk K, Minarovits J et al. The role of methylation in the phenotype-dependent modulation of Epstein-Barr nuclear antigen 2 and latent membrane protein genes in cells latently infected with Epstein-Barr virus. J Gen Virol 1989; 70:2989-3002.
36. Minarovits J, Hu LF, Marcsek Z et al. RNA polymerase III-transcribed EBER 1 and 2 transcription units are expressed and hypomethylated in the major Epstein-Barr virus-carrying cell types. J Gen Virol 1992; 73:1687-1692.
37. Altiok E, Minarovits J, Hu LF et al. Host-cell-phenotype-dependent control of the BCR2/BWR1 promoter complex regulates the expression of Epstein-Barr virus nuclear antigens 2-6. Proc Natl Acad Sci USA 1992; 89:905-909.
38. Arrand JR, Rymo L. Characterization of the major Epstein-Barr virus-specific RNA in Burkitt lymphoma-derived cells. J Virol 1982; 41:376-389.
39. Felton-Edkins ZA, Kondrashov A, Karali D et al. Epstein-Barr virus induces cellular transcription factors to allow active expression of EBER genes by RNA polymerase III. J Biol Chem 2006; 281:33871-33880.
40. Lerner MR, Andrews NC, Miller G et al. Two small RNAs encoded by Epstein-Barr virus and complexed with protein are precipitated by antibodies from patients with systemic lupus erythematosus. Proc Natl Acad Sci USA 1981; 78:805-809.
41. Toczyski DP, Matera AG, Ward DC et al. The Epstein-Barr virus (EBV) small RNA EBER1 binds and relocalizes ribosomal protein L22 in EBV-infected human B lymphocytes. Proc Natl Acad Sci USA 1994; 91:3463-3467.
42. Clarke PA, Schwemmle M, Schickinger J et al. Binding of Epstein-Barr virus small RNA EBER-1 to the double-stranded RNA-activated protein kinase DAI. Nucleic Acids Res 1991; 19:243-248.
43. Elia A, Vyas J, Laing KG et al. Ribosomal protein L22 inhibits regulation of cellular activities by the Epstein-Barr virus small RNA EBER-1. Eur J Biochem 2004; 271:1895-1905.
44. Komano J, Maruo S, Kurozumi K et al. Oncogenic role of Epstein-Barr virus-encoded RNAs in Burkitt's lymphoma cell line Akata. J Virol 1999; 73:9827-9831.
45. Ruf IK, Rhyne PW, Yang C et al. Epstein-Barr virus small RNAs potentiate tumorigenicity of Burkitt lymphoma cells independently of an effect on apoptosis. J Virol 2000; 74:10223-10228.
46. Ruf IK, Lackey KA, Warudkar S et al. Protection from interferon-induced apoptosis by epstein-barr virus small RNAs is not mediated by inhibition of PKR. J Virol 2005; 79:14562-14569.
47. Clemens MJ. Epstein-Barr virus: inhibition of apoptosis as a mechanism of cell transformation. Int J Biochem Cell Biol 2006; 38:164-169.
48. Iwakiri D, Zhou L, Samanta M et al. Epstein-Barr virus (EBV)-encoded small RNA is released from EBV-infected cells and activates signaling from Toll-like receptor 3. J Exp Med 2009; 206:2091-2099.
49. Sugden B, Warren N. A promoter of Epstein-Barr virus that can function during latent infection can be transactivated by EBNA-1, a viral protein required for viral DNA replication during latent infection. J Virol 1989; 63:2644-2649.
50. Jankelevich S, Kolman JL, Bodnar JW et al. A nuclear matrix attachment region organizes the Epstein-Barr viral plasmid in Raji cells into a single DNA domain. EMBO J 1992; 11:1165-1176.
51. Middleton T, Sugden B. Retention of plasmid DNA in mammalian cells is enhanced by binding of the Epstein-Barr virus replication protein EBNA1. J Virol 1994; 68:4067-4071.

52. White RE, Wade-Martins R, James MR. Sequences adjacent to oriP improve the persistence of Epstein-Barr virus-based episomes in B-cells. J Virol 2001; 75:11249-11252.
53. Wensing B, Stühler A, Jenkins P et al. Variant chromatin structure of the oriP region of Epstein-Barr virus and regulation of EBER1 expression by upstream sequences and oriP. J Virol 2001; 75.6235-6241
54. Levitskaya J, Sharipo A, Leonchiks A et al. Inhibition of ubiquitin/proteasome-dependent protein degradation by the Gly-Ala repeat domain of the Epstein-Barr virus nuclear antigen 1. Proc Natl Acad Sci USA 1997; 94:12616-12621.
55. Munz C. Epstein-barr virus nuclear antigen 1: from immunologically invisible to a promising T-cell target. J Exp Med 2004; 199:1301-1304.
56. Lunemann JD, Edwards N, Muraro PA et al. Increased frequency and broadened specificity of latent EBV nuclear antigen-1-specific T-cells in multiple sclerosis. Brain 2006; 129:1493-1506.
57. Rabson M, Gradoville L, Heston L et al. Non-immortalizing P3J-HR-1 Epstein-Barr virus: a deletion mutant of its transforming parent, Jijoye. J Virol 1982; 44:834-844.
58. Hammerschmidt W, Sugden B. Genetic analysis of immortalizing functions of Epstein-Barr virus in human B lymphocytes. Nature 1989; 340:393-397.
59. Ling PD, Rawlins DR, Hayward SD. The Epstein-Barr virus immortalizing protein EBNA-2 is targeted to DNA by a cellular enhancer-binding protein. Proc Natl Acad Sci USA 1993; 90:9237-9241.
60. Cordier M, Calender A, Billaud M et al. Stable transfection of Epstein-Barr virus (EBV) nuclear antigen 2 in lymphoma cells containing the EBV P3HR1 genome induces expression of B-cell activation molecules CD21 and CD23. J Virol 1990; 64:1002-1013.
61. Wang F, Tsang SF, Kurilla MG et al. Epstein-Barr virus nuclear antigen 2 transactivates latent membrane protein LMP1. J Virol 1990; 64:3407-3416.
62. Mannick JB, Cohen JI, Birkenbach M et al. The Epstein-Barr virus nuclear protein encoded by the leader of the EBNA RNAs is important in B-lymphocyte transformation. J Virol 1991; 65:6826-6837.
63. Harada S, Kjeff E. Epstein-Barr virus nuclear protein LP stimulates EBNA-2 acidic domain-mediated transcriptional activation. J Virol 1997; 71:6611-6618.
64. Nitsche F, Bell A, Rickinson A. Epstein-Barr virus leader protein enhances EBNA-2-mediated transactivation of latent membrane protein 1 expression: a role for the W1W2 repeat domain. J Virol 1997; 71:6619-6628.
65. Tomkinson B, Robertson E, Kieff E. Epstein-Barr virus nuclear proteins EBNA-3A and EBNA-3C are essential for B-lymphocyte growth transformation. J Virol 1993; 67:2014-2025.
66. Tomkinson B, Kieff E. Use of second-site homologous recombination to demonstrate that Epstein-Barr virus nuclear protein 3B is not important for lymphocyte infection or growth transformation in vitro. J Virol 1992; 66:2893-2903.
67. Waltzer L, Perricaudet M, Sergeant A et al. Epstein-Barr virus EBNA3A and EBNA3C proteins both repress RBP-J kappa-EBNA2-activated transcription by inhibiting the binding of RBP-J kappa to DNA. J Virol 1996; 70:5909-5915.
68. Robertson ES, Lin J, Kieff E. The amino-terminal domains of Epstein-Barr virus nuclear proteins 3A, 3B and 3C interact with RBPJ(kappa). J Virol 1996; 70:3068-3074.
69. Chen A, Zhao B, Kieff E et al. EBNA-3B- and EBNA-3C-regulated cellular genes in Epstein-Barr virus-immortalized lymphoblastoid cell lines. J Virol 2006; 80:10139-10150.
70. Smith P. Epstein-Barr virus complementary strand transcripts (CSTs/BARTs) and cancer. Semin Cancer Biol 2001; 11:469-476.
71. Al Mozaini M, Bodelon G, Karstegl CE et al. Epstein-Barr virus BART gene expression. J Gen Virol 2009; 90:307-316.
72. Sadler RH, Raab-Traub N. Structural analyses of the Epstein-Barr virus BamHI A transcripts. J Virol 1995; 69:1132-1141.
73. de Jesus O, Smith PR, Spender LC et al. Updated Epstein-Barr virus (EBV) DNA sequence and analysis of a promoter for the BART (CST, BARF0) RNAs of EBV. J Gen Virol 2003; 84:1443-1450.
74. He B, Raab-Traub N, Casali P et al. EBV-encoded latent membrane protein 1 cooperates with BAFF/BLyS and APRIL to induce T-cell-independent Ig heavy chain class switching. J Immunol 2003; 171:5215-5224.
75. Laux G, Dugrillon F, Eckert C et al. Identification and characterization of an Epstein-Barr virus nuclear antigen 2-responsive cis element in the bidirectional promoter region of latent membrane protein and terminal protein 2 genes. J Virol 1994; 68:6947-6958.
76. Sadler RH, Raab-Traub N. The Epstein-Barr virus 3.5-kilobase latent membrane protein 1 mRNA initiates from a TATA-less promoter within the first terminal repeat. J Virol 1995; 69:4577-4581.
77. Fennewald S, van Santen V, Kieff E. Nucleotide sequence of an mRNA transcribed in latent growth-transforming virus infection indicates that it may encode a membrane protein. J Virol 1984; 51:411-419.

78. Rechsteiner MP, Berger C, Weber M et al. Silencing of latent membrane protein 2B reduces susceptibility to activation of lytic Epstein-Barr virus in Burkitt's lymphoma Akata cells. J Gen Virol 2007; 88:1454-1459.
79. Rechsteiner MP, Berger C, Zauner L et al. Latent membrane protein 2B regulates susceptibility to induction of lytic Epstein-Barr virus infection. J Virol 2008; 82:1739-1747.
80. Swanson-Mungerson M, Longnecker R. Epstein-Barr virus latent membrane protein 2A and autoimmunity. Trends Immunol 2007; 28:213-218.
81. Tsai CL, Li HP, Lu YJ et al. Activation of DNA methyltransferase 1 by EBV LMP1 Involves c-Jun NH(2)-terminal kinase signaling. Cancer Res 2006; 66:11668-11676.
82. Hino R, Uozaki H, Murakami N et al. Activation of DNA methyltransferase 1 by EBV latent membrane protein 2A leads to promoter hypermethylation of PTEN gene in gastric carcinoma. Cancer Res 2009; 69:2766-2774.
83. Xia T, O'Hara A, Araujo I et al. EBV microRNAs in primary lymphomas and targeting of CXCL-11 by ebv-mir-BHRF1-3. Cancer Res 2008; 68:1436-1442.
84. Lung RW, Tong JH, Sung YM et al. Modulation of LMP2A expression by a newly identified Epstein-Barr virus-encoded microRNA miR-BART22. Neoplasia 2009; 11:1174-1184.
85. Lo AK, To KF, Lo KW et al. Modulation of LMP1 protein expression by EBV-encoded microRNAs. Proc Natl Acad Sci USA 2007; 104:16164-16169.
86. Barth S, Pfuhl T, Mamiani A et al. Epstein-Barr virus-encoded microRNA miR-BART2 down-regulates the viral DNA polymerase BALF5. Nucleic Acids Res 2008; 36:666-675.
87. Choy EY, Siu KL, Kok KH et al. An Epstein-Barr virus-encoded microRNA targets PUMA to promote host cell survival. J Exp Med 2008; 205:2551-2560.
88. Nachmani D, Stern-Ginossar N, Sarid R et al. Diverse herpesvirus microRNAs target the stress-induced immune ligand MICB to escape recognition by natural killer cells. Cell Host Microbe 2009; 5:376-385.
89. Niller HH, Wolf H, Minarovits J. Epigenetic dysregulation of the host cell genome in Epstein-Barr virus-associated neoplasia. Semin Cancer Biol 2009; 19:158-164.
90. Lunemann JD, Munz C. EBV in MS: guilty by association? Trends Immunol 2009; 30:243-248.
91. Pender MP. Infection of autoreactive B lymphocytes with EBV, causing chronic autoimmune diseases. Trends Immunol 2003; 24:584-588.
92. Wong M, Tsao BP. Current topics in human SLE genetics. Springer Semin Immunopathol 2006; 28:97-107.
93. Hewagama A, Richardson B. The genetics and epigenetics of autoimmune diseases. J Autoimmun 2009; 33:3-11.
94. Brooks WH, Le Dantec C, Pers JO et al. Epigenetics and autoimmunity. J Autoimmun 2010.
95. Ascherio A, Munger KL. Environmental risk factors for multiple sclerosis. Part I: the role of infection. Ann Neurol 2007; 61:288-299.
96. Ascherio A, Munger KL. Environmental risk factors for multiple sclerosis. Part II: Noninfectious factors. Ann Neurol 2007.
97. Poser CM. Notes on the pathogenesis of multiple sclerosis. Clin Neurosci 1994; 2:258-265.
98. Sutkowski N, Conrad B, Thorley-Lawson DA et al. Epstein-Barr virus transactivates the human endogenous retrovirus HERV-K18 that encodes a superantigen. Immunity 2001; 15:579-589.
99. Tai AK, O'Reilly EJ, Alroy KA et al. Human endogenous retrovirus-K18 Env as a risk factor in multiple sclerosis. Mult Scler 2008; 14:1175-1180.
100. Christensen T. Association of human endogenous retroviruses with multiple sclerosis and possible interactions with herpes viruses. Rev Med Virol 2005; 15:179-211.
101. Antony JM, van Marle G, Opii W et al. Human endogenous retrovirus glycoprotein-mediated induction of redox reactants causes oligodendrocyte death and demyelination. Nat Neurosci 2004; 7:1088-1095.
102. Alotaibi S, Kennedy J, Tellier R et al. Epstein-Barr virus in pediatric multiple sclerosis. JAMA 2004; 291:1875-1879.
103. Pohl D, Krone B, Rostasy K et al. High seroprevalence of Epstein-Barr virus in children with multiple sclerosis. Neurology 2006; 67:2063-2065.
104. Haahr S, Hollsberg P. Multiple sclerosis is linked to Epstein-Barr virus infection. Rev Med Virol 2006; 16:297-310.
105. Nielsen TR, Rostgaard K, Nielsen NM et al. Multiple sclerosis after infectious mononucleosis. Arch Neurol 2007; 64:72-75.
106. Rolls AE, Giovannoni G, Constantinescu CS et al. Multiple Sclerosis, Lymphoma and Nasopharyngeal Carcinoma: The Central Role of Epstein-Barr Virus? Eur Neurol 2009; 63:29-35.
107. DeLorenze GN, Munger KL, Lennette ET et al. Epstein-Barr virus and multiple sclerosis: evidence of association from a prospective study with long-term follow-up. Arch Neurol 2006; 63:839-844.
108. Nielsen TR, Pedersen M, Rostgaard K et al. Correlations between Epstein-Barr virus antibody levels and risk factors for multiple sclerosis in healthy individuals. Mult Scler 2007; 13:420-423.

109. Sundstrom P, Juto P, Wadell G et al. An altered immune response to Epstein-Barr virus in multiple sclerosis: a prospective study. Neurology 2004; 62:2277-2282.
110. Bray PF, Luka J, Bray PF et al. Antibodies against Epstein-Barr nuclear antigen (EBNA) in multiple sclerosis CSF and two pentapeptide sequence identities between EBNA and myelin basic protein. Neurology 1992; 42:1798-1804.
111. Cepok S, Zhou D, Srivastava R et al. Identification of Epstein-Barr virus proteins as putative targets of the immune response in multiple sclerosis. J Clin Invest 2005; 115:1352-1360.
112. Wucherpfennig KW, Strominger JL. Molecular mimicry in T-cell-mediated autoimmunity: viral peptides activate human T-cell clones specific for myelin basic protein. Cell 1995; 80:695-705.
113. Lang HL, Jacobsen H, Ikemizu S et al. A functional and structural basis for TCR cross-reactivity in multiple sclerosis. Nat Immunol 2002; 3:940-943.
114. Holmoy T, Vartdal F. Cerebrospinal fluid T-cells from multiple sclerosis patients recognize autologous Epstein-Barr virus-transformed B-cells. J Neurovirol 2004; 10:52-56.
115. Holmoy T, Kvale EO, Vartdal F. Cerebrospinal fluid CD4+ T-cells from a multiple sclerosis patient cross-recognize Epstein-Barr virus and myelin basic protein. J Neurovirol 2004; 10:278-283.
116. Gronen F, Ruprecht K, Weissbrich B et al. Frequency analysis of HLA-B7-restricted Epstein-Barr virus-specific cytotoxic T-lymphocytes in patients with multiple sclerosis and healthy controls. J Neuroimmunol 2006; 180:185-192.
117. Serafini B, Rosicarelli B, Franciotta D et al. Dysregulated Epstein-Barr virus infection in the multiple sclerosis brain. J Exp Med 2007; 204:2899-2912.
118. Ascherio A. Epstein-Barr virus in the development of multiple sclerosis. Expert Rev Neurother 2008; 8:331-333.
119. Franciotta D, Salvetti M, Lolli F et al. B-cells and multiple sclerosis. Lancet Neurol 2008; 7:852-858.
120. Salvetti M, Giovannoni G, Aloisi F. Epstein-Barr virus and multiple sclerosis. Curr Opin Neurol 2009; 22:201-206.
121. Willis SN, Stadelmann C, Rodig SJ et al. Epstein-Barr virus infection is not a characteristic feature of multiple sclerosis brain. Brain 2009; 132:3318-3328.
122. Peferoen LA, Lamers F, Lodder LN et al. Epstein Barr virus is not a characteristic feature in the central nervous system in established multiple sclerosis. Brain 2009.
123. Torkildsen O, Stansberg C, Angelskar SM et al. Upregulation of immunoglobulin-related genes in cortical sections from multiple sclerosis patients. Brain Pathol 2009.
124. Sawalha AH, Webb R, Han S et al. Common variants within MECP2 confer risk of systemic lupus erythematosus. PLoS ONE 2008; 3:e1727.
125. Sawalha AH, Jeffries M, Webb R et al. Defective T-cell ERK signaling induces interferon-regulated gene expression and overexpression of methylation-sensitive genes similar to lupus patients. Genes Immun 2008; 9:368-378.
126. Xiao C, Srinivasan L, Calado DP et al. Lymphoproliferative disease and autoimmunity in mice with increased miR-17-92 expression in lymphocytes. Nat Immunol 2008; 9:405-414.
127. Paschos K, Smith P, Anderton E et al. Epstein-barr virus latency in B-cells leads to epigenetic repression and CpG methylation of the tumour suppressor gene Bim PLoS Pathog 2009; 5:e1000492.
128. Harley JB, Harley IT, Guthridge JM et al. The curiously suspicious: a role for Epstein-Barr virus in lupus. Lupus 2006; 15:768-777.
129. James JA, Harley JB, Scofield RH. Epstein-Barr virus and systemic lupus erythematosus. Curr Opin Rheumatol 2006; 18:462-467.
130. James JA, Neas BR, Moser KL et al. Systemic lupus erythematosus in adults is associated with previous Epstein-Barr virus exposure. Arthritis Rheum 2001; 44:1122-1126.
131. James JA, Kaufman KM, Farris AD et al. An increased prevalence of Epstein-Barr virus infection in young patients suggests a possible etiology for systemic lupus erythematosus. J Clin Invest 1997; 100:3019-3026.
132. McClain MT, Heinlen LD, Dennis GJ et al. Early events in lupus humoral autoimmunity suggest initiation through molecular mimicry. Nat Med 2005; 11:85-89.
133. James JA, Gross T, Scofield RH et al. Immunoglobulin epitope spreading and autoimmune disease after peptide immunization: Sm B/B'-derived PPPGMRPP and PPPGIRGP induce spliceosome autoimmunity. J Exp Med 1995; 181:453-461.
134. Arbuckle MR, Reichlin M, Harley JB et al. Shared early autoantibody recognition events in the development of anti-Sm B/B' in human lupus. Scand J Immunol 1999; 50:447-455.
135. James JA, Harley JB. A model of peptide-induced lupus autoimmune B-cell epitope spreading is strain specific and is not H-2 restricted in mice. J Immunol 1998; 160:502-508.
136. Arbuckle MR, Gross T, Scofield RH et al. Lupus humoral autoimmunity induced in a primate model by short peptide immunization. J Investig Med 1998; 46:58-65.

137. James JA, Harley JB. Linear epitope mapping of an Sm B/B' polypeptide. J Immunol 1992; 148:2074-2079.

138. McClain MT, Poole BD, Bruner BF et al. An altered immune response to Epstein-Barr nuclear antigen 1 in pediatric systemic lupus erythematosus. Arthritis Rheum 2006; 54:360-368.

139. James JA, Scofield RH, Harley JB. Lupus humoral autoimmunity after short peptide immunization. Ann NY Acad Sci 1997; 815:124-127.

140. Sundar K, Jacques S, Gottlieb P et al. Expression of the Epstein-Barr virus nuclear antigen-1 (EBNA-1) in the mouse can elicit the production of anti-dsDNA and anti-Sm antibodies. J Autoimmun 2004; 23:127-140.

141. Kaufman KM, Kirby MY, Harley JB et al. Peptide mimics of a major lupus epitope of SmB/B'. Ann NY Acad Sci 2003; 987:215-229.

142. Incaprera M, Rindi L, Bazzichi A et al. Potential role of the Epstein-Barr virus in systemic lupus erythematosus autoimmunity. Clin Exp Rheumatol 1998; 16:289-294.

143. Sabbatini A, Bombardieri S, Migliorini P. Autoantibodies from patients with systemic lupus erythematosus bind a shared sequence of SmD and Epstein-Barr virus-encoded nuclear antigen EBNA I. Eur J Immunol 1993; 23:1146-1152.

144. Yamazaki M, Kitamura R, Kusano S et al. Elevated immunoglobulin G antibodies to the proline-rich amino-terminal region of Epstein-Barr virus nuclear antigen-2 in sera from patients with systemic connective tissue diseases and from a subgroup of Sjogren's syndrome patients with pulmonary involvements. Clin Exp Immunol 2005; 139:558-568.

145. Yu SF, Wu HC, Tsai WC et al. Detecting Epstein-Barr virus DNA from peripheral blood mononuclear cells in adult patients with systemic lupus erythematosus in Taiwan. Med Microbiol Immunol 2005; 194:115-120.

146. Moon UY, Park SJ, Oh ST et al. Patients with systemic lupus erythematosus have abnormally elevated Epstein-Barr virus load in blood. Arthritis Res Ther 2004; 6:R295-R302.

147. Kang I, Quan T, Nolasco H et al. Defective control of latent Epstein-Barr virus infection in systemic lupus erythematosus. J Immunol 2004; 172:1287-1294.

148. Gross AJ, Hochberg D, Rand WM et al. EBV and systemic lupus erythematosus: a new perspective. J Immunol 2005; 174:6599-6607.

149. Tsokos GC, Magrath IT, Balow JE. Epstein-Barr virus induces normal B-cell responses but defective suppressor T-cell responses in patients with systemic lupus erythematosus. J Immunol 1983; 131:1797-1801.

150. Berner BR, Tary-Lehmann M, Yonkers NL et al. Phenotypic and functional analysis of EBV-specific memory CD8 cells in SLE. Cell Immunol 2005; 235:29-38.

151. Yurasov S, Wardemann H, Hammersen J et al. Defective B-cell tolerance checkpoints in systemic lupus erythematosus. J Exp Med 2005; 201:703-711.

152. Wakabayashi C, Adachi T, Wienands J et al. A distinct signaling pathway used by the IgG-containing B-cell antigen receptor. Science 2002; 298:2392-2395.

153. Costenbader KH, Karlson EW. Epstein-Barr virus and rheumatoid arthritis: is there a link? Arthritis Res Ther 2006; 8:204.

154. Sawada S, Takei M, Inomata H et al. What is after cytokine-blocking therapy, a novel therapeutic target—synovial Epstein-Barr virus for rheumatoid arthritis. Autoimmun Rev 2007; 6:126-130.

155. Oliver JE, Silman AJ. Risk factors for the development of rheumatoid arthritis. Scand J Rheumatol 2006; 35:169-174.

156. Sanchez-Pernaute O, Ospelt C, Neidhart M et al. Epigenetic clues to rheumatoid arthritis. J Autoimmun 2008; 30:12-20.

157. Stastny P. Association of the B-cell alloantigen DRw4 with rheumatoid arthritis. N Engl J Med 1978; 298:869-871.

158. Gregersen PK, Silver J, Winchester RJ. The shared epitope hypothesis. An approach to understanding the molecular genetics of susceptibility to rheumatoid arthritis. Arthritis Rheum 1987; 30:1205-1213.

159. Jilg W, Bogedain C, Mairhofer H et al. The Epstein-Barr virus-encoded glycoprotein gp 110 (BALF 4) can serve as a target for antibody-dependent cell-mediated cytotoxicity (ADCC). Virology 1994; 202:974-977.

160. Saal JG, Krimmel M, Steidle M et al. Synovial Epstein-Barr virus infection increases the risk of rheumatoid arthritis in individuals with the shared HLA-DR4 epitope. Arthritis Rheum 1999; 42:1485-1496.

161. Dreyfus DH. Paleo-immunology: evidence consistent with insertion of a primordial herpes virus-like element in the origins of acquired immunity. PloS ONE 2009; 4:e5778.

162. Massa M, Mazzoli F, Pignatti P et al. Proinflammatory responses to self HLA epitopes are triggered by molecular mimicry to Epstein-Barr virus proteins in oligoarticular juvenile idiopathic arthritis. Arthritis Rheum 2002; 46:2721-2729.

163. Ray CG, Gall EP, Minnich LL et al. Acute polyarthritis associated with active Epstein-Barr virus infection. JAMA 1982; 248:2990-2993.

164. Blaschke S, Schwarz G, Moneke D et al. Epstein-Barr virus infection in peripheral blood mononuclear cells, synovial fluid cells and synovial membranes of patients with rheumatoid arthritis. J Rheumatol 2000; 27:866-873.
165. Balandraud N, Meynard JB, Auger I et al. Epstein-Barr virus load in the peripheral blood of patients with rheumatoid arthritis: accurate quantification using real-time polymerase chain reaction. Arthritis Rheum 2003; 48:1223-1228.
166. Takei M, Mitamura K, Fujiwara S et al. Detection of Epstein-Barr virus-encoded small RNA 1 and latent membrane protein 1 in synovial lining cells from rheumatoid arthritis patients. Int Immunol 1997; 9:739-743.
167. Agarwal V, Singh R, Chauhan S. Remission of rheumatoid arthritis after acute disseminated varicella-zoster infection. Clin Rheumatol 2007; 26:779-780.
168. Pomponi F, Cariati R, Zancai P et al. Retinoids irreversibly inhibit in vitro growth of Epstein-Barr virus-immortalized B lymphocytes. Blood 1996; 88:3147-3159.
169. Fox R, Sportsman R, Rhodes G et al. Rheumatoid arthritis synovial membrane contains a 62,000-molecular-weight protein that shares an antigenic epitope with the Epstein-Barr virus-encoded associated nuclear antigen. J Clin Invest 1986; 77:1539-1547.
170. Birkenfeld P, Haratz N, Klein G et al. Cross-reactivity between the EBNA-1 p107 peptide, collagen and keratin: implications for the pathogenesis of rheumatoid arthritis. Clin Immunol Immunopathol 1990; 54:14-25.
171. Kouri T, Petersen J, Rhodes G et al. Antibodies to synthetic peptides from Epstein-Barr nuclear antigen-1 in sera of patients with early rheumatoid arthritis and in preillness sera. J Rheumatol 1990; 17:1442-1449.
172. Baboonian C, Halliday D, Venables PJ et al. Antibodies in rheumatoid arthritis react specifically with the glycine alanine repeat sequence of Epstein-Barr nuclear antigen-1. Rheumatol Int 1989; 9:161-166.
173. Petersen J, Rhodes G, Roudier J et al. Altered immune response to glycine-rich sequences of Epstein-Barr nuclear antigen-1 in patients with rheumatoid arthritis and systemic lupus erythematosus. Arthritis Rheum 1990; 33:993-1000.
174. Roudier J, Petersen J, Rhodes GH et al. Susceptibility to rheumatoid arthritis maps to a T-cell epitope shared by the HLA-Dw4 DR beta-1 chain and the Epstein-Barr virus glycoprotein gp110. Proc Natl Acad Sci USA 1989; 86:5104-5108.
175. Tosato G, Steinberg AD, Blaese RM. Defective EBV-specific suppressor T-cell function in rheumatoid arthritis. N Engl J Med 1981; 305:1238-1243.
176. Toussirot E, Wendling D, Tiberghien P et al. Decreased T-cell precursor frequencies to Epstein-Barr virus glycoprotein Gp110 in peripheral blood correlate with disease activity and severity in patients with rheumatoid arthritis. Ann Rheum Dis 2000; 59:533-538.
177. Klatt T, Ouyang Q, Flad T et al. Expansion of peripheral CD8+ CD28- T cells in response to Epstein-Barr viurs in patients with rheumatoid arthritis. J Rheumatol 2005; 32:239-251.
178. David-Ameline J, Lim A, Davodeau F et al. Selection of T-cells reactive against autologous B lymphoblastoid cells during chronic rheumatoid arthritis. J Immunol 1996; 157:4697-4706.
179. Scotet E, David-Ameline J, Peyrat MA et al. T-cell response to Epstein-Barr virus transactivators in chronic rheumatoid arthritis. J Exp Med 1996; 184:1791-1800.
180. Baeten D, Peene I, Union A et al. Specific presence of intracellular citrullinated proteins in rheumatoid arthritis synovium: relevance to antifilaggrin autoantibodies. Arthritis Rheum 2001; 44:2255-2262.
181. Pratesi F, Tommasi C, Anzilotti C et al. Deiminated Epstein-Barr virus nuclear antigen 1 is a target of anti-citrullinated protein antibodies in rheumatoid arthritis. Arthritis Rheum 2006; 54:733-741.
182. Schellekens GA, Visser H, de Jong BA et al. The diagnostic properties of rheumatoid arthritis antibodies recognizing a cyclic citrullinated peptide. Arthritis Rheum 2000; 43:155-163.
183. Rantapaa-Dahlqvist S, de Jong BA, Berglin E et al. Antibodies against cyclic citrullinated peptide and IgA rheumatoid factor predict the development of rheumatoid arthritis. Arthritis Rheum 2003; 48:2741-2749.
184. Gu SY, Huang TM, Ruan L et al. First EBV vaccine trial in humans using recombinant vaccinia virus expressing the major membrane antigen. Dev Biol Stand 1995; 84:171-177.
185. Wolf HJ, Morgan AJ. Epstein-Barr Virus vaccines. In: Medveczky P, Friedman H, Bendinelli M, eds. Herpesviruses and Immunity. New York: Plenum Press, 1998:231-246.

CHAPTER 8

DOES GENOMIC IMPRINTING PLAY A ROLE IN AUTOIMMUNITY?

Cristina Camprubí and David Monk*

Imprinting and Cancer Group, Cancer Epigenetics and Biology Program (PEBC), Bellvitge Institute of Biomedical Investigation (IDIBELL), Barcelona, Spain
Corresponding Author: David Monk—Email: dmonk@iconcologia.net

Abstract: In the 19th century Gregor Mendel defined the laws of genetic inheritance by crossing different types of peas.[1] From these results arose his principle of equivalence: the gene will have the same behaviour whether it is inherited from the mother or the father. Today, several key exceptions to this principle are known, for example sex-linked traits and genes in the mitochondrial genome, whose inheritance patterns are referred to as 'non mendelian'. A third, important exception in mammals is that of genomic imprinting, where transcripts are expressed in a monoallelic fashion from only the maternal or the paternal chromosome. In this chapter, we discuss how parent-of-origin effects and genomic imprinting may play a role in autoimmunity and speculate how imprinted miRNAs may influence the expression of many target autoimmune associated genes.

INTRODUCTION

Discovery of Genomic Imprinting

The first evidence for imprinting came more than 25 years ago, from nuclear transfer experiments.[2,3] Mouse embryos were manipulated to contain either two maternal or paternal pronuclei, creating gynogenetic, or androgenetic embryos, respectively. Both sets of embryos failed to develop to term, with the gynogenetic embryos (containing only maternal chromosomes) developing a small embryo but with complete atrophy of extra-embryonic tissues. The androgenetic embryos (containing only paternal chromosomes) were characterised by overgrowth of the extra-embryonic tissues and

---

almost total absence of the embryo proper.[2] These pioneering experiments highlighted for the first time that the maternal and paternal genomes in a diploid cell are not functionally equivalent and therefore contain regions whose function is dependent on parental origin. The chromosomal regions of non-equivalence were identified in mice due to the existence of rare cases of uniparental disomy (UPD). UPD is the inheritance of both autosomal chromosomes from one parent and it was observed that inheritance of opposite parental UPDs resulted in different phenotypes that were often reciprocal.[4] It was almost a decade after the nuclear transfer experiments that the first imprinted gene was identified.[5] Since the discovery of *Igf2*, almost 100 imprinted genes have been identified in mice, with around half showing conserved monoallelic expression in humans (www.geneimprint.com). Imprinted genes have been shown to be important regulators of fetal and extra-embryonic growth and neurological development, through controlling cell signaling, cell cycle, metabolism and apoptosis.

Uniparental disomy also occurs in humans and for some human chromosomes are associated with disease due to the presence of imprinted genes on those chromosomes. The clearest example of reciprocal UPDs causing different phenotypes in humans is that of the behaviour syndromes Prader-Willi (PWS) and Angelman syndrome (AS), caused by a maternal or paternal UPD of chromosome 15, respectively.[6,7] It is also well known that UPDs affecting chromosome 14 cause different abnormal growth phenotypes that change according to the parental origin of the UPD.[8] Other examples are Beckwith-Wiedemann syndrome (BWS), where babies are macrosomic and Silver-Russell syndrome (SRS), where the babies are growth restricted. BWS is caused by a paternal UPD of chromosome 11 and SRS by a maternal UPD of chromosome 7.[9,10]

GENOMIC IMPRINTING

Genomic imprinting is the allele-specific expression of a gene depending on its parental origin. To date, most imprinted genes have been identified in mammalian species, however, the phenomenon is also observed in some flowering plants.[11] Since the two copies of autosomes in mammals are identical at the DNA sequence level, the difference in expression must be controlled by an epigenetic mechanism.[12] The term epigenetic refers to heritable changes that do not involve a change in the DNA nucleotide sequence. These include DNA methylation and posttranslational histone modifications that modify the status of chromatin, the molecule that eukaryotic DNA is packaged into. Chromatin consists of nucleosomes, formed by wrapping 146 base pairs of DNA around an octamer of four core histone proteins (H2A, H2B, H3 and H4). Depending on the methylation status of the DNA, combined with certain histone modifications, the chromatin can adopt an active or repressive status, named euchromatin and heterochromatin, respectively.

Genes subject to genomic imprinting constitute a particularly interesting example of epigenetic regulation, since there are active and repressed alleles of the same gene within a single cell. The allelic differences in transcriptional activity originate from the distinct patterns of chromatin structure, due to differential DNA methylation at CpG dinucleotides and covalent histone modifications.[13,14] The allele-specific epigenetic profile of imprinted genes is established in the male and female gametes and maintained throughout somatic development. Regions that display differential DNA methylation (DMRs) in the germ line are referred to as primary imprinting marks. If a DMR has been shown to be indispensable for monoallelic expression in gene targeting experiments, it is referred to as an Imprinting Control Region (ICR). Commonly, imprinted genes are grouped together in clusters, controlled in cis by a single ICR.

Epigenetic Mechanisms and Imprinting

DNA methylation is an essential modification to DNA, with established roles in gene regulation, genome defense through transcriptional silencing of retrotransposons and genome stability.[15] It is characterized by the transfer of methyl groups to the carbon 5 of cytosine molecules (5-mC) and leads to the recruitment of methyl-CpG binding domain and other transcriptional regulators. Methylated DNA tends to have a closed chromatin conformation and is associated with transcriptionally repressive histone modifications. This contrasts with unmethylated DNA, which is associated with permissive histone modifications and an open chromatin conformation.

DNA methylation is catalyzed by the DNA methyltransferases (DNMTs) that are classified into two families: DNMT1 and DNMT3.[16] The DNMT1 family includes the most abundant DNA methyltransferase in somatic cells, DNMT1, which is responsible for copying DNA methylation patterns to the daughter strands during DNA replication and repair. An oocyte specific DNMT1 (DNMT1o) is involved in maintenance of DNA-methylation at DMRs during early stages of embryo development.[17] The DNMT3 family includes two active forms, DNMT3A and DNMT3B and one regulatory factor, DNMT3-Like protein (DNMT3L). Both DNMT3A and DNMT3B have de novo methyltransferase activity enhanced by DNMT3L[18,19] although DNMT3A is the methyltranferase specifically required for DNA methylation of DMRs in the gametes.[20,21] Recently, it has been suggested that DNMT3 could also be associated with DNA methylation maintenance during DNA replication together with DNMT1.[22]

Histone Covalent Modification

Histone proteins, particularly in their N-terminal tails, are subject to a large number of posttranslational modifications.[23] Acetylation of lysines is generally associated with transcriptional activation. In contrast, the functional consequences of histone methylation, which can occur at lysines (K) and arginines (R), are more dependent on the specific site that is modified. For instance, methylation of H3K4 is closely linked to transcriptional competence, whereas methylation of H3K9 and K20 is associated with transcriptional repression. Further complexity comes from the fact that methylation at lysines can be in the form of either mono-, di- or trimethylation at lysines and mono- or dimethylation (asymmetric or symmetric) at arginines. Histone methylation marks at lysine and arginine residues are relatively stable and can carry epigenetic information from one somatic cell generation to the next.

Regions of differential DNA methylation with imprinted loci are often, but not exclusively, associated with differential chromatin modifications. Methylated alleles are coupled with repressive chromatin modifications such as H3K9me2/3, H4K20me3 and H2AK119u1.[24-27] This heritable repression is due to the coupling of the Polycomb group 1 (PcG) proteins and DNA methyltransferases to form a silencing complex.[28] Unmethylated regions are coupled with permissive chromatin modifications including H3K9ac and H3K4me2/3.[14] Recently it has been shown that certain imprinted genes, not associated with differential DNA methylation at their own promoters, have allelic histone modifications which are required for maintaining somatic imprinting.[24,25,29,30]

These general patterns of histone modifications at DMRs are maintained by the opposing actions of two sets of proteins, the histone acetyltransferases (HAT)/histone deacetylases (HDACs) and the histone methyltransferases (HMT)/histone demethylases (KDM).[31-33] These proteins specifically modify certain histone residues. In fact, the acquisition of differential DNA methylation in the maternal germ-line has recently been shown to require the finely tuned action of the H3K4 histone demethylase AOF1/KDM1B to remove H3K4me before the DNA can become methylated.[34] This process also demonstrates that the biochemical components associated with genomic imprinting are identical to those involved in cell differentiation. This suggests that imprinted regulation does not require unique modifiers to maintain allelic differences in chromatin structure and therefore may be equally prone to epigenetic deregulation during the development of disease states and cancer.

EXAMPLE OF AN IMPRINTED REGION: *H19/IGF2* LOCI—AN ANCIENT IMPRINTED DOMAIN

The first imprinted gene to be described was paternally expressed *Igf2*, which is crucial during murine embryogenesis and is implicated in the growth disorders Beckwith-Wiedemann syndrome (BWS) [MIM 130650], Silver-Russell syndrome (SRS) [MIM 180860] and tumorigenesis in humans.[35-37] The *H19/IGF2* locus is the best molecularly characterized imprinted domain in both humans and mice (see Fig. 1). In the mouse, dozens of targeted deletions have delineated the numerous *cis*-acting control elements and in humans characterization has been through the identification of specific epigenetic and cytogenetic defects.[38,39] To date, this gene cluster represents the most evolutionarily ancient imprinted locus identified.[40] The domain has two reciprocally expressed, imprinted transcripts, the maternally expressed, noncoding *H19* gene and the potent growth factor *IGF2*, which is expressed solely from the paternal allele.[41] Although the function of IGF2 as member of the insulin family of peptide growth factors is well known, the function of the *H19* noncoding RNA is still poorly understood.[42] Recently, this alternatively spliced, capped and polyadenylated RNA has been reported to be a pri-RNA for the microRNA miR-675.[40,43] This finding has important implications, as discussed later, suggesting that not all cellular responses due to epigenetic deregulation of this locus are caused by IGF2.

IMPRINTING REGULATION AT *H19/IGF2* DOMAIN

The expression of the *H19* and *Igf2* genes is controlled by the differential DNA methylation status of the *H19*-ICR (also known as the *H19* differentially methylated domain or DMD), which is located upstream of the *H19* transcription start site.[44] This ICR is one of the few known paternally DNA methylated ICRs in the genome. Regions of paternal DNA methylation, established somatically after fertilization, are also present at four additional specific sites; one overlapping the *H19* promoter and the remainder, DMR0, DMR1 and DMR2, spread throughout the *IGF2* gene (see Fig. 1).[45] Continued research into the imprinting control of this domain reveals a complicated regulatory mechanism that utilizes multiple enhancers, differentially methylated regions (DMRs), boundary elements, histone modifications and complex

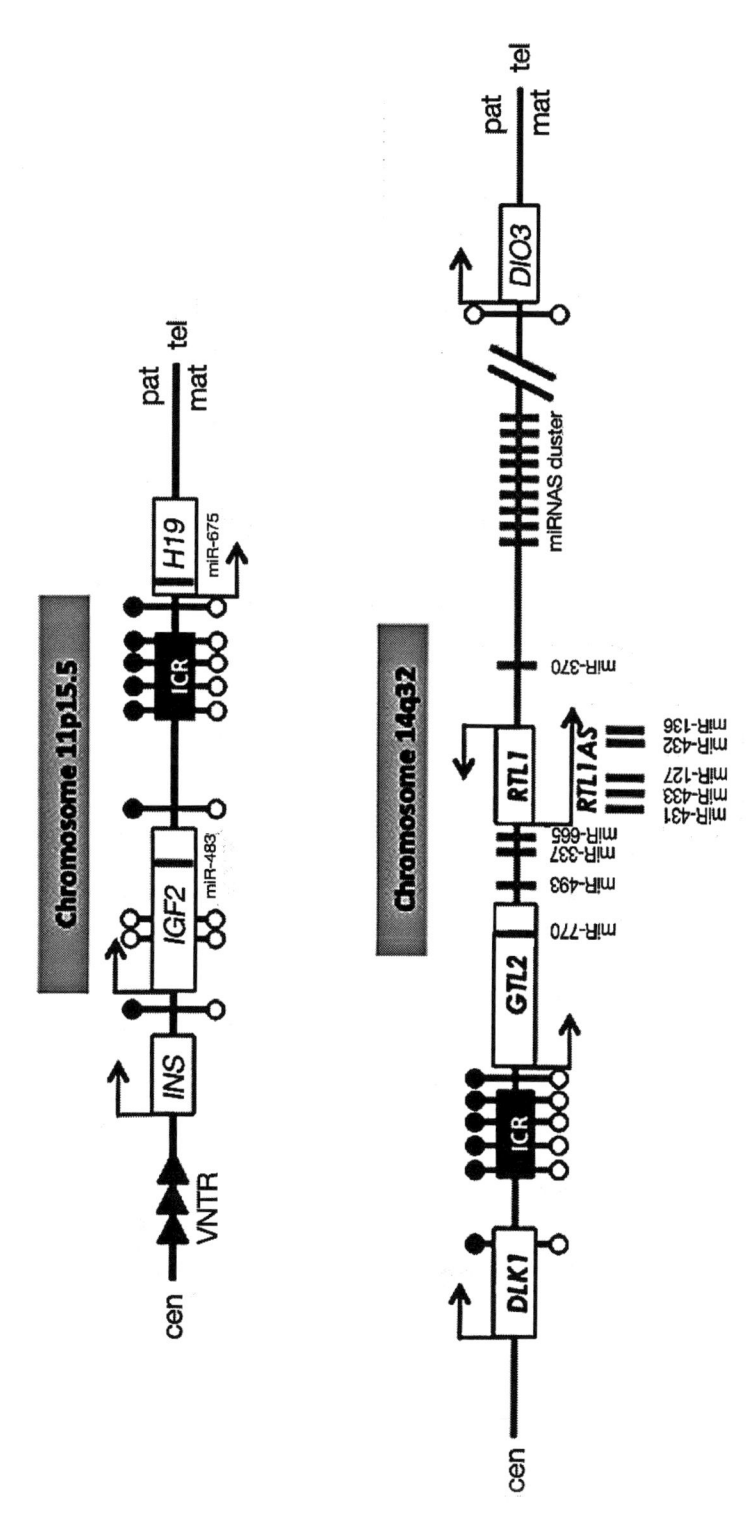

Figure 1. Genomic organization of the *H19-IGF2* and *DLK1-DIO3* imprinted domains on human chromosomes 11 and 14 respectively. The allelic expression in both domains is regulated by regions of paternal-allele DNA methylation. Both regions contain imprinted translated, untranslated and miRNA transcripts.

physical DNA looping, all of which are allele-specific and some species specific.[46,47] Briefly, the paternally DNA methylated germline ICR, located 2-4 kb upstream of the *H19* transcript, contains several CCCTC-binding factor (CTCF) binding sites.[48] These confer the ICR's function as a methylation-sensitive insulator between the multiple *Igf2* promoters and enhancers located downstream of *H19*. On the unmethylated maternal allele, CTCF binds to form a boundary that prevents the *Igf2* promoters interacting with the enhancers, whereas on the DNA methylated paternal allele, CTCF cannot bind and the *Igf2* promoters freely associate with the enhancer to bring about expression from the paternal allele only.[48,49] Using the chromatin confirmation capture technique (3C), it has been shown that on the maternal allele, CTCF binding mediates the formation of a tight, transcriptionally inactive loop around the *Igf2* gene. This involves interactions between the maternal allele of the *H19*-ICR, the matrix attachment region 3 (MAR3)[50] and *Igf2* DMR1, a region previously shown to be a methylation-sensitive silencer. On the paternal allele, the enhancer can form a methylation-sensitive, active chromatin domain through the interaction of the DNA methylated *H19*-ICR allele with the DNA methylated *Igf2* DMR2.[46,47]

Apart from the intrachromosomal interactions at the imprinted *H19-IGF2* locus, mediated by CTCF activity, it is notable that interchromosomal interactions have been reported that involve CTCF binding at the *H19*-ICR. The *H19*-ICR was shown to interact and colocalize with the non-imprinted *Wsb1/Nf1* genes on mouse chromosome 11.[51] This relationship is allele-specific, with the maternal unmethylated allele of the *H19*-ICR associating with the paternal *Wsb1/Nf1* domain. In addition, the maternal allele of the *H19*-ICR was shown to interact directly with the DMRs for the imprinted genes *Impact*, *Kcnq1* and *Napil5*.[52] More recently it has been reported that the *H19*-ICR forms interchromosomal interactions that control expression of several other imprinted genes to form an imprinted gene network, all of which contain CTCF sites.[53,54]

These higher order chromatin loops have been shown to require the sister chromatid cohesion protein, Cohesin. Cohesin binds to the same sites as CTCF, implicating a CTCF-Cohesin complex in regulating gene expression. Utilizing RNAi depletion, Nativio et al, have shown that a lack of SCC1, a cohesin subunit, results in deregulated *H19/IGF2* imprinting, implying that both CTCF and cohesin are required for appropriate monoallelic expression.[55] The CTCF-Cohesin complex is also known to be involved in V(D)J recombination during B lymphocyte development[56] and for appropriate T-helper cell expression of the *IFNG* gene,[57] but it is currently unknown whether the *H19*-ICR interacts with these additional CTCF-cohesin hubs during B- and T-cell differentiation.

AUTOIMMUNITY AND IMPRINTING

Autoimmune diseases are characterised by the failure of self-tolerance and a subsequent immune response against the body's own cells. There are currently eight distinct human phenotypes caused by mutations or epimutations in imprinted genes, with none of these specific disorders sharing features of autoimmune disease. However, as we discuss below, there is evidence that genomic imprinting may play a role in the development and progression of autoimmune disorders.

THE INVOLVEMENT OF IMPRINTED GENES IN TYPE 1 DIABETES

For many years it has been known that both B and T cells contribute to the pathogenesis of autoimmune diseases. It is therefore plausible that any gene that influences B- and T-cell differentiation or function may play a role. The paternally expressed *DLK1* gene maps to the IG-DMR regulated domain on human chromosome 14 (see Fig. 1). *DLK1* is involved in NOTCH dependent signaling that helps transitional B cells develop through cell-cell interactions with stromal cells. Mice that lack *Dlk1* expression have an increased number of early lineage B cells, but a decreased number of recirculated B cells in the bone marrow. In addition, *Dlk1* null mice show abnormal levels of preimmune serum immunoglobulin and an exaggerated antigen-specific humoral immune response.[58] In fitting with a potential role of *DLK1* in autoimmune disorders, DNA association studies using the human Genome-Wide Association (GWA) dataset has shown that paternal inheritance of a rs941576 SNP variant, located within the within the *DLK1-DIO3* locus, is a risk allele for Type 1 diabetes.[59] Insulin Type 1 diabetes mellitus (IDDM) is a multi-system metabolic disease resulting from impaired insulin function, which results in characteristic hyperglycemia and ketoacidosis. Several mechanisms are involved in its pathogenesis, including the delayed-type hypersensitivity reactions mediated by CD4+ TH1 cells that react with islet cell antigens, cytolytic T-lymphocyte mediated lysis of islet cells, production of cytokines TNK and IL-1 that damage the pancreas and production of autoantibodies against islet cells and insulin.

Multiple genes are involved in IDDM, with the majority of attention focusing on the human leukocyte antigen (HLA) genes. HLA genes encode antigen-presenting molecules that initiate T-lymphocyte proliferation after having bound "foreign" peptides and are key in selective loss of B cells. The HLA-DR2 and -DR4 loci are associated with increased susceptibility to IDDM in white Europeans.[60] It has been suggested that the genetics of HLA susceptibility show parent-of-origin effects, with the nontransmitting maternal HLA-DQ2 or -DQ8 alleles being a risk factor,[61] but these observations are disputed.[62,63] Non HLA genes also contribute to the disease. The first to be identified was the insulin gene (*INS*) itself, with the variable number tandem repeats (VNTR) in the 5'-upstream promoter region being associated with disease susceptibility. The *INS* gene is a paternally expressed imprinted gene,[64] and lies next to the paternally expressed *IGF2* gene (see Fig. 1). In rare cases it has been shown that *INS* transcription produces a polycystonic read through transcript that includes the *IGF2* exons,[65] but the function of this transcript is unknown. The expression level of *INS* is regulated by the VNTR. The shorter class I alleles correlate with higher expression in pancreas, but lower levels in thymus.[66,67] These shorter alleles are positively associated with IDDM, while the longer class III alleles are protective.[68] Two studies have suggested that the sensitization to insulin may occur during early life, as a result of ineffective tolerance induction by the decreased expression of insulin in the thymic epithelium in individuals with the VNTR class 1 allele. However, as tantalizing as this theory is, a study in 90 IDDM patients failed to show any association for insulin autoantibody levels with *INS*-VNTR genotype.[69]

PARENT-OF-ORIGIN ASSOCIATION WITH AUTOIMMUNE DISEASES

From the earliest genetic studies on twins, there has been strong evidence for a genetic component in the aetiology of autoimmunity.[70] Much has been learned about the genes involved in autoimmune disease by linkage analyses in families and genome-wide scans. Most autoimmne diseases are polygenic, with individuals inheriting polymorphisms that contribute to disease susceptibility and influence self-tolerance. Most susceptibility loci identified map to large chromosomal domains containing many genes, many of which overlap with regions identified for other numerous autoimmune diseases. Indeed, some HLA alleles within the MHC II region on human chromosome 6 show higher frequencies in various autoimmune patients than in controls. Psoriatic arthritis (PsA) is the combination of two recognised autoimmune diseases, severe arthritis and psoriasis,[71] which shows a less pronounced association with the MHC. Linkage analyses in 906 Icelandic PsA patients show some evidence for imprinted transmission at chromosome 16q. Higher LOD scores were observed when the study was restricted to pairs of affected relatives in whom the last transmission came from the father.[72] This is not the only report of nonMHC linkage in autoimmune phenotypes where LOD scores increased or decreased when the analysis was conditioned on parental transmission; this phenomenon has also been observed for both IDDM and Crohns disease.[73,74] Indeed, analysis of the UK genome-wide scan data revealed evidence for paternal association at D16S3098 in IDDM, which overlaps the region identified for PsA.[75]

IS LOSS-OF-IMPRINTING INVOLVED IN RHEUMATOID ARTHRITIS?

A joint linkage and imprinting analysis performed by Zhou et al on Genetic Analysis Workshop 15 (GAW15) data highlighted rheumatoid arthritis (RA) regions that might be imprinted, but the identified regions failed to withstand additional methods of data analysis.[76] This suggests that genomic imprinting is not involved in RA, however, reports have indicated that loss-of-imprinting (LOI) of *IGF2* occurs in synovial fibroblasts in RA patients[77] but whether this is the cause or consequence of the inflammation is unknown. In rheumatoid arthritis, the synovial membrane, which surrounds the joint space, becomes intensely cellular as a result of immunologic infiltration and increased number of synovial cells. This immune infiltrate contains a large number of T cells, mostly CD4+, that along with other cells express HLA-DR, indicative of activation by inflammation cytokines. These cytokines, that include IL-1 and TNF, are intense stimuli for resident synovial fibroblast (SF) activation. This activation results in the increased proliferation of SF cells to produce a pannus and the production of pro-inflammatory factors and matrix-degrading enzymes that destroy the underlying cartilage and bone.

Using large-scale gene expression profiling, Kasperkovitz et al, showed that RA SF cells show different gene expression profiles depending on the inflammatory status of the tissue from which they are derived.[78] Interestingly, RA SF cells derived from low-inflammatory tissue show high expression of *IGF2*. Subsequent work showed that this increase was due to LOI.[77,78] Thus, the disruption to *IGF2* might be involved in the aetiopathogenesis of RA by increasing the overall expression level of this potent mitogen.

Expression of *IGF2* has also been shown to be involved in aberrant T-cell activation.[79] The expression of *IGF2* in normal mononuclear cells in peripheral blood is imprinted, suggesting that the monoallelic paternal expression is maintained in differentiated

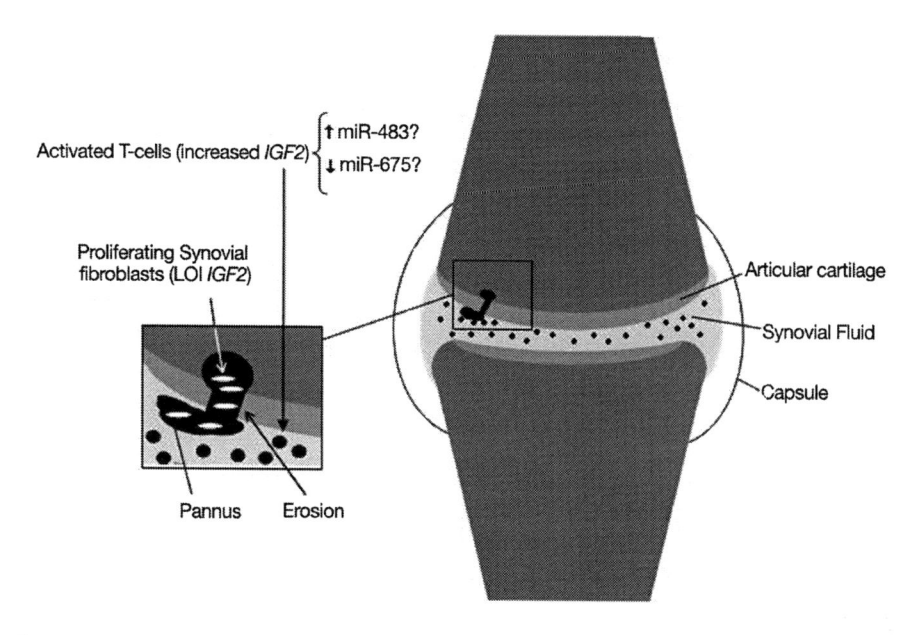

Figure 2. The involvement of *IGF2* in the aetiology of rheumatoid arthritis. Increased *IGF2* expression is observed T-cell activation, but it is currently unknown whether a concurrent increase in miR-483 also occurs. Loss-of-imprinting of *IGF2* is associated with proliferating synovial fibroblasts. These cells are responsible for pannus formation and ultimately joint erosion.

hematopoietic cells. However, one study observed LOI in all informative normal bone marrow samples, whereas corresponding peripheral blood shows normal monoallelic expression, suggesting that the high proliferation rates in the bone marrow cells requires a peak of IGF2 to stimulate division.[79] In unstimulated T cells, *IGF2* is monoallelically expressed, however, cultured lymphocytes exposed to PHA show LOI that persists for 72 hours, which results in a two-to six-fold increase of *IGF2* compared to resting T cells. This indicates that careful regulation of *IGF2* expression is required during both expansion in bone marrow, but also in T-cell stimulated proliferation (Fig. 2). However, this LOI of *IGF2* was not observed in lymphocytes isolated from RA patients.[80] It is therefore unclear whether LOI of *IGF2* in RA is maintained after T-cell activation in vivo, however, this mechanism maybe relevant in other, yet to be studied, autoimmune disorders.

FOOD FOR THOUGHT—IMPRINTED miRNAs INFLUENCING AUTOIMMUNE GENES?

MicroRNAs are small noncoding RNA molecules (22-23 nucleotides) that posttranscriptionally regulate gene expression by targeting the 3′ untranslated regions of specific messenger RNAs (mRNA) for degradation or translational repression. miRNA-mediated gene regulation is critical for normal cellular functions such as cell cycle, differentiation and apoptosis and if the process is compromised through genetic ablation of the miRNA machinery or the deregulation of individual miRNA, then this could lead to impaired immunological function and autoimmunity.

Table 1. A comprehensive list of imprinted miRNAs that potentially regulate genes involved in autoimmune diseases. All the miRNA-target gene interactions are catalogued in the TargetScan and miRBase databases

Autoimmune Disease	Candidate Gene	miRNA	miRNA Region
CeD	HLA-DQA1	miR-665	*DLK1-DIO3* (14q32)
MS	HLADRB1		
	HLA-B	miR-483	*IGF2-H19* (11p15.5)
Psoriasis	HLA-C	miR-665	*DLK1-DIO3* (14q32)
		miR-370	
	LCE3D	miR-296	*GNAS* (20q13.3)
Crohn's	IL23R		
	NOD2	miR-483	*IGF2-H19* (11p15.5)
		miR-431	*DLK1-DIO3* (14q32)
	CCR6	miR-433	
	TNFSF15	miR-127	
		miR-433	
		miR-432	
	CDKAL1	miR-335	*MEST* (7q32.2)
		miR-432	*DLK1-DIO3* (14q32)
		miR-296	*GNAS* (20q13.3)
RA	PTPN22	miR-335	*MEST* (7q32.2)
	HLADRB1	miR-665	*DLK1-DIO3* (14q32)
SLE	HLA-DQA1		
	BLK	miR-298	*GNAS* (20q13.3)
T1D	PTPN22	miR-335	*MEST* (7q32.2)
	C10orf59	miR-665	*DLK1-DIO3* (14q32)
	CTLA4	miR-432	
		miR-493	
	IL27	miR-296	GNAS (20q13.3)

It is estimated that almost 30% of all mRNAs are regulated by miRNAs, with each miRNA having multiple target mRNAs.[81] Additionally, roles for miRNAs in antigen receptor expression and successful lymphocyte-restricted gene expression are emerging.[82] A recent analysis of predicted miRNA-mediated regulation of 72 Lupus susceptibility genes in humans revealed numerous target sites for over 140 miRNAs conserved in mammals. These findings highlight the physiological need to control final protein products with enormous precision to maintain the balance between immunity and tolerance.[83] Overlap amongst targets of individual miRNAs is considerable, with the 11 miRNAs within the *DLK1-DIO3* imprinting cluster predicted to regulate 48 systemic lupus erythematosus (SLE) susceptibility genes. Indeed, this observation is not just limited to SLE, as when Royo et al extend the analysis to include all 19 miRNAs that map to imprinted loci,[84] it becomes evident that these imprinted miRNAs have seed target sites in many autoimmune associated genes, relating to many disorders (Table1).

CONCLUSION

A role for imprinted genes in B- and T-cell development and activation is becoming evident, however more research is required to confirm a direct role in the aetiology of autoimmune diseases. Recent studies have identified numerous imprinted miRNAs, the tissue-specific mRNA targets of which still have to be deciphered. It is therefore possible that any epigenetic disruption to the imprinting mechanism will affect the allelic expression of not only imprinted mRNAs but also the miRNAs, with the knock-on effect of altering the fine balance of their target gene expression in trans.

REFERENCES

1. Weiling F. Historical study: Johann Gregor Mendel 1822-1884. Am J Med Genet 1991; 40(1):1-25; discussion 26.
2. Surani MA, Barton SC, Norris ML. Development of reconstituted mouse eggs suggests imprinting of the genome during gametogenesis. Nature 1984; 308:548-550.
3. McGrath J, Solter D. Completion of mouse embryogenesis requires both the maternal and paternal genomes. Cell 1984; 37(1):179-183.
4. Cattanach BM, Kirk M. Differential activity of maternally and paternally derived chromosome regions in mice. Nature 1985; 315(6019): 496-498.
5. Giannoukakis N, Deal C, Paquette J et al. Parental genomic imprinting of the human IGF2 gene. Nat Genet 1993; 4(1):98-101.
6. Cassidy SB, Schwartz S. Prader-Willi and Angelman syndromes. Disorders of genomic imprinting. Medicine 1998; 77:140-151.
7. Cassidy SB, Dykens E, Williams CA. Prader-Willi and Angelman syndromes: sister imprinted disorders. Am J Med Genet 2000; 97(2):136-146.
8. Murphy SK, Wylie AA, Coveler KJ et al. Epigenetic detection of human chromosome 14 uniparental disomy. Hum Mutat 2003; 22(1):92-97.
9. Kotzot D, Schmitt S, Bernasconi F et al. Uniparental disomy 7 in Silver-Russell syndrome and primordial growth retardation. Hum Mol Genet 1995; 4(4):583-587.
10. Eggermann T, Eggermann K, Schönherr N. Growth retardation versus overgrowth: Silver-Russell syndrome is genetically opposite to Beckwith-Wiedemann syndrome. Trends Genet 2008; 24(4):195-204.
11. Feil R, Berger F. Convergent evolution of genomic imprinting in plants and mammals. Trends Genet 2007; 23(4): 192-199.
12. Verona RI, Mann MR, Bartolomei MS. Genomic imprinting: intricacies of epigenetic regulation in clusters. Annu Rev Cell Dev Biol 2003; 19: 237-259.
13. Ferguson-Smith AC, Sasaki H, Cattanach BM et al. Parental-origin-specific epigenetic modification of the mouse H19 gene. Nature 1993; 362(6422):751-755.
14. Gregory RI, Randall TE, Johnson CA et al. DNA methylation is linked to deacetylation of histone H3, but not H4, on the imprinted genes Snrpn and U2af1-rs1. Mol Cell Biol 2001; 21(16):5426-5436.
15. Bestor TH. The host defence function of genomic methylation patterns. Novartis Found Symp 1998; 214:187-195.
16. Cheng X, Blumenthal RM. Mammalian DNA methyltransferases: a structural perspective. Structure 2008; 16(3):341-350.
17. Cirio MC, Ratnam S, Ding F et al. Preimplantation expression of the somatic form of Dnmt1 suggests a role in the inheritance of genomic imprints. BMC Dev Biol 2008; 8:9.
18. Xie S, Wang Z, Okano M et al. Cloning, expression and chromosome locations of the human DNMT3 gene family. Gene 1999; 236(1):87-95.
19. Suetake I, Shinozaki F, Miyagawa J et al. DNMT3L stimulates the DNA methylation activity of Dnmt3a and Dnmt3b through a direct interaction. J Biol Chem 2004; 279(26):27816-27823.
20. Bourc'his D, Xu GL, Lin CS et al. Dnmt3L and the establishment of maternal genomic imprints. Science 2001; 294(5551):2536-2539.
21. Kaneda M, Okano M, Hata K et al. Essential role for de novo DNA methyltransferase Dnmt3a in paternal and maternal imprinting. Nature 2004; 429(6994):900-903.

22. Jones PA, Liang G. Rethinking how DNA methylation patterns are maintained. Nat Rev Genet 2009; 10(11):805-811.
23. Kouzarides T. Chromatin modifications and their function. Cell 2007; 128(4):693-705.
24. Umlauf D, Goto Y, Cao R et al. Imprinting along the Kcnq1 domain on mouse chromosome 7 involves repressive histone methylation and recruitment of Polycomb group complexes. Nat Genet 2004; 36(12):1296-1300.
25. Monk D, Arnaud P, Apostolidou S et al. Limited evolutionary conservation of imprinting in the human placenta. Proc Natl Acad Sci USA 2006; 103(17):6623-6628.
26. Delaval K, Govin J, Cerqueira F et al. Differential histone modifications mark mouse imprinting control regions during spermatogenesis. EMBO J 2007; 26(3):720-729.
27. Terranova R, Yokobayashi S, Stadler MB et al. Polycomb group proteins Ezh2 and Rnf2 direct genomic contraction and imprinted repression in early mouse embryos. Dev Cell 2008; 15(5):668-679.
28. Viré E, Brenner C, Deplus R et al. The Polycomb group protein EZH2 directly controls DNA methylation. Nature 2006; 439(7078):871-874.
29. Wagschal A, Sutherland HG, Woodfine K et al. G9a histone methyltransferase contributes to imprinting in the mouse placenta. Mol Cell Biol 2008; 28(3):1104-1113.
30. Monk D, Wagschal A, Arnaud P et al. Comparative analysis of human chromosome 7q21 and mouse proximal chromosome 6 reveals a placental-specific imprinted gene, TFPI2/Tfpi2, which requires EHMT2 and EED for allelic-silencing. Genome Res 2008; 18(8):1270-1281.
31. Lan F, Nottke AC, Shi Y. Mechanisms involved in the regulation of histone lysine demethylases. Curr Opin Cell Biol 2008; 20(3):316-325.
32. Selvi RB, Kundu TK. Reversible acetylation of chromatin: implication in regulation of gene expression, disease and therapeutics. Biotechnol J 2009; 4(3):375-390.
33. Spannhoff A, Hauser AT, Heinke R et al. The emerging therapeutic potential of histone methyltransferase and demethylase inhibitors. Chem Med Chem 2009; 4(10):1568-1582.
34. Ciccone DN, Su H, Hevi S et al. KDM1B is a histone H3K4 demethylase required to establish maternal genomic imprints. Nature 2009; 461(7262):415-418.
35. Weksberg R, Shen DR, Fei YL et al. Disruption of insulin-like growth factor 2 imprinting in Beckwith-Wiedemann syndrome. Nat Genet 1993; 5(2):143-150.
36. Ogawa O, Eccles MR, Szeto J et al. Relaxation of insulin-like growth factor II gene imprinting implicated in Wilms' tumour. Nature 1993; 362(6422):749-751.
37. Gicquel C, Rossignol S, Cabrol S et al. Epimutation of the telomeric imprinting center region on chromosome 11p15 in Silver-Russell syndrome. Nat Genet 2005; 37(9):1003-1007.
38. Sparago A, Cerrato F, Vernucci M et al. Microdeletions in the human H19 DMR result in loss of IGF2 imprinting and Beckwith-Wiedemann syndrome. Nat Genet 2004; 36(9):958-960.
39. Bliek J, Snijder S, Maas SM et al. Phenotypic discordance upon paternal or maternal transmission of duplications of the 11p15 imprinted regions. Eur J Med Genet 2009; 52(6):404-408.
40. Smits G, Mungall AJ, Griffiths-Jones S et al. Conservation of the H19 noncoding RNA and H19-IGF2 imprinting mechanism in therians. Nat Genet 2008; 40(8):971-976.
41. Tilghman SM, Bartolomei MS, Webber AL et al. Parental imprinting of the H19 and Igf2 genes in the mouse. Cold Spring Harb Symp Quant Biol 1993; 58:287-295.
42. Gabory A, Ripoche MA, Yoshimizu T et al. The H19 gene: regulation and function of a noncoding RNA. Cytogenet Genome Res 2006; 113(1-4):188-193.
43. Cai X, Cullen BR. The imprinted H19 noncoding RNA is a primary microRNA precursor. RNA 2007; 13(3):313-316.
44. Leighton PA, Ingram RS, Eggenschwiler J et al. Disruption of imprinting caused by deletion of the H19 gene region in mice. Nature 1995; 375(6526):34-39.
45. Lopes S, Lewis A, Hajkova P et al. Epigenetic modifications in an imprinting cluster are controlled by a hierarchy of DMRs suggesting long-range chromatin interactions. Hum Mol Genet 2003; 12(3):295-305.
46. Murrell A, Heeson S, Reik W. Interaction between differentially methylated regions partitions the imprinted genes Igf2 and H19 into parent-specific chromatin loops. Nat Genet 2004; 36(8):889-893.
47. Kurukuti S, Tiwari VK, Tavoosidana G et al. CTCF binding at the H19 imprinting control region mediates maternally inherited higher-order chromatin conformation to restrict enhancer access to Igf2. Proc Natl Acad Sci USA 2006; 103(28):10684-10689.
48. Hark AT, Schoenherr CJ, Katz DJ et al. CTCF mediates methylation-sensitive enhancer-blocking activity at the H19/Igf2 locus. Nature 2000; 405(6785):486-489.
49. Bell AC, Felsenfeld G. Methylation of a CTCF-dependent boundary controls imprinted expression of the Igf2 gene. Nature 2000; 405(6785):482-485.
50. Weber M, Hagège H, Murrell A et al. Genomic imprinting controls matrix attachment regions in the Igf2 gene. Mol Cell Biol 2003; 23(24):8953-8959.

51. Ling JQ, Li T, Hu JF et al. CTCF mediates interchromosomal colocalization between Igf2/H19 and Wsb1/Nf1. Science 2006; 312(5771):269-272.
52. Zhao Z, Tavoosidana G, Sjölinder M et al. Circular chromosome conformation capture (4C) uncovers extensive networks of epigenetically regulated intra- and interchromosomal interactions. Nat Genet 2006; 38(11):1341-1347.
53. Gabory A, Ripoche MA, Le Digarcher A et al. H19 acts as a trans regulator of the imprinted gene network controlling growth in mice. Development 2009;136(20):3413-3421.
54. Sandhu KS, Shi C, Sjölinder M et al. Nonallelic transvection of multiple imprinted loci is organized by the H19 imprinting control region during germline development. Genes Dev 2009; 23(22):2598-2603.
55. Nativio R, Wendt KS, Ito Y et al. Cohesin is required for higher-order chromatin conformation at the imprinted IGF2-H19 locus. PLoS Genet 2009; 5(11):e1000739.
56. Degner SC, Wong TP, Jankevicius G et al. Cutting edge: developmental stage-specific recruitment of cohesin to CTCF sites throughout immunoglobulin loci during B lymphocyte development. J Immunol 2009; 182(1):44-48.
57. Hadjur S, Williams LM, Ryan NK et al. Cohesins form chromosomal cis-interactions at the developmentally regulated IFNG locus. Nature 2009; 460(7253):410-413.
58. Raghunandan R, Ruiz-Hidalgo M, Jia Y et al. Dlk1 influences differentiation and function of B lymphocytes. Stem Cells Dev 2008; 17(3):495-507.
59. Wallace C, Smyth DJ, Maisuria-Armer M et al. The imprinted DLK1-MEG3 gene region on chromosome 14q32.2 alters susceptibility to type 1 diabetes. Nat Genet 2010; 42(1):68-71.
60. Lie BA, Todd JA, Pociot F et al. The predisposition to type 1 diabetes linked to the human leukocyte antigen complex includes at least one nonclass II gene. Am J Hum Genet 1999; 64(3):793-800.
61. Pani MA, Van Autreve J, Van der Auwera BJ et al. Non transmitted maternal HLA DQ2 or DQ8 alleles and risk of Type I diabetes in offspring: the importance of foetal or post partum exposure to diabetogenic molecules. Diabetologia 2002; 45(9):1340-1343.
62. Hermann R, Veijola R, Sipilä I et al. -to: Pani MA, Van Autreve J, Van Der Auwera BJ, Gorus FK, Badenhoop K (2002) Nontransmitted maternal HLA DQ2 or DQ8 alleles and risk of Type I diabetes in offspring: the importance of foetal or post partum exposure to diabetogenic molecules. Diabetologia 2003; 46(4):588-589.
63. Lambert AP, Gillespie KM, Bingley PJ et al. -to: Pani MA, Van Autreve J, Van Der Auwera BJ, Gorus FK, Badenhoop K (2002) Nontransmitted maternal HLA DQ2 or DQ8 alleles and risk of Type I diabetes in offspring: the importance of foetal or post partum exposure to diabetogenic molecules. Diabetologia 2003; 46(4):590-591.
64. Moore GE, Abu-Amero SN, Bell G et al. Evidence that insulin is imprinted in the human yolk sac. Diabetes 2001; 50(1):199-203.
65. Monk D, Sanches R, Arnaud P et al. Imprinting of IGF2 P0 transcript and novel alternatively spliced INS-IGF2 isoforms show differences between mouse and human. Hum Mol Genet 2006; 15(8):1259-1269.
66. Pugliese A, Zeller M, Fernandez A Jr et al. The insulin gene is transcribed in the human thymus and transcription levels correlated with allelic variation at the INS VNTR-IDDM2 susceptibility locus for type 1 diabetes. Nat Genet 1997; 15(3):293-297.
67. Vafiadis P, Bennett ST, Todd JA et al. Insulin expression in human thymus is modulated by INS VNTR alleles at the IDDM2 locus. Nat Genet 1997; 15(3):289-292.
68. Bennett ST, Lucassen AM, Gough SC et al. Susceptibility to human type 1 diabetes at IDDM2 is determined by tandem repeat variation at the insulin gene minisatellite locus. Nat Genet 1995; 9(3):284-292.
69. Pérez de Nanclares G, Bilbao JR et al. No association of INS-VNTR genotype and IAA autoantibodies. Ann NY Acad Sci 2004; 1037:127-130.
70. Worthington J, Silman AJ. Genetic control of autoimmunity, lessons from twin studies. Clin Exp Immunol 1995; 101(3):390-392.
71. Winchester R. Psoriatic arthritis. Dermatol Clin 1995; 13(4):779-792.
72. Karason A, Gudjonsson JE, Upmanyu R et al. A susceptibility gene for psoriatic arthritis maps to chromosome 16q: evidence for imprinting. Am J Hum Genet 2003; 72(1):125-131.
73. Akolkar PN, Gulwani-Akolkar B, Heresbach D et al. Differences in risk of Crohn's disease in offspring of mothers and fathers with inflammatory bowel disease. Am J Gastroenterol 1997; 92(12):2241-2244.
74. Alcolado JC, Laji K, Gill-Randall R. Maternal transmission of diabetes. Diabet Med 2002; 19(2):89-98.
75. Mein CA, Esposito L, Dunn MG et al. A search for type 1 diabetes susceptibility genes in families from the United Kingdom. Nat Genet 1998; 19(3):297-300.
76. Zhou X, Chen W, Swartz MD et al. Joint linkage and imprinting analyses of GAW15 rheumatoid arthritis and gene expression data. BMC Proc 2007; 1 Suppl 1:S53.

77. Martin-Trujillo A, van Rietschoten JG, Timmer TC et al. Loss of imprinting of IGF2 characterizes high IGF2mRNA-expressing type of Fibroblast-like Synoviocytes in Rheumatoid Arthritis. Ann Rheum Dis 2009 [Epub ahead of print].
78. Kasperkovitz PV, Timmer TC, Smeets TJ et al. Fibroblast-like synoviocytes derived from patients with rheumatoid arthritis show the imprint of synovial tissue heterogeneity: evidence of a link between an increased myofibroblast-like phenotype and high-inflammation synovitis. Arthritis Rheum 2005; 52(2):430-441.
79. Hofmann WK, Takeuchi S, Frantzen MA et al. Loss of genomic imprinting of insulin-like growth factor 2 is strongly associated with cellular proliferation in normal hematopoietic cells. Exp Hematol 2002; 30(4):318-323.
80. Möller B, Kerschbaumer G, Komor M et al. Genomic imprinting of insulin-like growth factor 2 (IGF-2) in chronic synovitis. Growth Horm IGF Res 2007; 17(6):500-505.
81. Wienholds E, Plasterk RH. MicroRNA function in animal development. FEBS Lett 2005; 579(26):5911-5922.
82. Chowdhury D, Novina CD. Potential roles for short RNAs in lymphocytes. Immunol Cell Biol 2005; 83(3):201-210.
83. Vinuesa CG, Rigby RJ, Yu D. Logic and extent of miRNA-mediated control of autoimmune gene expression. Int Rev Immunol 2009; 28(3-4):112-138.
84. Royo H, Cavaillé J. Noncoding RNAs in imprinted gene clusters. Biol Cell 2008; 100(3):149-166.

CHAPTER 9

A NEW EPIGENETIC CHALLENGE:
Systemic Lupus Erythematosus

Biola M. Javierre[1] and Bruce Richardson*[,2]

[1]Chromatin and Disease Group, Cancer Epigenetics and Biology Programme (PEBC), Bellvitge Biomedical Research Institute (IDIBELL), L'Hospitalet de Llobregat, Barcelona, Spain; [2]Department of Medicine, University of Michigan, Ann Arbor, Michigan, USA
*Corresponding Author: Bruce Richardson—Email: brichard@med.umich.edu

Abstract: In recent years, compelling evidence has been gathered that supports a role for epigenetic alterations in the pathogenesis of systemic lupus erythematosus (SLE). Different blood cell populations of SLE patients are characterized by a global loss of DNA methylation. This process is associated with defects in ERK pathway signalling and consequent DNMT1 downregulation. Hypomethylation of gene promoters has been described, which permits transcriptional activation and therefore functional changes in the cells and also hypomethylation of the ribosomal RNA gene cluster. Among the identified targets undergoing demethylation are genes involved in autoreactivity (ITGAL), osmotic lysis and apoptosis (PRF1, MMP14 and LCN2), antigen presentation (CSF3R), inflammation (MMP14), B- T-cell interaction (CD70 and CD40LG) and cytokine pathways (CSF3R, IL-4, IL-6 and IFNGR2). DNA methylation inhibitors are also known to induce autoreactivity in vitro and cause a lupus-like disease in vivo. Further, altered patterns of histone modifications have been described in SLE. CD4[+] lymphocytes undergo global histone H3 and H4 deacetylation and consequent skewed gene expression. Although multiple lines of evidence highlight the contribution of epigenetic alterations to the pathogenesis of lupus in genetically predisposed individuals, many questions remain to be answered. Attaining a deeper understanding of these matters will create opportunities in the promising area of epigenetic treatments.

Table 1. Symptoms described in SLE patients[1,6]

Affected Organ	Symptoms
Nonspecific	Fever, fatigue, weight loss
Circulatory system	Heart failure, pericarditis, endocarditis, myocarditis, coronary thrombosis
Cutaneous system	Rash, photosensitivity, alopecia, changes in pigmentation
Gastrointestinal system	Abdominal pain, peritonitis, pancreatitis, mesenteric vasculitis, nausea, dyspepsia
Haematological system	Leucopenia, lymphopenia, anaemia, thrombocytopenia
Musculoskeletal system	Arthralgia, myalgia, arthritis
Nervous system	Headache, mood, cognitive and movement disorders, psychosis, delirium, seizures
Pulmonary system	Pleuritis, dyspnea, serositis, pneumonitis, haemoptysis
Renal system	Glomerulonephritis, hypertension, haematuria, oedema, hyperlipidaemia.
Reproductive system	Miscarriage, pre-eclampsia, intrauterine growth restriction

INTRODUCTION

Systemic lupus erythematosus (SLE) is an autoimmune disorder characterized by the production of non-organ-specific autoantibodies against host components that generate inflammation and multisystem injury.[1,2] This disease can affect all sexes, ethnicities and ages although the highest prevalence is in women of African descent during their reproductive years.[1,3] The prevalence of SLE in Northern Europeans has been estimated at approximately 40 cases per 100,000 persons, in contrast to more than 200 per 100,000 persons among African-American populations.[4] Women are most commonly affected and the female to male ratio is 9:1. With respect to life expectancy, the 15-year survival rate is currently around 80% and the pattern of mortality is bimodal, with some dying earlier from consequences of the active autoimmune disease and others dying later from atherosclerotic cardiovascular disease.[5]

SLE is characterized by a broad range of clinical manifestations and unpredictable exacerbations and remissions. All systems and organs can be affected through autoantibody mediated inflammation. Cutaneous manifestations are the most common symptom of SLE, since 85% of patients develop various rashes, although there is a wide range of symptoms that do not include skin[1,6] (Table 1). The diagnosis of SLE is based on eleven criteria established by the American Rheumatism Association: malar rash, discoid rash, photosensitivity, oral ulcers, arthritis, serositis, renal disorder, neuropsychiatric alterations, haematological disorders, immunological alterations and the presence of antinuclear antibodies. At least four of these criteria are required to make the diagnosis with certainty.

The pathogenesis of SLE is complex and remains unclear. However, alterations of apoptotic processes and altered cytokine levels are two major mechanisms contributing to the loss of tolerance and consequent development of autoantibody production. Abnormalities in apoptosis are the source of autoantigens that induce inflammatory injury through autoantibody production. Moreover, this altered process may explain the fact that SLE autoantibodies mainly react with intracellular components. Defects in

Table 2. Main autoantibodies described in SLE patients

Autoantibody	Prevalence	Autoantigen	Antigen Location	Tissue Target
Anti-dsDNA	≈50-80%	Ds genetic material	Nuclear	Kidney and skin
Antinucleosomes	≈50-90%	Histones	Nuclear	Kidney and skin
Anti-Ro (SS-A)	≈25-40%	52 KDa or 60KDa proteins	Nuclear	Kidney, skin, foetal heart, lung
Anti-Sm	≈10-30%	Spliceosomal snRNP	Nuclear	Foetal heart
Anti-La (SS-B)	≈10-20%	48 KDa transcription terminator protein	Nuclear	Kidney
Anti-ribosomal-P	≈15%	60S ribosomal subunit phosphoproteins (P0,P1, P2)	Nuclear	Kidney, brain, liver
Anti-nRNP	≈23-40%	Spliceosomal snRNP	Nuclear	Muscles, circulatory system
Anti-Ku	≈20-40%	P70/p80 DNA reparation proteins	Nuclear	Joins, heart, lung
Anti-NMDA receptor	≈33-50%	NMDA Receptor	Membrane	Brain
Antiphospholipids	≈20-30%	Phospholipids	Membrane and extracellular	Circulatory system
Anti-α actinin	≈20%	α-actinin	Cytoplasm	Kidney
Anti-C1q	≈40-50%	C1q complement component	Extracellular	Kidney

Ds (double-stranded), Sm (Smith), nRNP (nuclear riboprotein), snRNP (small nuclear riboprotein), NMDA (N.-methyl-D-aspartate.[2,6,9,127-132]

apoptotic clearance and alterations of complement components related to phagocytosis have also been described.[7] Both alterations could lead to aberrant antigen uptake by antigen-presenting cells (APCs) and consequent presentation to B and T cells. On the other hand, a significant decrease of tingible body macrophages of the germinal centres (GCs) has been described in a subgroup of SLE patients. These phagocytes rarely contain apoptotic material. Mistakes in the elimination of apoptotic B cells induced after somatic mutation, or other cells undergoing apoptosis such as monocytes and macrophages, could be a source of autoantigen release. This apoptotic debris could then be presented by germinal node follicular dendritic cells (FDCs), providing survival and stimulatory signals for autoreactive B cells.[8] Autoantibody production against nuclear antigens is a hallmark of systemic lupus erythematosus. These antibodies are responsible for inflammatory injury through immune complex formation and are also useful for SLE diagnosis, prognosis and patient management. Moreover, these antibodies can bind to autoantigens or crossreact with other components blocking or increasing the functions of their targets. More than 50 autoantibody specificities have been described, most of which are to nuclear autoantigens and some are correlated with effects on tissues, disease manifestations and clinical stage (Table 2). For example, the anti-double-stranded DNA (anti-dsDNA) antibody is the most specific autoantibody in SLE since it is detected in 50-80% of lupus patients at some point during the course of the disorder, but in fewer than 0.5% of healthy people. However, the anti-dsDNA antibody is not very sensitive due in part to its transience. The presence of this autoantibody tends to be associated with clinical activity.[9] Indeed, in 80% of the SLE population, its first peak in serum presages the onset of clinical manifestations within five years.[10] Autoantibodies are also present in healthy people, where they have a nonpathological role.[11] The main difference between pathogenic SLE autoantibodies and those of healthy people is the high affinity of the pathogenic forms, which is due to the strong stimulation of B cells by CD4[+] lymphocytes that induces an antibody switch from IgM to IgG and a change in the molecular sequence of the secreted antibody.[2] Cytokines are also involved in SLE. Indeed, patients who suffer from lupus are characterized by the "interferon signature", due to overexpression of Type I interferons. Several cytokines and cytokine regulators are altered in SLE for genetic or epigenetic reasons. For example, a polymorphism of interferon regulatory factor 5 (IRF5) is an important risk factor for SLE development and a decrease of interleukin 2 production has been reported in T cells from SLE patients.[12,13] In contrast, increased serum interleukin 10 levels are associated with SLE activity.[14]

Currently, experts do not fully understand the aetiology of SLE. A combination of genetic risk and hormones is necessary but not sufficient to explain its development. The most widely accepted model of the disease highlights the importance of environmental events or factors in the onset of the pathology when the genetic context is predisposing. Genetic susceptibility is an important source of risk for developing SLE, as family aggregation and concordant twin research shows. One such study reported a concordance rate for SLE of over 25% in monozygotic twins compared with 2% in dizygotic siblings.[15] SLE is a multifactorial disease with complex genetics. Linkage and association studies have identified multiple loci that confer risk for lupus development[2,16,17] (Table 3). Some genes included in the disease susceptibility regions code for important immune system proteins, especially those of the cytokine signal transduction pathways, apoptosis and complement systems. Alterations of these genes can lead to a loss of tolerance and increased apoptosis of lymphocytes and monocytes. Hormonal and sexual genetic factors are also implicated in SLE aetiology, since ~85% of lupus patients are women, most of them of childbearing age. However there is also a greater prevalence of SLE in men with Klinefelter's syndrome suggesting that having 2 X chromosomes is also important for disease development.[18] Oral contraception increases the risk of SLE development and the number and severity of flares.[19] Conversely, menopause induces the opposite effects.[20] Hormonal analysis of women affected by SLE indicates an increase in prolactin levels and estradiol hydroxylation and a decrease in androgen levels in some patients.[21-24] The role of these hormones has been confirmed in studies using SLE mouse models, where prolactin and estrogens exacerbate the symptomatology in contrast to a suppressive effect of androgens.[25-27] Chimerism, the presence of cells from one individual in another person, is another potential aetiological factor in autoimmune disorders. Chimerism has been detected in a high percentage of women with SLE. Moreover, injection of chimeric cells into healthy mice induces a lupus-like disorder, indicating a potential role for this process in SLE aetiology.[28] Other evidence also suggests that viruses, such as Epstein-Barr virus

Table 3. Candidate risk loci in SLE development[2,16,17]

Name	Location	Function
ATG5	6q21	Apoptosis. Ubiquitination
BANK1	4q22-q24	B cell-specific scaffold. Immune adaptive system regulation.
BLK/ FAM167A	8p23-p22	Kinase. Immune adaptive system regulation/Unknown function.
C1q	1p36	Complement system member. Immune innate system regulation.
C2	6p11-21	Complement system member. Immune innate system regulation.
C4A	6p21.3	Complement system member. Immune innate system regulation.
C4B	6p11-21	Complement system member. Immune innate system regulation.
Chrom 8p21.1	8p21.1	Unknown function.
Chrom 5q33.3	5q33.3	Unknown function.
Chrom 1q25.1	1q25.1	Unknown function.
CRP	1q21-23	C-reactive protein. Clearing apoptotic debris. Immune innate system regulation.
FCGR2A	1q23	Receptor. Immune innate system regulation.
FCGR2B	1q22	Receptor. Immune innate system regulation.
FCGR3A	1q23	Receptor. Immune innate system regulation.
FCGR3B	1q23	Receptor. Immune innate system regulation.
HLA	6p11-21	Human leukocyte antigen. Immune adaptive system regulation.
ICA1	7p22	Unknown function.
IRAK1	Xq28	Kinase. IL1R pathway.
IRF5	7q32	TF. Interferon pathway. Apoptosis. Immune adaptive system regulation.
ITGAM	16p11.2	Adherence and phagocytosis. Immune innate system regulation
IKZF1	7p13-p11.1	TF. Lymphoid differentiation.
LYN	8q13	Kinase. Innate and adaptive immune system regulation.
MBL2	10q11-21	Mannose-binding lectin. Complement. Immune innate system regulation.
MECP2	Xq28	Methyl CpG binding protein
NMNAT2	1q25	Nicotinamide mononucleotide adenyltransferase
PARP	1q41-42	Apoptosis regulation.
PDCD1	2q37.3	B- and T-cell differentiation and apoptosis. Adaptive immune system regulation
PHRF1	11p15.5	Transcription.
PTPN22	1p13	Phosphatase. TCR pathway. Adaptive immune system regulation.
PXK	3p14.3	Kinase. Inflammatory response.
SCUBE1	22q13	Inflammatory response.

continued on next page

Table 3. Continued

Name	Location	Function
STAT4	2q32	TF. Cytokine response (IL12). CD4+ differentiation.
TLR5	1q41-42	Antigen receptor. Innate immune system regulation
TNFAIP3	6q23	TNF pathway. Apoptosis. Inflammation. Innate immune system regulation.
TNFSF4	1q25	Cytokine. T-cell-APC interaction. Adaptive immune system regulation.
TREX1	3q21	Exonuclease. Repair system. Granzyme A-mediated apoptosis
TYK2	19p13.2	Kinase. Cytokines and interferon pathway.
UBE2L3	22q11.21	Ubiquitination
XKR6	8p23.1	Unknown function
ZNF432	16q12	Transcription factor. Adaptive immune system regulation

Chrom (Chromosome), TCR (T-cell receptor), TF (transcriptional factor).

(EBV), or viral retro-elements, including human endogenous retrovirus (HERVs), are possible factors in SLE development through molecular mimicry or mutational mechanisms. In the particular case of EBV, increases in the percentage of infected B cells, in the viral load and in the viral gene expression have been described in SLE patients in comparison with healthy people. Such differences also occur between quiescent and active SLE in people.[29,30] In mice, immunization with the EBV nuclear antigen 1 (EBNA-1) induces production of Smith (Sm)-antibodies and anti-double-stranded DNA-antibodies.[31] The molecular mimicry of EBV may also be important because the Sm autoantigen is similar to EBNA-1 protein and both can induce lupus-like autoantibodies following direct immunization. Moreover, anti-Ro antibody crossreacts with EBNA-1 antigen.[32,33] Likewise, retrotransposable elements, mainly human endogenous retrovirus (HERVs), are implicated in SLE aetiology.[34] Molecular mimicry between retroviral proteins and autoantigens has been identified in SLE patients. For example the C-HERVs p30 *Gag* protein shares a homologous region and therefore crossreacts with human U1snRNP protein. Moreover, these repetitive sequences have the ability to deregulate immune genes in cis or trans, provoking loss of autotolerance. The MRL/lpr mouse model is a clear example in which the integration of a transposable element in the Fas gene alters the apoptosis process and induces SLE development by producing a nonfunctional Fas protein.[35] Finally, the environment plays a key role in SLE development. More than 100 drugs have been reported to cause a lupus-like disease and this disorder disappears after withdrawl of the compound. The drugs most commonly causing a lupus-like disease are hydalazine, quinidine, procainamide, phenytoin, isoniazid and d-penicillamine.[1] Exposure to sunlight, silica, mercury or pesticides are other common factors that unleash SLE development.[36] The majority of these drugs or exposures induce, directly or indirectly, changes in DNA methylation and histone modifications, highlighting the importance of epigenetics in SLE.

There is no permanent cure for SLE yet. Current treatments ameliorate symptoms by reducing inflammation and autoimmune activity. The use of anti-inflammatory drugs, such as nonsteroidal anti-inflammatory agents or corticosteroids, in combination with immunosuppressive medications such as mycophenolate mofetil or cyclophophamide, remains the most common treatment for SLE. In recent years, new strategies based on antibodies to immune cells, immunoadsorption and plasmapheresis, among others, have permitted some improvements in the treatment, although great efforts are still needed to find a cure for SLE. As discussed below, epigenetic therapy is an area that promises to help fulfil that objective.[1]

THE ROLE OF EPIGENETICS IN SLE

Epigenetics is one of the most rapidly expanding fields in biomedicine. Since Waddington defined epigenetics in 1939, great steps have been made in cell biology and disease pathogenesis, although much of the terrain remains unexplored.[37] Epigenetics, the study of reversible and potentially heritable changes in gene expression that do not depend on changes in DNA sequence, includes marks such as DNA methylation and histone modifications that define the cell transcriptome and ultimately the cell phenotype. Epigenetic regulation is essential for the normal development and function of the immune system and disruption of this regulatory mechanism can destroy the fine balance between a correctly functioning defence system and autoimmunity.[38]

Autoimmune diseases such as SLE arise when the immune system recognizes self-components of the body as damaged materials and reacts against them. Several lines of evidence indicate that environmental factors, including diet and lifestyle, can modulate the onset of SLE in a genetically predisposed person in part through epigenetic changes. For example, several drugs and ultraviolet light trigger a lupus-like disease in genetically predisposed people and twin studies reveal incomplete concordance (25-57%) between monozygotic siblings and a lower percentage among dizygotic ones (2-9%) indicating a requirement for exogenous triggers from the environment.[39,40]

In the following sections we review the most relevant publications in the field to give an overview of the implications of epigenetics in SLE pathogenesis and to summarize objectives for the near future.

CHANGES IN DNA METHYLATION OCCUR IN SLE

DNA Methylation: A Fundamental Epigenetic Mechanism

DNA methylation is the most extensively studied of the epigenetic mechanisms. In non-embryonic mammals, DNA methylation consists of the postsynthetic addition of a methyl group to the fifth carbon of the cytosine (C) pyrimidine ring located within a CpG dinucleotide.[41,42] CpG dinucleotides are statistically underrepresented in the genome due to spontaneous deamination of methylcytosines (mCs) to form thymidine during evolution.[43] In contrast, CpGs cluster in regions known as CpG islands that frequently coincide with gene regulatory sequences. With the exception of imprinted genes, X-chromosome genes and certain tissue-specific genes, CpG islands of healthy genomes are generally unmethylated and consequently permit transcription of the affected gene.[44] However, the majority of CpGs are located within intronic and intergenic DNA regions, particularly within the repetitive sequences and in normal cells these CpGs are methylated, thereby ensuring genomic stability and parasitic sequence silencing.[45,46] DNA methylation profiles are established during development by the de novo DNA methyltransferases (DNMTs) 3A and 3B and are maintained during mitosis by the

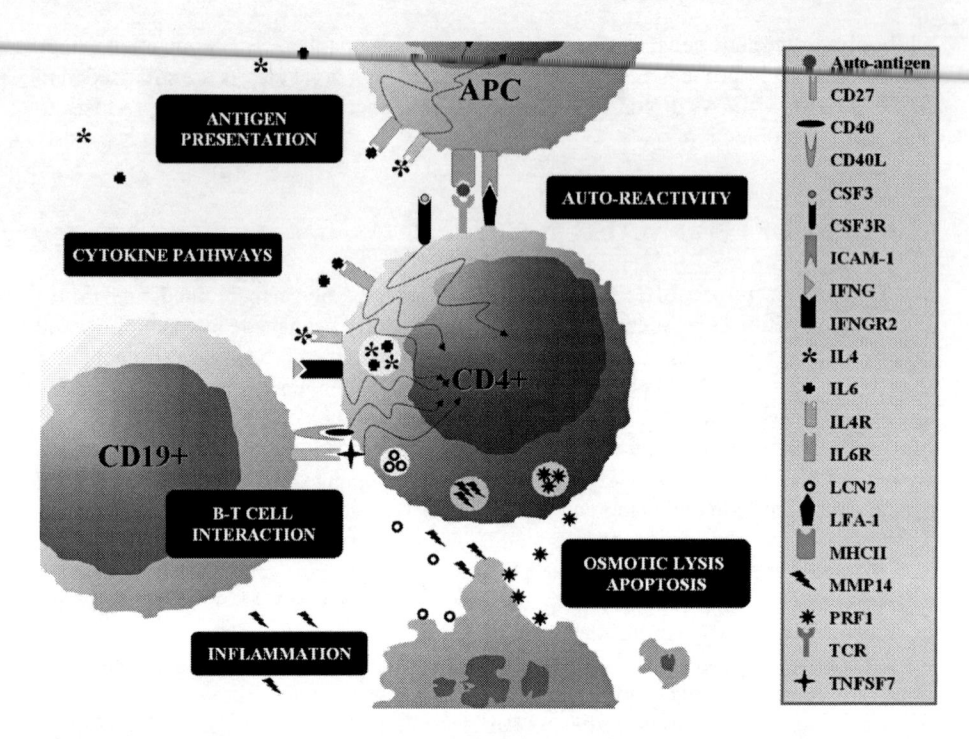

Figure 1. Altered immunological processes in SLE due to gene promoter demethylation. SLE is characterized by DNA methylation decrease in several gene promoters and this epigenetic deregulation induces autoreactivity (LFA-1), osmotic lysis and apoptosis (PRF1, MMP14 and LCN2), impaired antigen presentation (CSF3R) and inflammation (MMP14) as well as deregulated B-T-cell interaction (CD70 and CD40LG) and cytokine signalling (CSF3R, CD70, CD40LG IL-4, IL-6 and I FNGR2).

maintenance methyltransferase DNMT1.[47] DNA demethylation is also an epigenetic mechanism although its importance remains controversial. Unlike passive demethylation, the mechanism for active demethylation is still unclear, although it may be catalyzed by an enzymatic complex made up of a deaminase (AID), a glycosylase (MBD4) and gadd45α.[48]

Impaired DNA Methylation in SLE

The importance of DNA methylation in autoimmunity and especially in SLE, was established in the 1990s and has since been consolidated by many other observations. The first evidence of the involvement of DNA methylation in autoimmunity was the induction of self-reactivity in CD4+ T cells by 5-azacytidine (5-aza C). Human or mouse CD4+ T cells treated with 5-aza C or other DNA methylation inhibitors can be activated by autologous macrophages alone, responding to self-major histocompatibility complex (MHC) II molecules without the usual requirement for specific antigen.[49-53] Moreover, the adoptive transfer of CD4+ T cells treated with 5-aza C, procainamide or hydralazine into syngeneic mice induces a lupus-like disease. Notably, several medications, such as procainamide, hydralazine and 5-aza C and ultraviolet light, all inhibit DNA methylation, induce or aggravate SLE and trigger CD4+ T-cell autoreactivity in mice and humans.[52,54] Interestingly, mutations in the epigenetic machinery can cause other immune problems

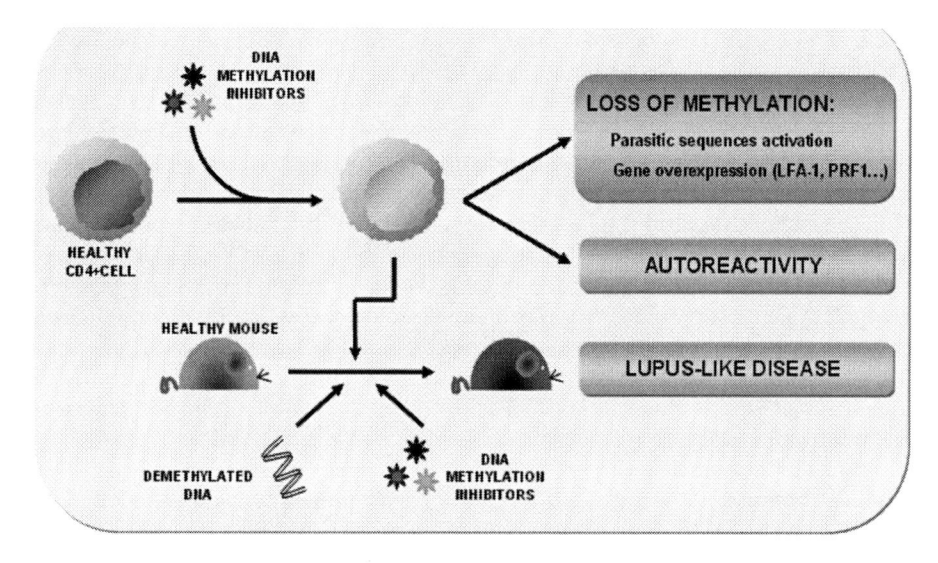

Figure 2. Relationship between DNA methylation and healthy biological systems. Treatment of human or mouse healthy CD4[+] T cells with DNA methylation inhibitors induces loss of global methylation, activation of parasitic sequences and gene overexpression. All of these epigenetic changes provoke CD4[+] T-cell autoreactivity and consequent self-tolerance break. Adoptive transference of these treated cells into healthy mice as well as administration of DNA methylation inhibitors or injection of hypomethylated DNA in this animal induces lupus-like disease.

as well. One example is the ICF (immunodeficiency, centromeric instability and facial abnormalities) syndrome, a disorder produced by a DNMT3B mutation and characterized by B cell immunodeficiency. Another is the mouse strain lacking a functional Gadd45α gene which develops lupus-like disease.[55] Interestingly, SLE is characterized by an increased apoptotic rate of peripheral monocytes, macrophages and lymphocytes coupled with impaired clearance of the resultant cellular debris, which provides a major source of autoantigens.[56,57] In addition, hypomethylated DNA, such as apoptotic or microbial DNA, is more antigenic than normal or necrotic DNA, which are characterized by a higher degree of methylation.[58,59] Thus, BALB/c mice immunized with apoptotic DNA develop a lupus-like disease, unlike mice immunized with necrotic or normal DNA. In addition, demethylation of necrotic or normal genetic material results in the induction of the pathogenic state.[60] These results suggest that circulating apoptotic DNA may mimic microbial DNA, potentially inducing autoimmunity.[61,62] Finally, a significant positive correlation between T-cell DNA hypomethylation, aging and increased probability of SLE development has been established.[63,64] Taking all these findings together, the importance of DNA methylation alterations in SLE pathogenesis is beyond doubt (Fig. 2).

A Global Decrease of DNA Methylation Characterizes SLE Individuals

The relationship between DNA hypomethylation and SLE pathogenesis was first proposed in the 1980s, but its direct involvement was not demonstrated until 1990 when Richardson and colleagues demonstrated impaired DNA methylation in SLE T cells.[65] These findings have been corroborated by multiple studies over recent years and similar results have been obtained from the analysis of subacute cutaneous lupus erythematosus (SCLE) patients.[66-68] These reports have also characterized the specific cell populations that undergo epigenetic alterations. In particular, a significant decrease in DNA methylation has been identified in CD4+ T cells but no differences have been detected in other peripheral blood populations.[68] Moreover, the methylation level of peripheral blood T cells from patients with active SLE is lower than that from patients with the inactive disease, emphasizing a direct relationship between lupus symptoms and DNA methylation.[65] The loss of global methylation can induce activation of endogenous retroviruses and dormant transposons, erase imprinting signals and deregulate gene expression, breaking immune-tolerance as the final consequence.[69] Regarding parasitic DNA activation, a controversial role for HERV in SLE aetiology due to molecular mimicry has been proposed. Indeed, the levels of transcription and translation of HERV clone 4-1 as well as of the production of antibodies against this retrovirus are significantly higher in SLE patients than in normal individuals.[70-72] In addition, the peptide p15E derived from the HERV clone 4-1 is able to induce the same immune abnormalities associated with SLE.[73] As mentioned above, DNA methylation is maintained by DNMT1, an enzyme regulated by the ras-MAPK pathway.[74] Similar to DNA methylation, CD4+ T cells of SLE patients also have lower DNMT1 activity levels and the decrease is associated with disease activity.[67,74,75] Recent studies have identified impaired protein kinase C (PKC) delta phosphorylation as being responsible for the ras-MAPK pathway alteration and subsequent decrease in DNMT1.[76] According to other reports, treating CD4+ T cells with hydralazine, which inhibits ERK pathway signalling by preventing PKC delta phosphorylation, also induces autoreactivity in vitro and lupus-like disease in vivo.[52,54] Similarly, the PKC delta knockout mouse model develops SLE[77](Fig. 3). Expression analysis of other epigenetic effector molecules, such as the methyl-CpG binding domain proteins (MBDs), have been performed in SLE patients although no compelling evidence has emerged due to the contradictory results.[66,68,78] Interestingly, several animal models have been used to study SLE because of the many clinical features they share with human lupus, and impaired DNA methylation has been reported in some of these. One example is the MRL/lpr mouse, in which insertion of an endogenous retrovirus into the Fas gene causes defective elimination of self-reactive T cells due to impaired apoptosis and lupus-like autoimmunity.[79] T cells in the lymphatic nodules and thymus of the MRL/lpr mouse are globally hypomethylated compared to the MRL+/+strain.[80] Moreover, changes in DNA methylation levels have been detected in different lymphatic tissues with aging in this mouse strain, correlating with SLE progression. Specifically, significant differences have not been detected in peripheral blood in contrast to the methylation loss detected in axillary lymph nodes and thymus and an increase in the spleen.[80] As in humans, DNMT1 expression is significantly lower in CD4+ T cells from 16-week-old MRL/lpr mice with active disease compared to younger mice in which autoimmunity has not yet been detected.[81] In contrast to SLE patients and other animal models, administration of 5-aza C to MRL/lpr mice has a protective effect, prolonging survival and reducing the splenomegaly, lymphadenopathy and autoantibody titers, although this may be due to DNA synthesis inhibition by 5-aza C, similar to other drugs used to treat human lupus, such as azathioprine or mycophenylate mofetil[82,83] (Fig. 4).

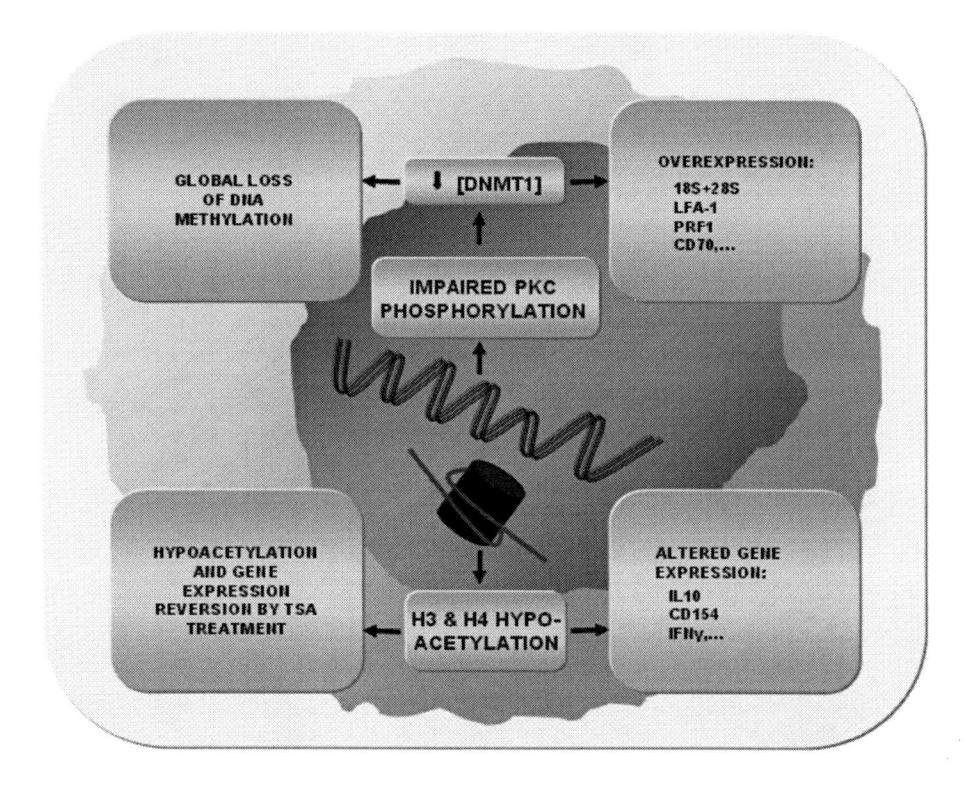

Figure 3. Epigenetic alterations of CD4⁺ T cells of SLE patients. Human SLE CD4⁺ T cells are characterized by global DNA hypomethylation and histone 3 and 4 loss of acetylation. Decreased DNA methylation results from the low level of expression of DNMT1 due to altered PKC phosphorylation and provokes gene and repetitive sequence overexpression. Global hypoacetylation induces skewed gene transcription and this altered expression profile can be reverted by HDAC inhibitors such as TSA DNMT1 (DNA methyltransferase 1), PKC (protein kinase C), H (histone), TSA (trichostatin A).

What Are the Specific DNA Sequences Undergoing Methylation Changes in SLE

As noted above, DNA methylation is an epigenetic modification that regulates gene expression and provides genomic stability in close collaboration with histone modifications. Basically, gene promoter methylation inhibits gene expression whereas the methylation of repetitive sequences allows silencing of parasitic elements and represses chromosomal recombination.[84] As promoter regions occupy a negligible genomic area compared with repetitive sequences, global methylation changes are mainly caused by the alteration of repetitive region methylation profiles. With respect to the repetitive sequences, recent data have identified the ribosomal RNA gene cluster as a region that is susceptible to the development of hypomethylation in SLE. The ribosomal gene is a repetitive sequence of about two megabases located in the short arms of acrocentric chromosomes.[85] The 18S and 28S regions undergo a loss of methylation and are overexpressed in SLE patients relative to healthy siblings.[67] These alterations can induce an increase in ribosomal particles that may provoke the synthesis of autoantibodies against them. Other repetitive sequences, such as D4Z4,

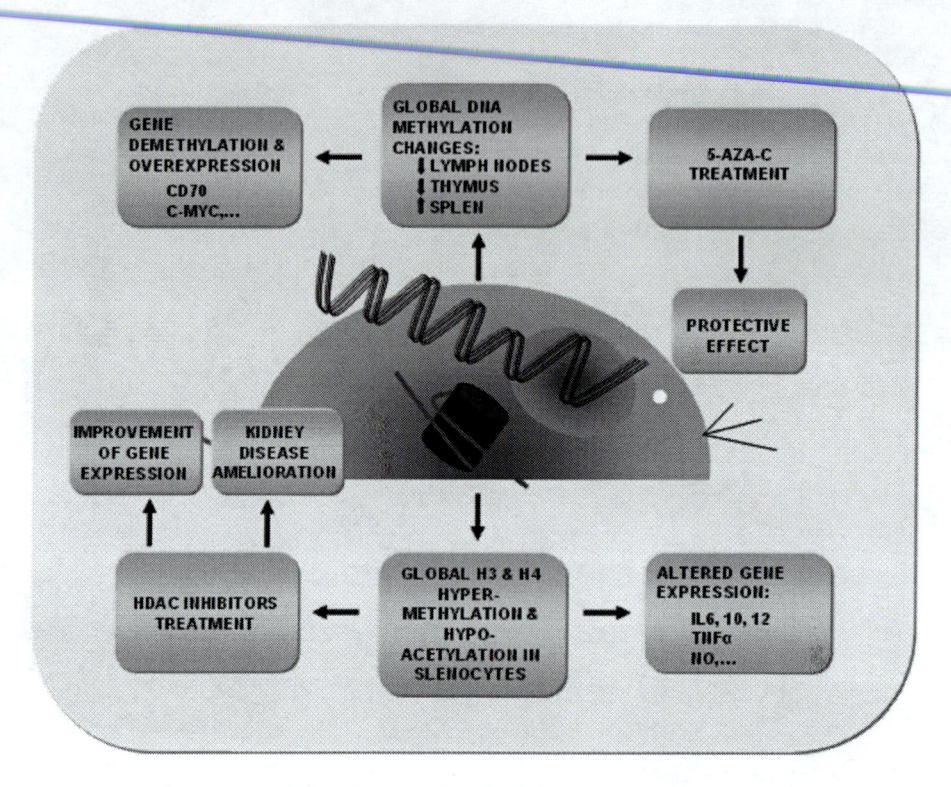

Figure 4. Epigenetic alterations of MRL/lpr SLE mouse model. The MRL/lpr model is characterized by global changes in DNA methylation and histone modifications compared with its mouse control. Lymph nodes and thymus DNA have low levels of methylation compared with spleen genomic material, which experiences methylation gain. These alterations correlate with altered gene expression. Unlike in humans, administration of DNMT inhibitors, such as 5-aza cytidine, has a protective effect. MRL/lpr splenocytes are characterized by global histone 3 and 4 hypermethylation and hypoacetylation and consequent altered gene expression. Administration of HDAC inhibitors improves kidney disease and gene expression profiles. 5-aza-C (5-aza cytidine), HDAC (histone deacetylases), H (histone).

NBL2, Alu, Satellite 2 or LINE-1, have been analysed, but no significant differences associated with SLE have been detected[67] (Fig. 3).

Even though repetitive sequence hypomethylation is the main factor responsible for the decrease in global DNA methylation, changes in gene promoters can also occur. Indeed, there is strong evidence of gene deregulation due to impaired DNA methylation; and T cells are particularly susceptible to gene promoter demethylation in lupus. One example of a gene characterized by loss of promoter methylation in SLE is CD11a. This gene (also called ITGAL) encodes one of the two proteins that comprise lymphocyte function-associated antigen-1 (LFA-1), an adhesion molecule of the integrin family involved in T-cell activation and signalling.[86,87] LFA-1 helps immunological synapse formation, conferring stability to the MHCII-TCR complex and costimulating T cells. Increases in the LFA-1 protein, such as occurs with CD11a overexpression, can break tolerance, possibly by overstablizing the lower affinity interaction of the T-cell antigen/MHC receptor with MHC molecules alone.[50] An upstream region of the ITGAL promoter enriched in Alu repeats is characterized by a loss of methylation that induces gene overexpression in CD4+ and CD8+ T cells of SLE patients.[51,88] Indeed, a direct correlation between disease activity and degree of CD11a promoter demethylation has been reported. Treatment with DNA demethylating drugs such as 5-aza C, procainamide or hydralazine induces a similar loss of methylation and stronger gene expression as well as conferring autoreactivity in vitro and lupus-like disease in vivo.[51] Moreover, the stable transfection of healthy T cells with an ITGAL expression construct induces the same effects.[53,62,88] Interestingly, this gene is damaged in a wide range of leukaemias and lymphomas.[89,90] Another example is the perforin (PRF1) gene,[91] a sequence that encodes a protein that integrates into target cell membranes, where it forms lethal pores.[92,93] PRF1 overexpression is positively correlated with disease activity in CD4+ T cells of SLE and SCLE patients as result of promoter hypomethylation.[91,94] The stronger expression may partly be responsible for the promiscuous T-cell-mediated killing of monocytes and macrophages that typifies SLE pathogenesis.[91] Similarly, CD4+ cells of healthy people become autoreactive killers of autologous monocytes after treatment with DNA methylation inhibitors and this property can be inhibited by adding the perforin inhibitor concanamycin A to the cells.[91] In addition to PRF1 and CD11a, CD70 and CD40LG are also methylation-sensitive genes in SLE. CD70, also known as TNFSF7 or CD27L, is a member of the tumour necrosis factor (TNF) family. This protein is a B cell costimulatory molecule mainly synthesized by activated B and T cells.[93] The CD70 promoter is hypomethylated in CD4+ T cells of SLE and SCLE patients and this loss of methyl groups causes an increase in transcription.[95-97] CD70 transfection of healthy CD4+ T cells or treating CD4+ cells with DNA methylation inhibitors also causes an increase in CD70 transcription and translation levels. Moreover, coculturing the treated or transfected cells with autologous B cells induces IgG overproduction, while the addition of antibodies against CD70 abrogates this increased production.[95] Similarly to CD70, CD40LG (also termed TNFSF5 or CD154) is also a B cell costimulatory molecule. Interestingly, it is encoded on the X-chromosome. For that reason, one copy in women is uniquely methylated and consequently silenced, while men have just one unmethylated copy. Indeed, the CD40LG regulatory region is hypomethylated in CD4+ T cells of women with active SLE, promoting overexpression of the molecule.[98,99] This could explain the striking propensity for females to develop SLE. Several interleukins, such as IL-4 and IL-6, can also be overexpressed due to DNA demethylation, similarly to the previous examples.[100] Although T cells are the best studied and most frequently altered cell type in SLE, other genes may be susceptible to impaired DNA methylation in other cell types. For example, one study of white blood cells identified 49 genes that were differently methylated in five pairs of monozygotic twins discordant for SLE. Extending the study to a larger and more diverse population, the loss of methylation of eight gene promoters (IFNGR2, MMP14, LCN2, CSF3R, PECAM1, CD9, AIM2 AND PDX1) was confirmed and the first five of these genes were shown to have significantly reduced expression[67] (Figs. 1 and 3).

Mouse models are also used to study SLE pathogenesis and thereby detect genes that are deregulated by epigenetic mechanisms. For example, MRL/lpr mice share the impaired CD70 methylation profile with SLE patients, confirming an important role for this gene in lupus pathogenesis.[81] Conversely, the proto-oncogene c-myc is exclusively overexpressed due to gene promoter demethylation in this mouse model, unlike in humans[101,102](Fig. 4).

In conclusion, important genes are characterized by impaired DNA methylation in SLE, which gives rise to increased autoreactivity (ITGAL), osmotic lysis and apoptosis (PRF1, MMP14, LCN2) and inflammation (MMP14), as well as deregulating antigen presentation (CSF3R), B- T-cell interaction (CD70, CD40LG) and cytokine signalling (CSF3R, IL-4, IL-6, IFNGR2)(Fig. 1).

CHANGES IN HISTONE MODIFICATIONS ARE ALSO INVOLVED IN SLE PATHOGENESIS

The Epigenetic Contribution of Histone Modifications

Histones are nuclear proteins that associate with DNA to form nucleosomes, enabling it to be packaged into the nucleus and regulating its expression. Histones have tails that protrude from the nucleosome and can be modified by the covalent addition of chemical moieties such as methyl, phosphate or acetyl groups, among others.[103,104] The combination of these added modifications in different amino acids of the histone tails in part determines the affinity between DNA and histones and also generates or eliminates protein-binding sites, regulating accessibility to different regulatory proteins.[105,106]

Histone Modification Patterns Are Also Altered in SLE

As mentioned above, an increased apoptotic rate coupled with impaired clearance of apoptotic debris characterizes SLE.[56] During apoptosis, chromatin is cleaved by caspases, endonucleases and granzyme B as well as undergoing the addition or elimination of histone modifications. All of these changes can create new epitopes potentially recognized by the immune system, aggravating or inducing SLE development.[107] There is compelling evidence for specific binding of SLE autoantibodies to apoptotically modified antigens. For example, the lupus mouse-derived monoclonal antibody KM-2 mainly recognizes acetylated lysine 8, 12 and 16 in histone H4. Four hours after inducing apoptosis, the affected cells exhibit increased histone acetyl transferase (HAT) expression and reduced levels of histone deacetylases (HDAC), allowing H4 acetylation.[108] Moreover, the apoptosis-induced acetylation on lysine 12 of H2B is a target for predisease lupus mouse antibodies.[109]

Changes in histone modifications occur not only during apoptosis but in other situations as well. Histone alterations are also detected in SLE cells and correlate with aberrant gene expression patterns that may be associated with lupus pathogenesis. The first evidence for impaired histone modifications in lupus emerged from the use of epigenetic drugs in SLE mouse models. In vivo administration of HDAC inhibitors, such as trichostatin A (TSA), suberoylanilide hydroxamic acid (SAHA) and others, ameliorates kidney disease in MRL/lpr mice without changing autoantibody titers.[110,111] Administration of HDAC inhibitors to MRL/lpr splenocytes reduces the expression of various cytokines, including IL-6, IL-10, IL-12, or TNF-α.[110,111] Indeed, a mouse model characterized by an HDAC p300 mutation exclusively in B cells develops lupus-like disease.[112] A recent study has also analyzed H3 and H4 methylation and acetylation levels in splenocytes of MRL/lpr mice. Global hypoacetylation and hypermethylation (excluding H3K4 methylation) relative to the control MRL/MPJ mouse model has been reported and novel histone modifications characterize the SLE model. Administration of TSA reverts the impaired histone modifications and improves the disease course in this model[113](Fig. 4).

Histone modifications have also been studied in people with SLE. Similar to MRL/lpr splenocytes, CD4+ T cells of SLE patients with active disease are characterized by global H3 and H4 hypoacetylation and disease activity correlates inversely with H3 acetylation.[114] This T cell subset overexpresses IL-10 and CD154 and underproduces IFN-γ. Further, treating SLE CD4+ cells with TSA reverses the skewed gene expression.[115] Monocytes also develop changes in histone modifications in SLE. Using ChIP on chip analysis, 179 genes have been characterized as likely to undergo H4 hyperacetylation in monocytes of SLE patients. The acetylation-enriched genes mainly affect macrophage activation, cell proliferation, central nervous system toxicity and antiviral immunity and they also have potential IRF1 binding sites within the 5 Kb upstream region. Although many genes are hyperacetylated, only twelve of them are known to exhibit expression changes. Moreover, treating these macrophages with IFNα increased expression of the 179 selected genes and induced acetylation of histones located in 199 promoter genes.[116] These results not only confirm the role of altered histone modifications in SLE but also suggest the possibility of using them in epigenetic treatments (Fig. 3).

POTENTIAL USE OF EPIGENETIC DRUGS FOR SLE TREATMENT

Progress in the field of epigenetics has been faster than in any other discipline, reflecting its extensive involvement in different diseases. Compelling evidence demonstrating a role for epigenetic dysregulation in SLE emerged several years ago, is now widely accepted and holds promise for therapeutic applications. One of the most important aspects of epigenetic regulation is the possibility of reversion through the use of drugs that inhibit the epigenetic machinery. In fact, some of these compounds are already being used in preclinical and clinical phases for the treatment of haematological malignancies following their approval by the US Food and Drug Administration.[117] The effects of DNMTs and histone modification enzyme inhibition summarised above support the potential for using these inhibitors for disease amelioration. Indeed, studies based on treatments with HDAC inhibitors highlight the ability of these drugs to reverse the skewed gene expression associated with lupus and to modulate immune system activity and reduce inflammation.[118,119] Before designing a therapeutic approach, an in-depth understanding is required of the epigenetic alterations of each cell type associated with the disease. To this end, we need to develop and use SLE animal models as well as create cell lines in which to test the agents. Problems associated with human studies can be resolved using in vitro and animal models, although one must always bear in mind their limitations and corroborate the results in SLE patients. In addition, a more exhaustive study of the relationship between cancer and autoimmunity will help us extrapolate our extensive knowledge of epigenetic deregulation in cancer to SLE.[120] Further, a new gene expression regulator, known as microRNA (miRNA), is attracting attention because of its involvement in many disorders.[121,122] miRNAs are noncoding RNA molecules, around 22 nucleotides long, that regulate the expression of target genes through various posttranscriptional mechanisms.[123] The current finding that a set of miRNAs are differentially expressed in lupus patients and normal controls together with a recent description of their epigenetic regulation (including DNA methylation-dependent regulation of miRNA expression) suggests a potential role for epigenetic dysregulation of miRNA in SLE.[124-126] For this reason, miRNAs are potential players in SLE pathogenesis as well as potential therapeutic targets and diagnosis biomarkers.[121]

CONCLUSION

In conclusion, a deeper and more specific understanding of the epigenetic alterations at the level of DNA methylation and histone modifications of gene promoters, repetitive sequences and miRNAs that occur in lupus and the exhaustive study of the epigenetic connections between cancer and autoimmunity are the new epigenetic aims in the fight against SLE in the immediate future.

REFERENCES

1. D'Cruz DP, Khamashta MA, Hughes GR. Systemic lupus erythematosus Lancet, 2007; 369(9561):587-596.
2. Rahman A, Isenberg DA. Systemic lupus erythematosus. N Engl J Med 2008; 358(9):929-939.
3. Cooper GS, Dooley MA, Treadwell EL et al. Hormonal and reproductive risk factors for development of systemic lupus erythematosus: results of a population-based, case-control study. Arthritis Rheum 2002; 46(7):1830-1839.
4. Johnson AE, Gordon C, Palmer RG et al. The prevalence and incidence of systemic lupus erythematosus in Birmingham, England. Relationship to ethnicity and country of birth. Arthritis Rheum; 1995; 38(4):551-558.
5. Urowitz MB, Bookman AA, Koehler BE et al. The bimodal mortality pattern of systemic lupus erythematosus. Am J Med 1976; 60(2):221-225.
6. Rothfield N, Sontheimer RD, Bernstein M. Lupus erythematosus: systemic and cutaneous manifestations. Clin Dermatol 2006; 24(5):348-362.
7. Munoz LE, Gaipl US, Franz S, et al. SLE—a disease of clearance deficiency? Rheumatology (Oxford) 2005; 44(9):1101-1107.
8. Baumann I, Kolowos W, Voll RE et al. Impaired uptake of apoptotic cells into tingible body macrophages in germinal centers of patients with systemic lupus erythematosus. Arthritis Rheum 2002; 46(1):191-201.
9. Isenberg DA, Manson JJ, Ehrenstein MR, et al. Fifty years of anti-ds DNA antibodies: are we approaching journey's end? Rheumatology (Oxford) 2007; 46(7):1052-1056.
10. Ng KP, Manson JJ, Rahman A et al. Association of antinucleosome antibodies with disease flare in serologically active clinically quiescent patients with systemic lupus erythematosus. Arthritis Rheum 2006; 55(6):900-904.
11. Avrameas S. Natural autoantibodies: from 'horror autotoxicus' to 'gnothi seauton'. Immunol Today 1991; 12(5):154-159.
12. Fujii Y, Fujii K, Tanaka Y. Attempt to correct abnormal signal transduction in T-lymphocytes from systemic lupus erythematosus patients. Autoimmun Rev 2006; 5(2):143-144.
13. Graham RR, Kozyrev SV, Baechler EC et al. A common haplotype of interferon regulatory factor 5 (IRF5) regulates splicing and expression and is associated with increased risk of systemic lupus erythematosus. Nat Genet 2006; 38(5):550-555.
14. Houssiau FA, Lefebvre C, Vanden Berghe M et al. Serum interleukin 10 titers in systemic lupus erythematosus reflect disease activity. Lupus 1995; 4(5):393-395.
15. Sullivan KE. Genetics of systemic lupus erythematosus. Clinical implications. Rheum Dis Clin North Am 2000; 26(2):229-256, v-vi.
16. Rhodes B, Vyse TJ. The genetics of SLE: an update in the light of genome-wide association studies. Rheumatology (Oxford) 2008; 47(11):1603-1611.
17. Moser KL, Kelly JA, Lessard CJ et al. Recent insights into the genetic basis of systemic lupus erythematosus. Genes Immun 2009; 10(5):373-379.
18. Jacobson DL, Gange SJ, Rose NR et al. Epidemiology and estimated population burden of selected autoimmune diseases in the United States. Clin Immunol Immunopathol 1997; 84(3):223-243.
19. Sanchez-Guerrero J, Karlson EW, Liang MH et al. Past use of oral contraceptives and the risk of developing systemic lupus erythematosus. Arthritis Rheum 1997; 40(5):804-808.

20. Mok CC, Lau CS, Ho CT et al. Do flares of systemic lupus erythematosus decline after menopause? Scand J Rheumatol 1999; 28(6):357-362.
21. Lahita RG, Bradlow HL, Ginzler E,et al. Low plasma androgens in women with systemic lupus erythematosus. Arthritis Rheum 1987; 30(3):241-248.
22. Lahita RG, Bradlow L, Fishman J et al. Estrogen metabolism in systemic lupus erythematosus: patients and family members. Arthritis Rheum 1982; 25(7):843-846.
23. Folomeev M, Dougados M, Beaune J et al. Plasma sex hormones and aromatase activity in tissues of patients with systemic lupus erythematosus. Lupus 1992; 1(3):191-195.
24. Jara LJ, Lavalle C, Espinoza LR. Does prolactin have a role in the pathogenesis of systemic lupus erythematosus? J Rheumatol 1992; 19(9):1333-1336.
25. Roubinian JR, Talal N, Greenspan JS et al. Effect of castration and sex hormone treatment on survival, anti-nucleic acid antibodies and glomerulonephritis in NZB/NZW F1 mice. J Exp Med 1978; 147(6):1568-1583.
26. Roubinian JR, Papoian R, Talal N. Androgenic hormones modulate autoantibody responses and improve survival in murine lupus. J Clin Invest 1977; 59(6):1066-1070.
27. Elbourne KB, Keisler D, McMurray RW. Differential effects of estrogen and prolactin on autoimmune disease in the NZB/NZW F1 mouse model of systemic lupus erythematosus. Lupus 1998; 7(6):420-427.
28. Kremer Hovinga IC, Koopmans M, de Heer E et al. Chimerism in systemic lupus erythematosus—three hypotheses. Rheumatology (Oxford) 2007; 46(2):200-208.
29. James JA, Harley JB, Scofield RH. Epstein-Barr virus and systemic lupus erythematosus. Curr Opin Rheumatol 2006; 18(5):462-467.
30. Gross AJ, Hochberg D, Rand WM et al. EBV and systemic lupus erythematosus: a new perspective. J Immunol 2005; 174(11):6599-6607.
31. Sundar K, Jacques S, Gottlieb P et al. Expression of the Epstein-Barr virus nuclear antigen-1 (EBNA-1) in the mouse can elicit the production of anti-dsDNA and anti-Sm antibodies. J Autoimmun 2004; 23(2):127-140.
32. Poole BD, Scofield RH, Harley JB et al. Epstein-Barr virus and molecular mimicry in systemic lupus erythematosus. Autoimmunity 2006; 39(1):63-70.
33. Kaufman KM, Kirby MY, Harley JB et al. Peptide mimics of a major lupus epitope of SmB/B'. Ann N Y Acad Sci 2003; 987:215-229.
34. Balada E, Ordi-Ros J, Vilardell-Tarres M. Molecular mechanisms mediated by human endogenous retroviruses (HERVs) in autoimmunity. Rev Med Virol 2009; 19(5):273-286.
35. Chu JL, Drappa J, Parnassa A et al. The defect in Fas mRNA expression in MRL/lpr mice is associated with insertion of the retrotransposon, ETn. J Exp Med 1993; 178(2):723-730.
36. Cooper GS, Parks CG, Treadwell EL et al. Occupational risk factors for the development of systemic lupus erythematosus. J Rheumatol 2004; 31(10):1928-1933.
37. Portela A, Esteller M. Epigenetic modifications and their relevance to disease Nat Biotech., 2010.
38. Strickland FM, Richardson BC. Epigenetics in human autoimmunity. Epigenetics in autoimmunity—DNA methylation in systemic lupus erythematosus and beyond. Autoimmunity 2008; 41(4):278-286.
39. Rao T, Richardson B. Environmentally induced autoimmune diseases: potential mechanisms. Environ Health Perspect 1999; 107 Suppl 5:737-742.
40. Jarvinen P, Aho K. Twin studies in rheumatic diseases. Semin Arthritis Rheum 1994; 24(1):19-28.
41. Singal R, Ginder GD. DNA methylation. Blood 1999; 93(12):4059-4070.
42. Lister R, Pelizzola M, Dowen RH et al. Human DNA methylomes at base resolution show widespread epigenomic differences. Nature 2009; 462(7271):315-322.
43. Bird A. Molecular biology. Methylation talk between histones and DNA. Science 2001; 294(5549):2113-2115.
44. Cedar H. DNA methylation and gene activity. Cell 1988; 53(1):3-4.
45. Ehrlich M, Gama-Sosa MA, Huang LH et al. Amount and distribution of 5-methylcytosine in human DNA from different types of tissues of cells. Nucleic Acids Res 1982; 10(8):2709-2721.
46. Tuck-Muller CM, Narayan A, Tsien F et al. DNA hypomethylation and unusual chromosome instability in cell lines from ICF syndrome patients. Cytogenet Cell Genet 2000; 89(1-2):121-128.
47. Klose RJ, Bird AP. Genomic DNA methylation: the mark and its mediators. Trends Biochem Sci 2006; 31(2):89-97.
48. Rai K, Huggins IJ, James SR et al. DNA demethylation in zebrafish involves the coupling of a deaminase, a glycosylase and gadd45. Cell 2008; 135(7):1201-1212.
49. Richardson B. Effect of an inhibitor of DNA methylation on T-cells. II. 5-Azacytidine induces self-reactivity in antigen-specific T4+ cells. Hum Immunol 1986; 17(4):456-4570.
50. Yung R, Powers D, Johnson K et al. Mechanisms of drug-induced lupus. II. T-cells overexpressing lymphocyte function-associated antigen 1 become autoreactive and cause a lupuslike disease in syngeneic mice. J Clin Invest 1996; 97(12):2866-2871.

51. Richardson BC, Strahler JR, Pivirotto TS et al. Phenotypic and functional similarities between 5-azacytidine-treated T-cells and a T-cell subset in patients with active systemic lupus erythematosus. Arthritis Rheum 1992; 35(6):647-662.

52. Cornacchia E, Golbus J, Maybaum J et al. Hydralazine and procainamide inhibit T-cell DNA methylation and induce autoreactivity. J Immunol 1988; 140(7):2197-2200.

53. Quddus J, Johnson KJ, Gavalchin J et al. Treating activated CD4+ T-cells with either of two distinct DNA methyltransferase inhibitors, 5-azacytidine or procainamide, is sufficient to cause a lupus-like disease in syngeneic mice. J Clin Invest 1993; 92(1):38-53.

54. Yung R, Chang S, Hemati N et al. Mechanisms of drug-induced lupus. IV. Comparison of procainamide and hydralazine with analogs in vitro and in vivo. Arthritis Rheum 1997; 40(8):1436-1443.

55. Salvador JM, Hollander MC, Nguyen AT et al. Mice lacking the p53-effector gene Gadd45a develop a lupus-like syndrome. Immunity 2002; 16(4):499-508.

56. Emlen W, Niebur J, Kadera R. Accelerated in vitro apoptosis of lymphocytes from patients with systemic lupus erythematosus. J Immunol 1994; 152(7):3685-3692.

57. Kaplan MJ, Lewis EE, Shelden EA et al. The apoptotic ligands TRAIL, TWEAK and Fas ligand mediate monocyte death induced by autologous lupus T-cells. J Immunol 2002 169(10):6020-6029.

58. Yu D, Zhu FG, Bhagat L et al. Potent CpG oligonucleotides containing phosphodiester linkages: in vitro and in vivo immunostimulatory properties. Biochem Biophys Res Commun 2002; 297(1):83-90.

59. Messina JP, Gilkeson GS, Pisetsky DS. The influence of DNA structure on the in vitro stimulation of murine lymphocytes by natural and synthetic polynucleotide antigens. Cell Immunol 1993; 147(1):148-157.

60. Wen ZK, Xu W, Xu L et al. DNA hypomethylation is crucial for apoptotic DNA to induce systemic lupus erythematosus-like autoimmune disease in SLE-nonsusceptible mice. Rheumatology (Oxford) 2007; 46(12):1796-1803.

61. Krieg AM. CpG DNA: a pathogenic factor in systemic lupus erythematosus? J Clin Immunol 1995; 15(6):284-292.

62. Yung RL, Quddus J, Chrisp CE et al. Mechanism of drug-induced lupus. I. Cloned Th2 cells modified with DNA methylation inhibitors in vitro cause autoimmunity in vivo. J Immunol 1995; 154(6):3025-3035.

63. Golbus J, Palella TD, Richardson BC. Quantitative changes in T-cell DNA methylation occur during differentiation and ageing. Eur J Immunol 1990; 20(8):1869-1872.

64. Zhang Z, Deng C, Lu Q et al. Age-dependent DNA methylation changes in the ITGAL (CD11a) promoter. Mech Ageing Dev 2002; 123(9):1257-1268.

65. Richardson B, Scheinbart L, Strahler J et al. Evidence for impaired T-cell DNA methylation in systemic lupus erythematosus and rheumatoid arthritis. Arthritis Rheum 1990; 33(11):1665-1673.

66. Luo Y, Li Y, Su Y et al. Abnormal DNA methylation in T-cells from patients with subacute cutaneous lupus erythematosus. Br J Dermatol 2008; 159(4):827-833.

67. Javierre BM, Fernandez AF, Richter J et al. Changes in the pattern of DNA methylation associate with twin discordance in systemic lupus erythematosus. Genome Res 2010; 20(2):170-179.

68. Lei W, Luo Y, Lei W et al. Abnormal DNA methylation in CD4+ T-cells from patients with systemic lupus erythematosus, systemic sclerosis and dermatomyositis. Scand J Rheumatol 2009;1-6.

69. Okada M, Ogasawara H, Kaneko H et al. Role of DNA methylation in transcription of human endogenous retrovirus in the pathogenesis of systemic lupus erythematosus. J Rheumatol 2002; 29(8):1678-1682.

70. Knight SJ, Flannery AV, Hirst MC et al. Trinucleotide repeat amplification and hypermethylation of a CpG island in FRAXE mental retardation. Cell 1993; 74(1):127-134.

71. Sekigawa I, Okada M, Ogasawara H et al. Lessons from similarities between SLE and HIV infection. J Infect 2002; 44(2):67-72.

72. Sekigawa I, Ogasawara H, Kaneko H et al. Retroviruses and autoimmunity. Intern Med 2001; 40(2):80-86.

73. Naito T, Ogasawara H, Kaneko H et al. Immune abnormalities induced by human endogenous retroviral peptides: with reference to the pathogenesis of systemic lupus erythematosus. J Clin Immunol 2003; 23(5):371-376.

74. Deng C, Kaplan MJ, Yang J et al. Decreased Ras-mitogen-activated protein kinase signaling may cause DNA hypomethylation in T-lymphocytes from lupus patients. Arthritis Rheum 2001; 44(2):397-407.

75. Ogasawara H, Okada M, Kaneko H et al. Possible role of DNA hypomethylation in the induction of SLE: relationship to the transcription of human endogenous retroviruses. Clin Exp Rheumatol 2003; 21(6):733-738.

76. Kammer GM, Perl A, Richardson BC et al. Abnormal T-cell signal transduction in systemic lupus erythematosus. Arthritis Rheum 2002; 46(5):1139-1154.

77. Miyamoto A, Nakayama K, Imaki H et al. Increased proliferation of B-cells and auto-immunity in mice lacking protein kinase Cdelta. Nature 2002; 416(6883):865-869.

78. Balada E, Ordi-Ros J, Vilardell-Tarres M. DNA methylation and systemic lupus erythematosus. Ann N Y Acad Sci 2007; 1108:127-136.

79. Wu J, Zhou T, He J et al. Autoimmune disease in mice due to integration of an endogenous retrovirus in an apoptosis gene. J Exp Med 1993; 178(2):461-468.
80. Mizugaki M, Yamaguchi T, Ishiwata S et al. Alteration of DNA methylation levels in MRL lupus mice. Clin Exp Immunol 1997; 110(2):265-269.
81. Sawalha AH, Jeffries M. Defective DNA methylation and CD70 overexpression in CD4+ T-cells in MRL/lpr lupus-prone mice. Eur J Immunol 2007; 37(5):1407-1413.
82. Yoshida H, Yoshida M, Merino R et al. 5-Azacytidine inhibits the lpr gene-induced lymphadenopathy and acceleration of lupus-like syndrome in MRL/MpJ-lpr/lpr mice. Eur J Immunol 1990; 20(9):1989-1993.
83. Schauenstein K, Csordas A, Krömer G et al. In-vivo treatment with 5-azacytidine causes degeneration of central lymphatic organs and induces autoimmune disease in the chicken. Int J Exp Pathol 1991; 72(3):311-318.
84. Guil S, Esteller M. DNA methylomes, histone codes and miRNAs: tying it all together. Int J Biochem Cell Biol 2009; 41(1):87-95.
85. Huang S, Rothblum LI, Chen D. Ribosomal chromatin organization. Biochem Cell Biol 2006; 84(4):444-449.
86. Lu Q, Kaplan M, Ray D et al. Demethylation of ITGAL (CD11a) regulatory sequences in systemic lupus erythematosus. Arthritis Rheum 2002; 46(5):1282-1291.
87. Hogg N, Laschinger M, Giles K et al. T-cell integrins: more than just sticking points. J Cell Sci 2003; 116(Pt 23):4695-4705.
88. Richardson B, Powers D, Hooper F et al. Lymphocyte function-associated antigen 1 overexpression and T-cell autoreactivity. Arthritis Rheum 1994; 37(9):1363-1372.
89. Robillard N, Pellat-Deceunynck C, Bataille R. Phenotypic characterization of the human myeloma cell growth fraction. Blood 2005; 105(12):4845-4848.
90. Puig-Kroger A, Sanchez-Elsner T, Ruiz N et al. RUNX/AML and C/EBP factors regulate CD11a integrin expression in myeloid cells through overlapping regulatory elements. Blood 2003; 102(9):3252-3261.
91. Kaplan MJ, Lu Q, Wu A et al. Demethylation of promoter regulatory elements contributes to perforin overexpression in CD4+ lupus T-cells. J Immunol 2004; 172(6):3652-3661.
92. van den Broek MF, Hengartner H. The role of perforin in infections and tumour surveillance. Exp Physiol 2000; 85(6):681-685.
93. Kobata T, Jacquot S, Kozlowski S et al. CD27-CD70 interactions regulate B-cell activation by T-cells. Proc Natl Acad Sci USA 1995; 92(24):11249-11253.
94. Luo Y, Zhang X, Zhao M et al. DNA demethylation of the perforin promoter in CD4(+) T-cells from patients with subacute cutaneous lupus erythematosus. J Dermatol Sci 2009; 56(1):33-36.
95. Oelke K, Lu Q, Richardson D et al. Overexpression of CD70 and overstimulation of IgG synthesis by lupus T-cells and T-cells treated with DNA methylation inhibitors. Arthritis Rheum 2004; 50(6):1850-1860.
96. Luo Y, Zhao M, Lu Q. Demethylation of promoter regulatory elements contributes to CD70 overexpression in CD4+ T-cells from patients with subacute cutaneous lupus erythematosus. Clin Exp Dermatol 2009.
97. Lu Q, Wu A, Richardson BC. Demethylation of the same promoter sequence increases CD70 expression in lupus T-cells and T-cells treated with lupus-inducing drugs. J Immunol 2005; 174(10):6212-6219.
98. Lu Q, Wu A, Tesmer L et al. Demethylation of CD40LG on the inactive X in T-cells from women with lupus. J Immunol 2007; 179(9):6352-6358.
99. Zhou Y, Yuan J, Pan Y et al. T-cell CD40LG gene expression and the production of IgG by autologous B cells in systemic lupus erythematosus. Clin Immunol 2009; 132(3):362-370.
100. Mi XB, Zeng FQ. Hypomethylation of interleukin-4 and -6 promoters in T-cells from systemic lupus erythematosus patients. Acta Pharmacol Sin 2008; 29(1):105-112.
101. Evans JL, Boyle WJ, Ting JP. Molecular basis of elevated c-myb expression in the abnormal L3T4-, Lyt-2- T-lymphocytes of autoimmune mice. J Immunol 1987; 139(10):3497-3505.
102. Eleftheriades EG, Boumpas DT, Balow JE et al. Transcriptional and posttranscriptional mechanisms are responsible for the increased expression of c-myc protooncogene in lymphocytes from patients with systemic lupus erythematosus. Clin Immunol Immunopathol 1989; 52(3):507-515.
103. Strahl BD, Allis CD. The language of covalent histone modifications. Nature 2000; 403(6765):41-45.
104. Peterson CL, Laniel MA. Histones and histone modifications. Curr Biol 2004;14(14):R546-R551.
105. Santos-Rosa H, Caldas C. Chromatin modifier enzymes, the histone code and cancer. Eur J Cancer 2005; 41(16):2381-2402.
106. Matouk CC, Marsden PA. Epigenetic regulation of vascular endothelial gene expression. Circ Res 2008; 102(8):873-887.
107. Boix-Chornet M, Fraga MF, Villar-Garea A et al. Release of hypoacetylated and trimethylated histone H4 is an epigenetic marker of early apoptosis. J Biol Chem 2006; 281(19):13540-13547.
108. Dieker JW, Fransen JH, van Bavel CC et al. Apoptosis-induced acetylation of histones is pathogenic in systemic lupus erythematosus. Arthritis Rheum 2007; 56(6):1921-1933.
109. van Bavel CC, Dieker J, Muller S et al. Apoptosis-associated acetylation on histone H2B is an epitope for lupus autoantibodies. Mol Immunol 2009; 47(2-3):511-516.

110. Mishra N, Reilly CM, Brown DR et al. Histone deacetylase inhibitors modulate renal disease in the MRL-lpr/lpr mouse. J Clin Invest 2003; 111(4):539-552.
111. Reilly CM, Mishra N, Miller JM et al. Modulation of renal disease in MRL/lpr mice by suberoylanilide hydroxamic acid. J Immunol 2004 173(6):4171-4178.
112. Forster N, Gallinat S, Jablonska J et al. p300 protein acetyltransferase activity suppresses systemic lupus erythematosus-like autoimmune disease in mice. J Immunol 2007; 178(11):6941-6948.
113. Garcia BA, Busby SA, Shabanowitz J et al. Resetting the epigenetic histone code in the MRL-lpr/lpr mouse model of lupus by histone deacetylase inhibition. J Proteome Res 2005 ; 4(6):2032-2042.
114. Hu N, Qiu X, Luo Y et al. Abnormal histone modification patterns in lupus CD4+ T-cells. J Rheumatol 2008; 35(5):804-810.
115. Mishra N, Brown DR, Olorenshaw IM et al. Trichostatin A reverses skewed expression of CD154, interleukin-10 and interferon-gamma gene and protein expression in lupus T-cells. Proc Natl Acad Sci USA 2001; 98(5):2628-2633.
116. Zhang Z, Song L, Maurer K et al. Global H4 acetylation analysis by ChIP-chip in systemic lupus erythematosus monocytes. Genes Immun, 2009.
117. Yoo CB, Jones PA. Epigenetic therapy of cancer: past, present and future. Nat Rev Drug Discov 2006; 5(1):37-50.
118. Adcock IM. HDAC inhibitors as anti-inflammatory agents. Br J Pharmacol 2007; 150(7):829-831.
119. Brogdon JL, Xu Y, Szabo SJ et al. Histone deacetylase activities are required for innate immune cell control of Th1 but not Th2 effector cell function. Blood 2007; 109(3):1123-1130.
120. Javierre BM, Esteller M, Ballestar E. Epigenetic connections between autoimmune disorders and haematological malignancies. Trends Immunol 2008; 29(12):616-623.
121. Pauley KM, Cha S, Chan EK. MicroRNA in autoimmunity and autoimmune diseases. J Autoimmun 2009; 32(3-4):189-194.
122. Wang Y, Liang Y, Lu Q. MicroRNA epigenetic alterations: predicting biomarkers and therapeutic targets in human diseases. Clin Genet 2008; 74(4):307-315.
123. Bartel DP. MicroRNAs: genomics, biogenesis, mechanism and function. Cell 2004; 116(2):281-297.
124. Lujambio A, Calin GA, Villanueva A et al. A microRNA DNA methylation signature for human cancer metastasis. Proc Natl Acad Sci USA, 2008. 105(36):13556-13561.
125. Dai Y, Huang YS, Tang M et al. Microarray analysis of microRNA expression in peripheral blood cells of systemic lupus erythematosus patients. Lupus 2007; 16(12):939-946.
126. Tang Y, Luo X, Cui H et al. MicroRNA-146A contributes to abnormal activation of the type I interferon pathway in human lupus by targeting the key signaling proteins. Arthritis Rheum 2009; 60(4):1065-1075.
127. Sawalha AH, Harley JB. Antinuclear autoantibodies in systemic lupus erythematosus. Curr Opin Rheumatol 2004; 16(5):534-540.
128. Mannik M, Merrill CE, Stamps LD et al. Multiple autoantibodies form the glomerular immune deposits in patients with systemic lupus erythematosus. J Rheumatol 2003; 30(7):1495-1504.
129. Amoura Z, Koutouzov S, Chabre H et al. Presence of antinucleosome autoantibodies in a restricted set of connective tissue diseases: antinucleosome antibodies of the IgG3 subclass are markers of renal pathogenicity in systemic lupus erythematosus. Arthritis Rheum 2000; 43(1):76-84.
130. Kowal C, Degiorgio LA, Lee JY et al. Human lupus autoantibodies against NMDA receptors mediate cognitive impairment. Proc Natl Acad Sci USA 2006; 103(52):19854-19859.
131. Becker-Merok A, Kalaaji M, Haugbro K et al. Alpha-actinin-binding antibodies in relation to systemic lupus erythematosus and lupus nephritis. Arthritis Res Ther 2006; 8(6):R162.
132. Siegert CE, Daha MR, Swaak AJ et al. The relationship between serum titers of autoantibodies to C1q and age in the general population and in patients with systemic lupus erythematosus. Clin Immunol Immunopathol 1993; 67(3 Pt 1):204-209.

CHAPTER 10

EPIGENETIC DEREGULATION IN RHEUMATOID ARTHRITIS

Emmanuel Karouzakis, Renate E. Gay, Steffen Gay and Michel Neidhart*

Center for Experimental Rheumatology, University Hospital Zurich, Gloriastrasse, Zurich, Switzerland
Corresponding Author: Michel Neidhart—Email: michel.neidhart@usz.ch

Abstract: In this chapter, we discuss the current understanding of the possible epigenetics changes that occur in rheumatoid arthritis. In particular, we describe that deregulation of DNA methylation and histone modifications can occur in the immune system and lead to rheumatoid arthritis. In addition, we discuss the role of rheumatoid arthritis synovial fibroblasts in autoimmunity. Examples of changes in DNA methylation and histone modification occurring in synovial fibroblasts during the disease process are reviewed in this chapter. In conclusion, we discuss the possible use of epigenetic therapy and describe future experiments that can elucidate further the epigenetic changes observed in the disease.

INTRODUCTION

Rheumatoid arthritis (RA) is a chronic systemic inflammatory disorder of unknown etiology that causes joint destruction. It is known as an autoimmune disease and is characterised by polyarticular pain, swelling, morning stiffness, malaise and fatigue. The disease does not have specific features and develops over a period of time. Arthritis usually affects the metacarpophalangeal (MCP) and proximal interphalangeal (PIP) joints of both hands, as the most characteristic early clinical feature. Classification criteria for RA were drafted in 1956 by the American College of Rheumatology (ACR) and revised in 1987 in order to provide guidelines for clinical trials.

The etiology of RA remains still unknown. It has been hypothesised that infectious agents such as viruses and bacteria cause a chronic inflammatory response that targets

Epigenetic Contributions in Autoimmune Disease, edited by Esteban Ballestar.
©2011 Landes Bioscience and Springer Science+Business Media.

components of the joints.[1] Environmental factors have also been implicated in the development of RA such as smoking. The genetic predisposition to RA of individuals with HLADRB1 "shared epitope" has raised the possibility of a specific autoantigen that triggers a T-cell clonal response.[2]

However, to cause autoimmunity other factors are also required. In contrast to genetic alterations, epigenetic changes are defined as changes in gene expression that do not involve a change in the DNA sequence. In this chapter, we will mainly consider two epigenetic mechanisms, namely DNA methylation and histone modifications. Epigenetic alterations play a role in numerous diseases, including cancer and developmental diseases.[3]

The epigenetic modification of DNA with 5-methylcytosine is an important regulatory event involved in chromatin structure, genomic imprinting, inactivation of the X chromosome, transcription and retrotransposon silencing. This modification is catalyzed and maintained by the DNA methyltransferases (DNMTs) and is interpreted by the methyl-CpG binding proteins. DNA methyltransferases are not limited to catalyzing DNA methylation, but also take part in the regulation of gene expression through interactions with other proteins that repress transcription and modify chromatin structure. Importantly, the replication of DNA methylation marks during mitosis is sensitive to the environment and exogenous agents that decreases S-adenosylmethionine levels, or decrease DNA methyltransferase 1 (DNMT1) levels or enzyme activity, result in failure to replicate the patterns. Errors will be accumulated over successive cell divisions. In this model, this causes aberrant expression of genes normally silenced by DNA methylation. In addition, histone modifications—acetylation, methylation, etc.—serve as signals, referred as the histone code, that renders the genome accessible to the transcription initiation machinery. For example, histone acetylation reflects a balance between histone acetyltransferases (HAT) and histone deacetylases (HDAC) that is sensitive to environmental stimuli. DNA methylation and histone modifications may be functionally linked, in order to silence or allow the expression of specific genes. Environmental insults trigger a response of the immune system and local activation of cells, e.g., fibroblasts, allowing tissue repair. This reaction is dependent on the genetic predisposition and epigenetic settings and is the response of a healthy organism (Fig. 1).

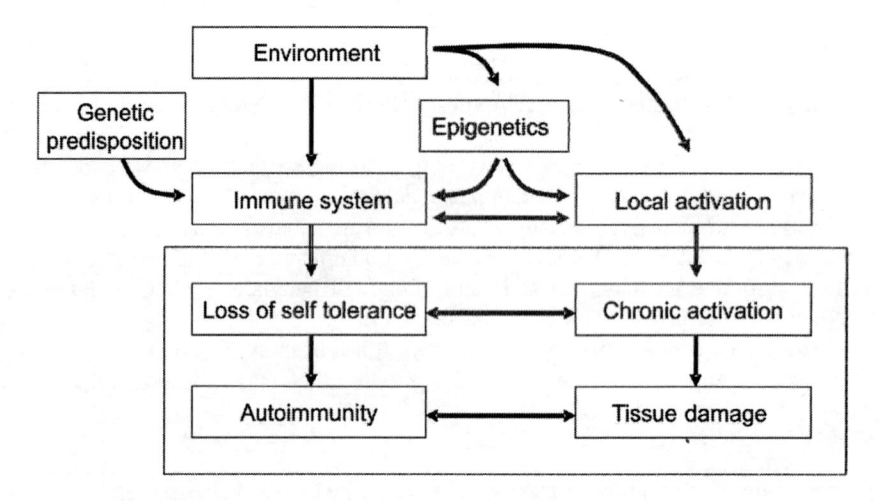

Figure 1. Central role of epigenetics in the pathogenesis of rheumatoid arthritis.

Loss of self tolerance leads to autoimmunity and rheumatoid arthritis. The chronic activation of local cells finally is responsible for the synovial tissue damage.

GENETICS AND ENVIRONMENT

Rheumatoid arthritis (RA) is a systemic disease affecting approximately 1% of the population worldwide. It is characterized by inflammation, infiltration of cells of the immune system, a hyperplastic synovial tissue and destruction of the joints by synovial fibroblasts and osteoclasts (Fig. 2). Family and twin studies suggest a 50% genetic contribution to RA and a high concordance rate in monozygotic twins (12-30%).[4] The HLA genes at 6p21 show the strongest linkage to RA. In particular, HLA-DRB1 allele variants are associated to increased susceptibility.[5] However, familial risk due to the HLA genes has been estimated to be only 15-30%, suggesting that other genes or factors play a significant role. Other genes include PTPN22 (1858T variant) and PADI-4.[6,7]

The limited historical descriptions of RA before industrialization suggest that changing environmental influences might be important in the etiology. An examination of 800 medieval skeletons in the United Kingdom failed to show any evidence of RA, while the disorder is now present in 1% of the population.[8] This has been confirmed in Italy and Egypt. Increased urbanization has been associated with an increased prevalence of RA. Another hypothesis is that RA was a New World disease which subsequently spread to the old World. If so, perhaps definition of its original location and spread would allow identification of the cause.[9] Investigation of the skeletons of American Indians revealed that RA did exist in the New World prior to the voyages of Columbus and even those

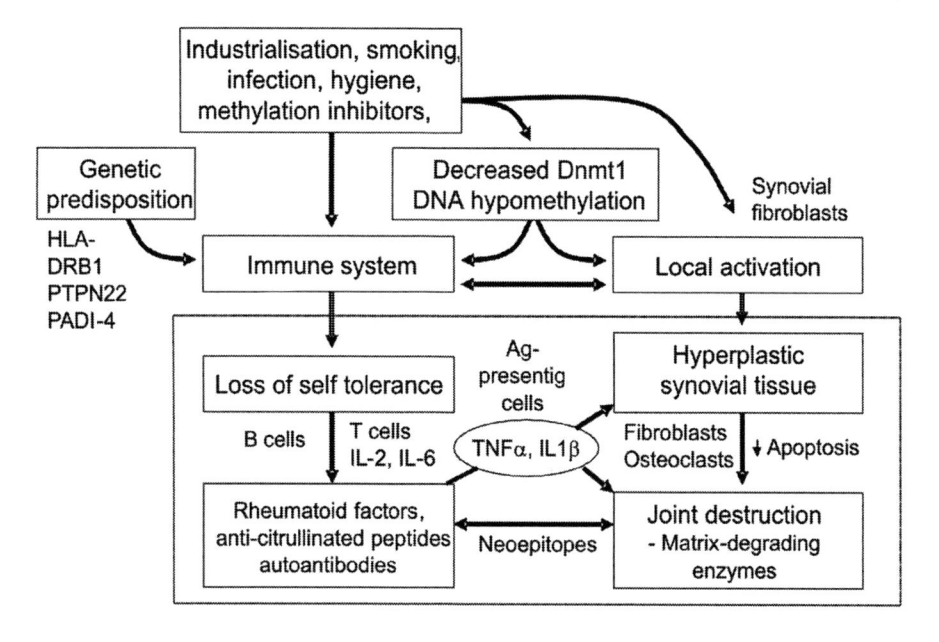

Figure 2. Pathogenesis of rheumatoid arthritis. T cells and synovial fibroblasts show global hypomethylation.

attributed to the Vikings. The arthritis in ancient American Indians of Tennessee (more than 4,000 years ago) is indistinguishable from contemporary RA. The female predominance (3:1), nature of bone involvement, X-ray appearance and distribution of joint involvement are identical to that found in living patients. According to this hypothesis, RA started as a disease of American Indians, who are still predisposed to this potentially crippling disease. The study of over 20,000 skeletons has identified its spread in North America and subsequently to Europe. These data indicate the presence of RA in a very small area of southwestern Kentucky, west-central Tennessee and northwestern Alabama in the archaic period (5000-500 BC). This was followed by a minor spread to Ohio in the Woodland period (500 BC-1000 AD). Finally, an explosive spread occurred after the late 18th century. Interestingly, in parallel, the first documented case of RA appeared in Europe at that time (Paris 1785). The nature of the disease may have altered at that time. Either the expression changed and it became more severe or the incidence of disease increased.[10] If this is true, American Indians should have old recepies against arthritides. Indeed, this is the case. Mashed yucca root mixed with water and swallowed is an American Indian arthritis remedy. The Cherokee Indians took the powered root of Aralia racemosa ("spikenard") as a tea for RA. They also pounded the root and applied it as a poultice to painful areas of the body. The spreading of the disease in the 18th century would suggest an infectious origin. Current models of RA propose that the initiating event is a T-cell response to an agent acquired from the environment, but the nature of this trigger is uncertain. Potential candidates implicated in an infectious etiology include Mycobacterium tuberculosis, Escherichia coli, Proteus mirabilis, Epstein-Barr virus, Parvovirus B19 and retroviruses. This was suggested to be supported by increased antibody titers to the infectious organism in RA or the possibility of molecular mimicry. A bacterial life form, *E. insidiosa*, can produce RA in deer, swine and dogs and a number of animals, including man, birds and fish might be infected by the organism. Examination of Cherokee folk beliefs suggests that they had some recognition of the connection between this infection and arthritis.[11] The importance of environmental factors in RA is suggested for example by the lower prevalence in rural Africans than in their counterparts who migrated to the towns.[12]

Early events in the infant development could influence the later occurrence of RA. Thus, high birth weight is positively associated and breast-feeding is negatively associated with RA.[13] High weight at one year of age is associated with occurrence of rheumatoid factors (RF).[14] RF are autoantibodies (IgA, IgM or IgG) that recognize the Fc parts of other antibodies and thus form immune complexes.

In addition, a significant association exists between infant hygiene and RF status among adult women. Sharing a bedroom during childhood is associated with a lower risk of being RF positive.[15] Thus, it appears that higher growth and less exposure to infections may increase the likelihood of developing RA and the RA-associated autoantibody RF. Parallels exist between an effect of hygiene on RF production and the effect of hygiene on allergy and asthma.

Such observations gave rise to the so-called "hygiene-hypothesis": Decreased infectious exposure is associated with increased allergy in the developed world.[16] This could be also the case for RA. It has been concluded that a developing immune system exposed to improved standards of hygiene is more likely to produce RF and perhaps begin the pathological process that leads to RA. Common mechanisms may be shared between autoimmune and allergic disease whereby infections at critical periods of development produce permanent and ultimately damaging changes in immune functioning. These, in conjunction with specific genetic background and other environmental factors may lead to disease.

Smoking is associated with an increased risk for developing RA and a more severe disease outcome.[17] The presence of risk factor PTPN22 (R620W variant) interacts with heavy cigarette smoking in a synergistic manner in RA.[7] Sirtuins (SIRTs) that deacetylate proteins, including histones and the subsequent influence on NF-kappaB-dependent gene expression could represent a link between smoking and epigenetics.[18,19] Infection and nutrition also were proposed to play a role in the disease.[20,21]

EPIGENETIC CONTROL OF IMMUNE SYSTEM IN RHEUMATOID ARTHRITIS

The use of HDAC inhibitors as therapeutic agents has been explored in RA.[22] In the RA synovial tissue, however, the balance of HAT and HDAC activities appears clearly in favour of HATs or a loss of HDAC activity.[23] The expression of the different HDACs has to be studied in the various subpopulations. Possibly, the effect of HDAC inhibitors could be mediated by nonhistone substrates. For example, TSA may inhibit NO production.[24]

Autoantibodies against citrullinated proteins are very specific for RA and can be found in 50-80% of the patients. In the presence of calcium ions, peptidylarginine deiminase (PADI) enzymes catalyze the posttranslational modification reaction generating citrulline residues. Mammalian PADI enzymes are involved in a number of regulatory processes during cell differentiation and development such as skin keratinization, myelin maturation and histone deimination. PADI-4, localized in the nucleus, is overexpressed in RA synovial tissues.[25] This enzyme could represent a link between high risk to develop RA and production of autoantibodies against citrullinated peptides.[5] Whether histone deimination is involved in the disease, however, is unknown. PADIs could play a role also in multiple sclerosis, in which the PADI-2 promoter is hypomethylated and the protein is overexpressed.[26] PADI-2 catalyses the myelin basic protein citrullination that results in a loss of myelin stability.

T- cell DNA is demethylated in RA and as in SLE, this may result in the generation of autoreactive T cells.[27] Interleukin-2 and Tumor Necrosis Factor alpha (TNFα) are regulated by epigenetics, their promoters being demethylated in activated T cells and in mature monocytes respectively. More relevant in the context of the disease was the report of a single unmethylated CpG motif in the 5′ regulatory region of the interleukin-6 (IL-6) gene in peripheral blood mononuclear cells taken from patients with RA.[28] The effector cells of joint destruction, however, are mainly the synovial fibroblasts. They produce matrix-degrading enzymes which lead to a progressive destruction of cartilage and bone.[29]

The main function of the normal synovial tissue is to supply the fluid which lubricates and amortises the joint to minimize the friction. In RA, the synovial tissue overgrows as a result of infiltration by cells of the immune system, activation and increased survival rate of the resident cells.

EPIGENETIC CONTROL OF RHEUMATOID ARTHRITIS SYNOVIAL FIBROBLASTS

Synovial fibroblasts origin from mesenchymal stem cells, which are undifferentiated, multipotent cells that reside in various human tissues and have the potential to differentiate into osteoblasts, chondrocytes, adipocytes or fibroblasts.[30] They are readily available reservoirs of reparative cells that are capable of mobilizing, proliferating and differentiating into the appropriate cell type in response to certain environmental signals. The development of mesenchymal stem cells is dependent on the microenvironment, such as stimulation from growth factors. Fibroblasts are metabolically active cells that have critical roles in the regulation of extracellular matrices, interstitial fluid volume and pressure as well as wound healing. During tissue repair, for instance, fibroblasts undergo a change in state from their normal, relatively quiescent phenotype, in which they are involved in the slow turnover of the extracellular matrix, to a proliferative and contractile phenotype termed myofibroblasts. Furthermore, fibroblasts are thought to develop specific characteristics in response to their microenvironment. To produce such characteristics, certain genes are silenced in fibroblasts in some tissues but expressed in those in other tissues. In the synovial tissue, as it is the case in other compartments, tissue-specific genes are expressed. These patterns of gene expression are, in large part, under epigenetic control (Fig. 3).

The activated phenotype of synovial fibroblasts in RA could be an intrinsic property of these cells. When co-implanted with human cartilage into severe, combined immunodeficient (SCID) mice, they are invasive even in the absence of other cells of the

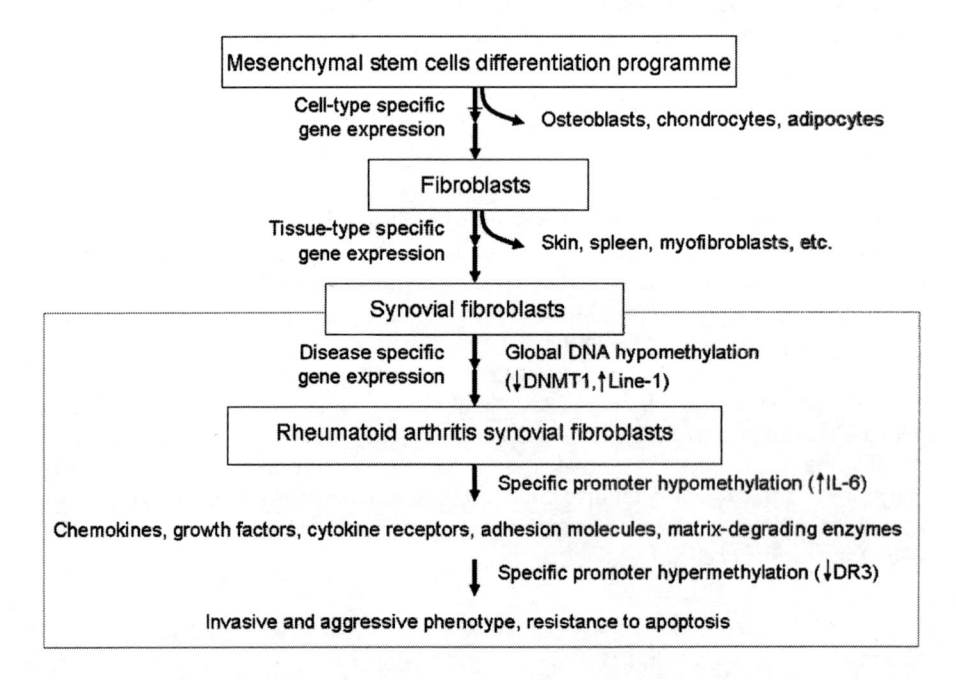

Figure 3. Epigenetic control of synovial fibroblast differentiation into aggressive cells in rheumatoid arthritis. Global hypomethylation and specific promoter hypermethylation are responsible for the aggressive phenotype and the resistance to apoptosis.

human immune system.[31] This concept is reflected in vitro by, for example, the increased production of matrix-degrading enzymes and adhesion molecules. The "imprinted" aggressive and invasive phenotype of synovial fibroblasts in RA could be determined by genetic and/or epigenetic modifications.

Synovial fibroblasts, more than other types of fibroblasts, acquire phenotypic characteristics commonly associated with transformed cells.[32] Synovial fibroblasts from patients with RA show "spontaneous" activities, associated with aggressive behavior and different from the synovial fibroblasts of patients with osteoarthritis or normal synovial fibroblasts. For example, RASF up-regulate proto-oncogenes, specific matrix degrading enzymes, adhesion molecules and produce cytokines, including interleukin-6 (IL-6).[33-36] These observations of an intrinsically activated cellular phenotype prompted us to search for epigenetic modifications.

The first evidence that epigenetics may play a role in the aggressive behavior of synovial fibroblasts in RA was the observation that the endogenous retroviral element LINE-1 is reactivated in the RA synovial lining and at sites of cartilage and bone invasion.[37-39] The expression of LINE-1 proteins in RA synovial tissues is associated with a partially hypomethylated promoter region.[40] In normal cells, repetitive sequences such as LINE-1, Alu and α-satellite repeats are silenced by methylation and their expression can reflect global DNA hypomethylation. This general cellular mechanism has important consequences in RA synovial fibroblasts because methylation markers are not correctly transmitted from mother to daughter cells. The incorrect methylation patterns induce either cellular dedifferentiation or a completely new phenotype. The cause could be a deficient production of DNMT1 in proliferating and activated RA synovial fibroblasts. Other diseases have also been associated with decreased activity of Dnmts. For example, ICF (immunodeficiency, centromeric region instability and facial anomalies) syndrome is an autosomal-recessive disease that is associated with abnormal DNA methylation and mutations in the catalytic domain of DNMT3b.[41] The disease causes immunodeficiency as a result of reduced immunoglobulin levels and involves chromosomal instability due to hypomethylation of satellite repeats.

With regard to the potential role of genomic hypomethylation in generating aggressive SFs, we hypothesized that the RASF phenotype could be mimicked in normal SFs by inhibition of DNMT1, for example by chronic treatment with a nontoxic dose of the DNA methyltransferase inhibitor 5-azacytidine.[40] In this study, about 200 genes were found to be chronically upregulated more than twofold by DNA hypomethylation, which was associated with enhanced protein expression in most cases. Furthermore, hypomethylation led to irreversible phenotypic changes in normal synovial fibroblasts, so that they resembled activated RA synovial fibroblasts. Proinflammatory cytokines such as tumor necrosis factor alpha, interleukin-1 beta and IL-6 have multiple and profound influences on the pathogenesis of RA. These cytokines can affect genomic methylation.[30,42-43] Pro-inflammatory cytokines and growth factors accelerate the cell cycle. During DNA replication, normal synovial fibroblasts recruit DNMT1 to interact with proliferating cell nuclear antigen (PCNA) at the DNA replication fork to ensure the correct setting of methylation markers. In RA synovial fibroblasts, however, DNMT1 is deficient and that results in a gradual genomic hypomethylation, a process that would worsen with each cell cycle. Alternatively, the ability to demethylate DNA actively has been attributed to various factors, including growth arrest and the p53-effector protein Gadd45a, a small p38 mitogen-activated protein kinase-binding molecule.[44] Interestingly, mice lacking the gene encoding Gadd45a develop autoimmunity.[45] Possibly, disruption in the p53-dependent cascade leads to increased invasiveness of RA synovial fibroblasts and may also transform normal synovial fibroblasts into cells that display an aggressive, RA-like behaviour.[46]

This raises also the question whether the global genomic hypomethylation is accompanied, or followed by specific promoter hypermethylation, as this is the case in various tumors. At least one example is reported in the literature, i.e., by silencing the death receptor 3, which could, at least in part, explain the relative resistance to apoptosis reported for RA synovial fibroblasts in certain patients.[47]

X-CHROMOSOME INACTIVATION

Worldwide, 0.8% of the population has RA, with 80% of patients developing their condition between 35 and 50 years of age; 67% of people with rheumatoid arthritis are women. The predominance of females among patients with autoimmune diseases suggests possible involvement of a defective X chromosome inactivation. X chromosome inactivation is an epigenetic event resulting in multiple levels of control for modulation of the expression of X-linked genes in normal female cells such that there remains only one active X chromosome in the cell. The extent of this control is unique among the chromosomes and has the potential for problems when regulation is disrupted.[48] Chromosome-wide inactivation is initiated by the expression of the long nonprotein-coding Xist RNA. This RNA is transcribed from the Xic gene on the future inactive X chromosome and accumulates over this chromosome triggering transcriptional silencing. Autoantibodies against structures of the inactivated X chromosome, colocalized with the Xist RNA, were reported in serum of patients with SLE.[49]

Xist RNA expression, however, is not sufficient for initiating gene repression. X chromosome inactivation is a multistep process that comprises an ordered series of chromatin modifications that occur in a developmentally regulated manner. Recruitment of Polycomb group proteins, which are known to be required for maintaining the repression of homeobox (Hox) genes, has been implicated in the transition from the initiation phase to the maintenance phase of X chromosome inactivation. HOX genes are transcription regulators involved in cell type-specific differentiation and patterning of the body plan in vertebrates. Particularly, the Hox D family is involved in limb formation in mice and chicks. Both Hox 4C and Hox D9 are over-expressed in RA synovial tissues.[50-51]

Compared to the active chromosome, the inactivated X chromosome has high levels of DNA methylation, low levels of histone acetylation, low levels of histone H3 K4 trimethylation and high levels of histone H3 K9 trimethylation, all of which are associated with gene silencing. In RA synovial tissues, high levels of histone acetylation is reported.[23]

Nonrandom X chromosome inactivation could be a factor in the development of autoimmune diseases. Hypothesized was that, in young females, the presentation of self-antigens could be biased by antigen-presenting cells during thymic development of tolerance for self-antigens. If self-antigens from the inactivated parentally derived X chromosome were not represented, then negative selection of auto-reactive T cells towards those self-antigens could not occur.[52] Evidence linking skewed X chromosome inactivation to autoimmunity was reported in RA.[53]

An important factor in RA is the abnormal pattern of methylation. 5-methylcytosine residues in the DNA are formed from the transfer of the methyl group from S-adenosylmethionine to the C-5 position of cytosine by the DNMts. A hypothesis has

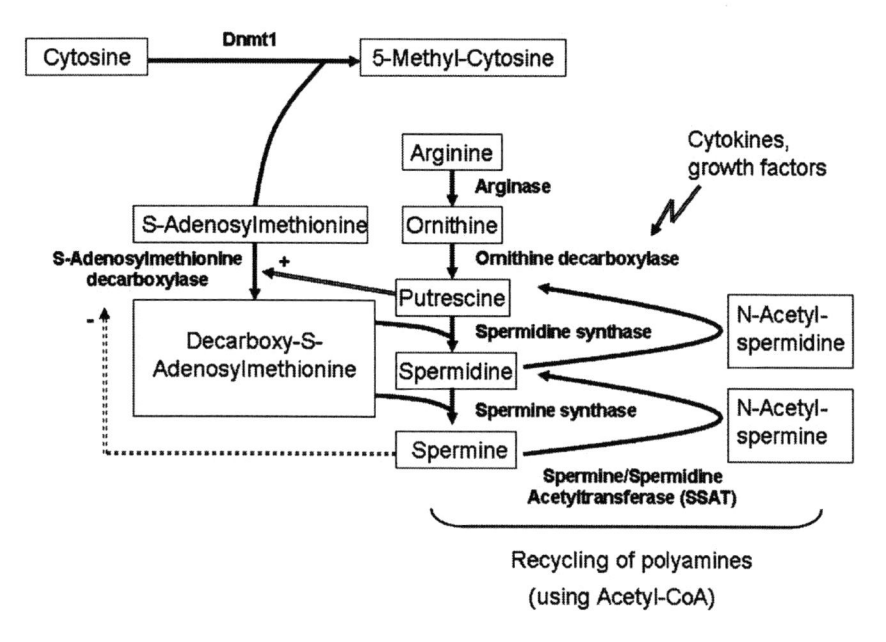

Figure 4. Biosysnthesis and recycling of polyamines, competition with dimethyltransferases for the pool of S-adenonsylmethionine.

been proposed that explains some autoimmune diseases as occurring due to loss of dosage compensation of X-linked polyamine genes at Xp22.1, which impact on intracellular methylation.[54] In this regard it is of interest that the polyamines, spermidine and spermin, are produced from ornithine after activation of the enzyme ornithine decarboxylase, which is responsive to various growth and inflammatory stimuli. S-Adenosylmethionine is required for the conversion into polyamines (putrescine, spermidine and spermine) (Fig. 4). The genes related to Xp22.1 are spermine synthase, which catalyse the conversion of spermidine into spermine and spermidine/spermine–N1–acetyltransferase (SSAT1), which recycles spermine and spermidine into putrescine. The expression of these enzymes is up-regulated in RA synovial fibroblasts by interleukin-1.[55-56] Thereby, free putrescine levels in synovial fluid were found to be significantly elevated in RA, compared to OA.[57] In accordance with the hypothesis of an increased polyamine recycling, urinary polyamine levels were also detected to be significantly elevated in patients with RA, compared to OA or healthy controls; they correlated to the degree of joint functional damage and radiological progression.[58] An over-expression of SSAT1 may result in a decrease of S-adenosylmethionine, the cell's methyl donor. This could account for an insufficient DNA methylation, in addition to the relative deficiency of DNMT1 during proliferation.[40]

AGING, EPIGENETICS AND AUTOIMMUNITY

Various epidemiological studies support the increasing risk of RA during aging. The immune system undergoes significant changes during aging which may lead to autoimmune disease. For example, rheumatoid factor increases during aging.[59] The expansion of the T-cell population of CD4+ CD28- is linked to aging and is tought to be associated with RA.[60] These cells are autoreactive, resistant to apoptosis and secrete large amounts of pro-inflammatory cytokines. The increased numbers of these cells correlate with the severity of RA. Also, B- cells of elderly persons produce antibodies that have lower affinity for antigen than young persons. Experimental data have shown that the increase of pro-inflammatory cytokines such as IL-6, TNF-alpha, C-reactive protein (CRP) occurred in elderly healthy persons.[61] In addition, the transcription factor NFk-beta that regulates the expression of a variety of pro-inflammatory genes increases with aging.[62] Therefore, chronic inflammation is more frequent during aging and might be associated with rheumatoid arthritis. Deregulation of the epigenome could be a consequence of changes in the immune system. Epigenetic studies in monozygotic twins showed that DNA methylation and histone modifications increase during aging.[63] Most importantly, the twins had large differences in epigenetic marks if they have developed a disease or they lived in different environments. An interesting study using monozygotic twins for SLE identified that the global 5-methylcytosine content is decreased in the identical twin with SLE, when compared with the healthy twin.[64] Also in the same study the authors observed changes in CpG areas and expression of ribosomal RNA genes. Other studies have measured the global DNA methylation levels and the methylation of CpG marks in Alu repeats and found that they are reduced during aging.[65] Furthermore, recent studies showed that certain genes become either hypermethylated or hypomethylated in animals depending on their age.[66] These changes have been shown to be tissue specific. Thus, changes in epigenetic marks occurring during aging should be taken into consideration in studies investigating DNA methylation in rheumatoid arthritis.

CONCLUSION AND OUTLOOK

The pathogenesis of rheumatoid arthritis as described in this chapter is poorly understood; clearly, it has both genetic and environmental components. How environmental factors contribute to the development of this disease is still largely unknown. However, convincing evidence emerged recently that the environment modifies the disease susceptibility (and perhaps even severity) through epigenetic mechanisms. In this regard, the investigation of the discordance in disease between monozygotic twins could be of special interest. Monozytic twins accumulate epigenetic differences during their lifetime that can be attributed to environmental factors, such as smoking, infections, nutrition, reproduction and exposition to xenobiotics.

Recent data have demonstrated that global genomic hypomethylation might play a role in the pathogenesis of RA, not only in T cells, but also regarding synovial fibroblasts, the effector cells of joint damage; genes overexpressed in this context contribute to the activated phenotype of RA synovial fibroblasts. The genomic location which allows such a general activation of the cell is still not known; possibly, methylation-sensitive transcription factors are involved. It can be expected that in some cases, global DNA hypomethylation is followed by a specific gene hypermethylation, as it has been described in numerous cancers. However, the hypomethylated cells often showed a decreased expression of DNMT1 that represent a strategy to avoid transformation, i.e., a random methylation of genes due to a deficient DNA template during replication that at the end results in tumor cells in the case that genes of the cell cycle or in the regulation of apoptosis are affected. Unclear is also whether epigenetic changes or the disease come first. The timing and the hierarchy of the events need to be investigated. A whole epigenome approach would be useful, using e.g., tiling arrays. The cause of epigenetic disorders could be multiple, from environmental stimuli, the inflammatory milieu, to an increased degradation of DNMT1 and/or an increased recycling of polyamines. Reversing DNA hypomethylation could be a challenge for the future, for example by a treatment with S-adenosylmethionine and inhibiting the recycling of polyamines. However, inhibiting SSAT1 also might be necessary to block the increased consumption of S-adenosylmethionine. Clearly, different mechanisms of deregulation probably account for each of the diseases, including various causes of DNA hypomethylation and modifications in the histone code. Regarding therapies on an epigenetic basis, it is interesting to note that HDAC inhibitors have selective anti-inflammatory and immune modulating activities. Many of them (e.g., phenylbutyrate, TSA, FK288, SAHA, MS-275) were found beneficial in animal models. However, it will be important to develop inhibitors selective for HDAC isoenzymes. Chromatin immunoprecipitation in conjunction with microarray hybridization or coupled with high-throughput sequencing, using specific antibodies against different histone modifications will help to elucidate the sequential changes in the histone modification profile. Finally, the role of other components of the nucleus, such as HMG1 (high-mobility group box 1) and methyl binding proteins, that can regulate gene transcription in RA should be investigated.

REFERENCES

1. Ebringer A, Wilson C, Tiwana H. Is rheumatoid arthritis a form of reactive arthritis? J Rheumatol 2000; 27:559-563.
2. Nepom GT, Byers P, Seyfried C et al. HLA genes associated with rheumatoid arthritis. Identification of susceptibility alleles using specific oligonucleotide probes. Arthritis Rheum 1989; 32:15-21.
3. Robertson KD. DNA methylation and human disease. Nat Rev Genet 2005; 6(8):597-610.
4. Alercon-Segovia D, Alecon-Riquelme ME, Cardiel MH et al. Famillial aggregation of sistemi lupus erythematosus, rheumatoid arthritis and other autoimmune diseases in 1,177 lupus patients from the GLADEL color. Arthritis Rheum 2005; 52:1138-1147.
5. Orozco G, Rueda B, Martin J. Genetic basis of rheumatoid arthritis. Biomed Pharmacother 2006; 60:656-662.
6. Orozco G, Pascual-Salcedo D, Lopez-Nevot MA et al. Auto-antibodies, HLA and PTPN22: susceptibility markers for rheumatoid arthritis. Rheumatology 2008; 47:138-141.
7. Costenbader KL, Chang SC, De Vivo I et al. Genetic polymorphisms in PTPN22, PADI-4 and CTLA-4 and risk for rheumatoid arthritis in two longitudinal cohort studies: evidence of gene-environment interactions with heavy cigarette smocking. Arthritis Res Ther 2008; 10:R52.
8. Rogers J, Dieppe P. Skeletal palaeopathology and the rheumatic diseases: where are we now? Ann Rheum Dis 1990; 49:885-886.
9. Rothschild BM. Tennessee origin of rheumatoid arthritis. Res Notes 1991; 5, F.H. McClung Museum.
10. Gunnell D, Roggers J, Dieppe P. Height and health: predicting longevity from bone length in archaeological remains. J Epidemiol Community Health 2001; 55:505-507.
11. Bridges PS. Prehistoric arthritis in the Americas. Ann Rev Anthropology 1992; 21:67-91.
12. Wordsworth P, Bell J. Polygenic susceptibility in rheumatoid arthritis. Ann Rheum Dis 1991; 50:343-346.
13. Jacobsson LT, Jacobsson ME, Askling J et al. Perinatal characteristics and risk of rheumatoid arthritis. Brit Med J 2003; 326:1068-1069.
14. Walker-Bone K, Farrow S. Rheumatoid arthritis. Clin Evid (Online) 1 2007; pii:1124.
15. Edwards CJ, Goswami R, Goswami P et al. Growth and infectious exposure during infancy and the risk of rheumatoid factor in adult life. Ann Rheum Dis 2006; 65:401-404.
16. Strachan DP. Hay fever, hygiene and household size. Brit Med J 1989; 299:1259-1260.
17. Klareskog L, Stolt P, Lundberg K et al. A new model fo an etiology of rheumatoid arthritis : smoking may trigger HLA-DR (shared epitope)-restricted immune reactions to autoantigens modified by citrullination. Arthritis Rheum 2006; 54:38-46.

18. Yang SR, Wright J, Bauter M et al. Sirtuin regulates cigarette smoke-induced proinflammatory mediator release via RelA/p65 NF-kappaB in macrophages in vitro and in rat lungs in vivo: implication for chronic inflammation and aging. Am J Physiol Lung Cell Mol Physiol 2007; 292:L567-576.

19. Kawahara TL, Mischishita F, Adler AS et al. SIRT6 links histone H3 lysine 9 deacetylation to NF-kappaB-dependant gene expression and organismal life span. Cell 2009; 136:62-74.

20. Smith JB, Haynes MK. Rheumatoid arthritis—a molecular understanding. Ann Intern Med 2002; 136:908-922.

21. Ermann J, Fathman CG. Autoimmune diseases: genes, bugs and failed regulation. Nat Immunol 2001; 2:759-761.

22. Grablec AM, Tak PP, Reedquist KA. Trageting histone deacetylase activity in rheumatoid arthritis and asthma as prototypes of inflammatory disease: should we keep our HATs on? Arthritis Res Ther 2008; 10:226.

23. Huber LC, Brock M, Hemmtazad H et al. Histone deacetylase/acetylase activity in total synovial tissue derived from rheumatoid arthritis and osteoarthritis patients. Arthritis Rheum 2007; 56:1087-1093.

24. Garcia BA, Busby SA, Shabanowitz J et al. Resetting the epigenetic histone code in the MRL-lpr/lpr mouse model of lupus by histone deacetylase inhibition. J Proteome Res 2005; 4:2032-2042.

25. Chang X, Zhao Y, Sun S et al. The expression of PADI4 in synovium of rheumatoid arthritis. Rheumatol Int 2009; 29:1411-1416.

26. Moscarello MA, Mastronardi FG, Wood DD. The role of citrullinated proteins suggests a novel mechanism in the pathogenesis of multiple sclerosis. Neurochem Res 2007; 32:251-256.

27. Richardon B, Scheinbart L, Strahler J et al. Evidence of impaired T-cell DNA methylation in systemic lupus erythematosus and rheumatoid arthritis. Arthritis Rheum 1990; 33:1665-1673.

28. Nile CJ, Read RC, Akil M et al. Methylation status of a single CpG site in the IL6 promoter is related to IL6 messenger RNA levels and rheumatoid arthritis. Arthritis Rheum 2008; 58:2686-2693.

29. Karouzakis E, Neidhart M, Gay RE et al. Molecular and cellular basis of rheumatoid joint destruction. Immunol Lett 2006; 106:8-13.

30. Karouzakis E, Gay RE, Gay S. Epigenetic control in rheumatoid arthritis synovial fibroblasts. Nat Rev Rheumatol 2009; 5:266-272.

31. Muller-Ladner U, Pap T, Gay RE et al. Mechanisms of disease: the molecular and cellular basis of joint destruction in rheumatoid arthritis. Nat Clin Pract Rheumatol 2005; 1:102-110.

32. Lafyatis R, Remmers EF, Roberts AB et al. Anchorage-independent growth of synoviocytes from arthritic and normal joints. Stimulation by exogenous platelet-derived growth factor and inhibition by transforming growth factor-beta and retinoids. J Clin Invest 1989; 83:1267-1276.

33. Müller-Ladner U, Kriegsmann J, Gay RE et al. Oncogenes in rheumatoid arthritis. Rheum Dis Clin North Am 1995; 21:675-690.

34. Konttinen YT, Ainola M, Valleala H et al. Analysis of 16 different matrix metalloproteinases (MMP-1 to MMP-20) in the synovial membrane: different profiles in trauma and rheumatoid arthritis. Ann Rheum Dis 1999; 58:691-697.

35. Rinaldi N, Schwarz-Eywill M, Weis D et al. Increased expression of integrins on fibroblast-like synoviocytes from rheumatoid arthritis in vitro correlates with enhanced binding to extracellular matrix proteins. Ann Rheum Dis 1997; 56:45-51.

36. Firestein GS, Alvaro-Gracia JM, Maki R. Quantitative analysis of cytokine gene expression in rheumatoid arthritis. J Immunol 1990; 144:3347-3353.

37. Neidhart M, Rethage J, Kuchen S et al. Retrotransposable L1 elements expressed in rheumatoid arthritis synovial tissue: association with genomic hypomethylation and influence on gene expression. Arthritis Rheum 2000; 43:2634-2647.

38. Ali M, Veale DJ, Reece RJ et al. Overexpression of transcripts containing LINE-1 in the synovia of patients with rheumatoid arthritis. Ann Rheum Dis 2003; 62:663-666.

39. Kuchen S, Seemayer CA, Rethage J et al. The L1 retroelement-related p40 protein induces p38delta MAP kinase. Autoimmunity 2004; 37:57-65.

40. Karouzakis E, Gay RE, Michel BA et al. DNA hypomethylation in rheumatoid arthritis synovial fibroblasts. Arthritis Rheum 2009; 60(12):3613-3622.

41. Xu GL, Bestor TH, Bourc'his D et al. Chromosome instability and immunodeficiency syndrome caused by mutations in a DNA methyltransferase gene. Nature 1999; 402:187-191.

42. Hmadcha A, Bedoya FJ, Sobrino F et al. Methylation-dependent gene silencing induced by interleukin 1 β via nitric oxide production. J Exp Med 1999; 190:1595-1604.

43. Wehbe H, Henson R, Meng F et al. Interleukin-6 contributes to growth in cholangiocarcinoma cells by aberrant promoter methylation and gene expression. Cancer Res 2006; 66:10517-10524.

44. Barreto G, Schäfer A, Marhold J et al. Gadd45a promotes epigenetic gene activation by repair-mediated DNA demethylation. Nature 2007; 445:671-675.

45. Salvador JM, Hollander MC, Nguyen AT et al. Mice lacking the p53-effector gene Gadd45a develops a lupus-like syndrome. Immunity 2002; 16:499-508.

46. Pap T, Aupperle KR, Gay S et al. Invasiveness of synovial fibroblasts is regulated by p53 in the SCID mouse in vivo model of cartilage invasion. Arthritis Rheum 2001; 44:676-681.
47. Takami N, Osawa K, Miura Y et al. Hypermethylated promoter region of DR3, the death receptor 3 gene, in rheumatoid arthritis synovial cells. Arthritis Rheum 2006; 54:779-787.
48. Yin X, Latif R, Tomer Y et al. Thyroid epigenetics: X chromosome inactivation in patients with autoimmune thyroid disease. Ann NY Acad Sci 2007; 1110:193-200.
49. Hong B, Reeves P, Panning B. Identification of an autoimmune serum containing antibodies against the Barr body. Proc Natl Acad Sci USA 2001; 98:8703-8708.
50. Xue C, Hasunuma T, Asahara H et al. Transcriptional regulation of the HOX4C gene by basic fibroblast growth factor on rheumatoid synovial fibroblasts. Arthritis Rheum 1997; 40:1628-1635.
51. Nguyen NC, Hirose T, Nakazawa M et al. Expression of HOXD9 in fibroblast-like synoviocytes from rheumatoid arthritis patients. Int J Mol Med 2002; 10:41-48.
52. Brooks WH. X chromosome inactivation and autoimmunity. Clinic Rev Allergy Immunol 2009; in press.
53. Brix TH, Knudsen GP, Kristiansen M et al. High frequency of skewed X-chromosome inactivation in females with autoimmune thyroid disease: a possible explanation for the female predisposition to thyroid autoimmunity. J Clin Endocrinol Metab 2005; 90:5949-5953.
54. Ozbalkan Z, Bagişlar S, Kiraz S et al. Skewed X chromosome inactivation in blood cells of women with scleroderma. Arthritis Rheum 2005; 52:1564-1570.
55. Furumitsu Y, Yukioka K, Yukioka M et al. Interleukin-1beta induces elevation of spermidine/spermine N1-acetyltransferase activity and an increase in the amount of putrescine in synovial adherent cells from patients with rheumatoid arthritis. J Rheumatol 2000; 27:1352-1357.
56. Andreas K, Lübke C, Häupl T et al. Key regulatory molecules of cartilage destruction in rheumatoid arthritis: an in vitro study. Arthritis Res Ther 2008;10:R9.
57. Yukioka K, Yukioka K, Kojima A et al. Polyamine levels in synovial tissues and synovial fluids of patients with rheumatoid arthritis. J Rheumatol 1992; 19:689-692.
58. Furumitsu Y, Yukioka K, Kojima A et al. Levels of urinary polyamines in patients with rheumatoid arthritis. J Rheumatol 1993; 20:1661-1665.
59. Hasler P, Zouali M. Immune receptor signaling, aging and autoimmunity. Cell Immunol 2005; 233(2):102-108.
60. Goronzy JJ, Weyand CM. Aging, autoimmunity and arthritis: T-cell senescence and contraction of T-cell repertoire diversity—catalysts of autoimmunity and chronic inflammation. Arthritis Res Ther 2003; 5(5):225-234.
61. Johnson TE. Recent results: biomarkers of aging. Exp Gerontol 2006; 41(12):1243-1246.
62. Adler AS, Sinha S, Kawahara TL. Motif module map reveals enforcement of aging by continual NF-kappaB activity. Genes Dev 2007; 21(24):3244-3257.
63. Fraga MF, Ballestar E, Paz MF. Epigenetic differences arise during the lifetime of monozygotic twins. Proc Natl Acad Sci USA 2005; 102(30):10604-10609.
64. Javierre BM, Fernandez AF, Richter J. Changes in the pattern of DNA methylation associate with twin discordance in systemic lupus erythematosus. Genome Res 2010; 20(2):170-179.
65. Wilson VL, Smith RA, Ma S. Genomic 5-methyldeoxycytidine decreases with age. J Biol Chem 1987; 262(21):9948-9951.
66. Maegawa S, Hinkal G, Kim HS. Widespread and tissue specific age-related DNA methylation changes in mice. Genome Res 2010; 20(3):332-340.

CHAPTER 11

PROSPECTS FOR EPIGENETIC COMPOUNDS IN THE TREATMENT OF AUTOIMMUNE DISEASE

Nadine Chapman-Rothe and Robert Brown

Department of Surgery and Cancer, Hammersmith Hospital Campus, Imperial College London, London, UK
Emails: Nadine Chapman-Rothe—nadine.rothe04@imperial.ac.uk; Robert Brown—b.brown@imperial.ac.uk

Abstract: There is growing evidence for a role for epigenetic mechanisms in the development of autoimmune diseases. In most cases of autoimmune disease the precise epigenetic mechanism involved remains to be resolved, however DNA hypomethylation accompanied by hypoacetylation of histone H3/H4 is commonly observed. Due to the reversible nature of epigenetic marks their maintenance enzymes such as DNA methyltransferases (DNMTs), histone deacetylases (HDACs) and histone lysine methyltransferases (HKMT) are attractive drug targets. Small molecule inhibitors of histone modification and DNA methylation maintenance are increasingly becoming available and will be useful chemical biological tools to dissect epigenetic mechanisms in these diseases. However, although epigenetic therapies used in cancer treatment are a promising starting point for the exploration of autoimmune disease treatment, there is a requirement for more specific and less toxic agents for these chronic diseases or for use as chemopreventative agents.

INTRODUCTION

The finding that malignant cancer cells display a multitude of epigenetic alterations, has triggered extensive research into epigenetic drug development. Since research into autoimmune diseases has also revealed that epigenetic mechanisms contribute to the development of autoimmune diseases, epigenetic therapies from the cancer arena seem to be a promising starting point for the exploration of autoimmune disease treatment. Due to the reversible nature of epigenetic marks their maintenance enzymes such as DNA methyltransferases (DNMTs), histone deacetylases (HDACs) and histone lysine methyltransferases (HKMT) are attractive drug targets. So far, a few promising compounds that target such epigenetic maintenance enzymes are in cancer clinical trials or registered for use against certain malignancies. Although in most cases of autoimmune disease the precise epigenetic mechanism involved remains to be resolved, it appears that one common feature is DNA hypomethylation which is accompanied by hypoacetylation of histone H3/H4. Options for epigenetic therapies are so far limiting, however we will discuss one of the most promising druggable targets: histone deacetylases (HDACs). Since the epigenetic mechanisms of most autoimmune diseases have not been fully resolved yet, additional epigenetic targets and future perspectives will also be discussed.

THE CLASSES OF HDACs AND THEIR INHIBITORS

The enzymes removing acetyl-groups of histone tails are known as histone deacetylases (HDACs) and are presented by two distinct protein classes, the SIR2 family of NAD+-dependent HDACs (Class III) and the classical HDAC family. The latter consists of two different phylogenetic groups, namely Class I and Class II whose action is zinc dependent.[1] The HDACs of Class I are most closely related to the *S. cerevisiae* transcriptional regulator RPD3, whereas class II HDACs share homology with HDAC1, another yeast deacetylase (see ref. 2). HDAC functions and main targets are presented in Table 1.

As shown in Table 1 each HDAC regulates its own more or less specific substrates or pathways, potentially making each HDAC a specific target for inhibition. However, to date there are few specific inhibitors against individual HDACs and most available compounds inhibit an entire class.[3] Despite these hurdles, investigations are underway and the subsequent paragraph introduces the most common HDAC inhibitors (HDACi) and their targeted classes. Interest in further HDACi development for cancer therapy has been fuelled by the over-expression of HDAC1 in colon and several other tumor types and the suppression of tumor growth following knock-down of formerly over-expressed HDACs.[4]

HDAC inhibitors have demonstrated antitumor activity in clinical trials and one drug of this class, Vorinostat (SAHA), is US Food and Drug Administration approved for the treatment of cutaneous T-cell lymphoma. The hydroxamic acid moiety of inhibitors such as Vorinostat directly interact with the zinc ion at the base of the catalytic pocket.[5] Due to fundamental epigenetic differences of normal and tumor cells, HDACi are proposed to selectively kill tumor cells at lower concentrations than normal cells, suggesting the existence of an optimal therapeutic window.[6] Although the majority of HDACi drug development has focused on the treatment of cancer, their potential as anti-inflammatory agents has been proposed.[7] Recent studies have shown the potential anti-inflammatory action of several HDACi in animal studies and therefore opened a new path for the treatment of autoimmune diseases.[8] Such animal model studies have suggested that HDACi may be a promising experimental chemical tool, especially for the treatment of chronic immune and inflammatory disorders such as rheumatoid arthritis (RA), psoriasis, inflammatory bowel disease (IBD), multiple sclerosis and systemic lupus erythematosus (SLE).[8]

The following Table 2 gives a brief overview of different HDACi classes and their compounds which are currently either in clinical studies or approved.

HDACs interact with multiple protein complexes as well as histones, have multiple additional protein targets, some of which can be found listed in Table 3. Therefore, the efficacy of HDACis in autoimmune diseases may be due not only to their effect on the histone acetylation status itself, but also on other acetylated proteins in the cell. For example, acetylation of p53 is required for its transcription independent functions associated with activation of the pro-apoptotic gene (BAX), reactive oxygen species production and apoptosis in response to HDACis. For instance, the acetylation of p53 prevented the formation of the Ku70-BAX complex, thereby enhancing apoptosis.[9]

HDACi can selectively alter gene transcription, partly through chromatin remodelling and partly through changes in the structure of proteins in transcription factor complexes.[10] It is worth emphasizing that important regulatory proteins such as hormone receptors,

Table 1. Histone deacetylases families and their known functions

HDAC Class	Name	Function
HDAC class I	HDAC1 and HDAC2	Complex dependent; found in Sin2, NuRD and Co-REST, can act directly on DNA-binding proteins (YY1, Rb binding protein 1 and SP1), phosphorylation required for function
	HDAC3	SMRT and N-CoR are necessary for activity, is able to form oligomers with other HDACs like HDAC4 and 5, but mostly it interacts with itself, may have role in cell cycle progression
	HDAC8	Similar to HDAC3, probably very low abundance of expression
HDAC class II	HDAC6	Exhibits two catalytical domains in tandem, has signal for ubiquitination, probably particularly prone to degradation, functions as tubulin deacetylase but it is also found in the nucleus together with HDAC11
	HDAC10	Exists in two splice variants, interacts with HDAC1, 2, 3, 4, 5 and 7
	HDAC4	Exhibits binding domains for CTBP, MEF2; amongst others it shows interaction with BCL6, CBX5, MAPK1, RbAP40 and HDAC3
	HDAC5	Interacts only with HDAC3 and MEF2. Deacetylates core histones (H2A, H2B, H3 and H4); is also involved in muscle maturation by repressing transcription of myocyte enhancer MEF2C
	HDAC7	Deacetylates core histones (H2A, H2B, H3 and H4), also involved in muscle maturation by repressing transcription of myocyte enhancer factors such as MEF2A, MEF2B and MEF2C. May be involved in Epstein-Barr virus (EBV) latency, possibly by repressing the viral BZLF1 gene
	HDAC9a, 9b, HDRP	Are splice variants, HRDP lacks the catalytic domain but it is able to recruit HDAC3. All three interact with MEF2 indicating a function in muscle differentiation

continued on next page

Table 1. Continued

HDAC Class	Name	Function
HDAC11	HDAC11	More closely related to class I than to class II, not present in any known HDAC complex
HDAC class III—SIR2 family	SIRT1	Deacetylates histones (preference for H4K16), PCAF/MyoD, EP300, TAF168, HTATSF1, TP53, XRCC6, NKRF and forkhead proteins. Regulation of insulin and glucose homeostasis, fat reduction and neuron survival
	SIRT2	Predominantly cytoplasmatic, deacetylates -tubulin and histones, overexpression delays mitosis, SIRT2 colocalises with chromatin during G2/M transition, preference for H4K16 in vitro
	SIRT3	Localized to mitochondrial matrix, deacetylates in vitro, multiple substrates including histones and tubulin, may be important under conditions of energy limitations
	SIRT4	Localized to mitochondria and lacks detectable deacetylase activity but shows ADP-ribosyltransferase activity
	SIRT5	Localized to mitochondria with weak deacetylase activity and no apparent ADP-ribosyltransferase activity
	SIRT6	Nuclear protein, regulates DNA repair, role in aging
	SIRT7	Localized to nucleolus and promotes rRNA transcription, associated with RNA pol I, so far, no deacetylase activity measured, but activity NAD-dependent

chaperon proteins and cytoskeleton proteins, which regulate cell proliferation, immune response and cell death, are nonhistone protein targets of HDACi. The acetylation status of several important gene regulator and transcription factors associated with cellular immunity is well known, such as E2F1, p53, STAT1, STAT3 and NF-κB and importantly all of those genes have been shown to respond to HDACi treatment.[11-16] STAT1, STAT3 and NF-κB are often considered to be "master immune" regulatory transcription factors and since their activity is directly regulated by acetylation, HDACi treatment can lead to changes of their downstream targets such as changes in cytokine levels and effects on immune cell functions.[17] Thus, the expression of downstream target genes might be affected following HDACi treatment through hyperacetylation of STAT1, STAT3 and NF-κB, rather than through histone hyperacetylation affecting transcription of these genes. Furthermore, increasing evidence supports a role for acetylation of transcription factors in mediating the selective induction of apoptotic genes in response to DNA damage such as the acetylation of p53 following DNA damage.[18] Lastly, HDACi treatments are also known to elevate reactive oxygen species (ROS) levels, which can induce cell death in a manner independent of caspase activation (see ref. 3).

Table 2. Classes and names of common HDAC inhibitors, their targets and clinical trial status. HDAC, histone deacetylase; HDACi, HDAC inhibitors. N/A, not available.

Class of HDACi	Compounds	HDAC Target	Clinical Trials
Hydroxamate	Suberoylanilide hydroxamic acid (SAHA, Vorinostat)	Class I, II	Approved for advanced T cell lymphoma
	PXD101, LAQ824, LBH589	Class I, II	Phase II
	Trichostatin (TSA),	Class I, II	N/A
	Oxamflatin, Scriptaid, Suberic bishydroxamic acid (SBHA), Azelaic bishydroxamic acid (ABHA), CG-1521	N/A	N/A
	Pyroxamide	Class I, unknown effect on class II	Phase I
	SK-7041, SK-7068	HDACs1 and 2	N/A
	Tubacin	HDAC6	N/A
Alipathic acid	Phenylbutyrate, Valproic acid (VPA)	Class I, II	Phase I, II
	AN-9 (prodrug), Savicol	N/A	N/A
	Baceca	Class I	Phase I, II
Benzamide	MS-275	HDACs 1, 2, 3 and slightly 8	Phase I, II
	MGCD0103	HDAC1, 2, 3, 11	Phase I, II
Cyclic peptide	Depsipeptide (FK228)	Class I	Phase I, II
	Trapoxin A	Class I, II	N/A
	Apicidin	HDAC 1, 3	N/A
	CHAPs	Class I	N/A

Reproduced from: Chapman-Rothe N, Brown R. Future Med Chem 2009; 1(8):1481-1495;[67] with permission of Future Science Ltd.

A number of animal experiments in a range of autoimmune disease models point towards HDACi efficacy in reducing common symptoms of arthritis.[19] One example is rheumatoid arthritis (RA).[20] In RA, the HDACs antirheumatic properties are proposed as being due to the inhibition of the nuclear factor kappa B (NF-κB), leading to the suppression of a variety of pro-inflammatory cytokines and matrix metalloproteases (MMPs), with subsequent inhibition of rheumatoid arthritis synovial fibroblast (RASF) proliferation.[8] Interestingly, in the human cartilage, matrix lying chondrocytes also responded well to the HDACis Trichostatin-A (TSA) and butyrate, showing suppressed pro-inflammatory mediator expression[21] and decreased expression of MMPs, thereby preventing the degradation of collagen and aggrecan.[22] Furthermore, in a rat adjuvant-induced arthritis model p16 and p21 in RASFs were induced following Phenylbutyrate and TSA treatment, which has been suggested to be linked to preventing further pannus formation, cartilage and bone destruction and also to reduced joint swelling.[23] TSA treatment also sensitized RASFs for TRAIL-induced apoptosis[24] and in combination with ultrasound induced RASFs specific apoptosis.[25]

Table 3. Proteins targeted by histone deacetylases

Function	Proteins
DNA binding transcriptional factors	P53, c-Myc, AML1, BCL-6, E2F1, E2F2, E2F3, GATA-1, GATA-2, GATA-3, GATA-4, Ying Yang 1 (YY1), NF-κB, MEF2, CREB, HIF-1a, BETA2, POP-1, IRF-2, IRF-7, SRY, EKLF
Steroid receptors	Androgen receptor, estrogen receptor a, glucocorticoid receptor
Transcription coregulators	RB, DEK, MSL-3, HMGI(Y)/HMGA1, CtBP2, PGC-1α
Signalling mediators	STAT3, Smad7, β-catenin, IRS-1
DNA repair enzymes	Ku70, WRN, TDG, NEIL2, FEN1
Nuclear import	Rch1, importin-α7
Chaperon protein	HSP90
Structural protein	α-tubulin
Inflammation mediator	HMGB1
Viral proteins	E1A, L-HDAg, S-HDAg, T-antigen, HIV Tat

Table adapted from Bolden et al, 2006.[3]

Similarly, in preclinical rodent models of Type-II collagen-induced arthritis, HDACis Vorinostat and Entinostat soothed paw swelling and decreased bone erosion and bone resorption which are key complications of the disease.[26] Comparable results were achieved with Romidepsin which suppressed joint swelling, synovial inflammation and bone and cartilage destruction in a mouse autoantibody-induced arthritis model.[27] Romidepsin also inhibited angiogenesis and significantly decreased TNFα and IL-1 levels in synovial tissues mainly through the re-expression of p16 and p21.[28] Comparable results were achieved with the ITF-2357 inhibitor.[29]

The inhibition of NF-κB activation in macrophages through the local administration of butyrate also proved beneficial for the treatment of ulcerative colitis in an inflammatory bowel mouse diseases (IBD) model.[30,31] Moreover in preclinical mouse disease models the administration of Vorinostat and Valporate improved colitis induced via a clear inhibition of colonic pro-inflammatory cytokines.[32] The administration of HDACis also proved beneficial in mouse models resembling systemic lupus erythematosus (SLE). SLE is characterized by increased cytokine levels, deregulated autoantibody production and renal inflammation. Here, TSA and Vorinostat evoked a reduction in proteinuria, glomerulonephritis and spleen weight which was accompanied by suppression of proinflammatory cytokines and reduction of auto-antibodies.[33] In an animal model resembling multiple sclerosis (MS), TSA reduced spinal cord inflammation and neuronal axonal loss. Here, TSA also improved the disability in the relapsing phase of experimental autoimmune encephalomyelitis (EAE), a widely-employed rodent model of MS.[34,35] Lastly, a recent report showing the over-expression of HDAC1 in psoriatic skin, points towards another possible application range for HDACis.[36]

As promising as the available HDAC inhibitors are, their great disadvantage is the lack of specificity. So far, except for tubacln which specifically targets HDAC6, usually an entire class rather than a specific enzyme is inhibited by the majority of HDACi undergoing clinical evaluation.[18] Although it is likely that more specific inhibitors will become available, these will require complete re-evaluation for safety and efficacy. While pan-HDACis have proven useful in the treatment of certain cancers, where they are given over a short time period to a life-threatening disease, their use to treat chronic conditions over extended periods of time raises different issues. HDAC inhibitors are generally well tolerated with limited hematological toxicity, however dose dependent toxicities that have been consistently observed including nausea, fatigue and flushing. Cardiac toxicity is also a consistent feature, with asymptomatic T wave changes being a frequent finding. Significant dysrhythmias however are seen only rarely. This T wave flattening has been observed with all the pan-HDACi studied and despite the different chemical properties of these drugs suggesting a drug class effect common to all pan-HDACis. It remains uncertain whether more specific drugs targeting a specific HDAC will avoid these toxicities while retaining efficacy, or whether alternative targets, with reduced toxicity when inhibited, will have to be considered.

DNMT INHIBITORS

Although so far there is no evidence for a global hypermethylation occurring in autoimmune diseases, patients suffering from the inflammatory bowel disease (IBD) appear to gain aberrant methylation in some of the WNT signalling genes during disease progression. This progressive feature starts at an early event in the disease and seems to be limited to the methylation of WNT signalling genes during the development of IBD-associated neoplasis. Moreover, methylation of APC1A, APC2, SFRP1 and SFRP2 appears to mark the progression of IBD colitis to IBD-associated neoplasia.[37]

One of the most studied and advanced drug class of epigenetic therapies are DNMT inhibitors (DNMTis). At present DNMTis are either based on cytidine derivatives, nucleosides which are incorporated into DNA during DNA replication, or small molecule compounds directly targeting DNMTs, such as catalytic site inhibitors.[38] Once derivatives are incorporated into DNA, due to the replacement of the N at position 5 of cytidine as in 5-azacytosine (Vidaza) and 5-aza-2'-deoxycytidine (Decitabine/Dacogen), they impede the resolution of a covalent reaction intermediate, preventing the release of the DNMT.[39] Through the degradation of DNMT adducts methyltransferase activity is eventually depleted. Subsequent cell divisions will lead to an increasing loss of DNA methylation. In haematological cancer both drugs restored activity of epigenetically silenced tumor suppressor genes (see ref. 40). An increasing number of putative nonnucleoside DNMTis are now being examined for demethylating activity.[38] However, their demethylating activity and ability to induce gene re-expression remains controversial and bench marking studies have shown substantially lower activity of the nonnucleoside inhibitors compared to nucleoside inhibitors.[41,42] Another alternative to nucleoside DNMTis is the oligonucleotide (20mer) antisense inhibitor of DNMT1, MG98. Although this second-generation inhibitor down-regulates DNMT1 in vitro and there is evidence of suppression of DNMT1 expression in some patients treated with MG98, a downstream effect of DNA demethylation was not detectable in tumor or surrogate tissues comparable to that observed for nucleoside DNMTis.[43,44]

Despite encouraging efficacy of certain DNMTi in haematological cancers, their usefulness for autoimmune disease and IDB in specific remains uncertain. A major limitation of DNMTi use for IBD will be the lack of specificity to specific genes and incorporation into DNA inducing DNA damage, both of which most likely will lead to unwanted side effects in patients. Their toxicity, such as myelosuppression, will be dose limiting and limit their biological effectiveness.[45] Furthermore, nucleoside DNMTs are unlikely to be of value in the treatment of chronic diseases or if used as a preventative agent, where repeat treatments over prolonged periods of time are required. Nucleoside inhibitors such as Azacytidine are suspected human carcinogens based on induction of malignant tumors at multiple tumor sites in multiple species of experimental animal.[46] This emphasizes the need for more gene specific agents which then should have less nonspecific toxicity.

Another approach to target methylation dependent silencing at CpG islands could be to inhibit the mediators of DNA methylation's effects on gene expression, rather than the mark itself. So far, there are three domains known to target methylated DNA. Methyl-CpG binding domain proteins (MBDs) are represented by MBD1, MBD2, MBD4 and MECP2; a zinc-finger motif specifically recognizing methylated DNA has been found in KAISO and lastly the SRA-domain proteins UHRF1 and UHRF2 recognize hemi-methylated DNA.[47,48] All three classes of proteins have a crucial role in linking DNA methylation with transcriptional silencing. Their binding to methylated (or hemi-methylated) DNA allows the recruitment of protein complexes which include chromatin modifying enzymes such as HDACs, which in turn can lead to epigenetic silencing. Recently, the role of UHRF1 as a drug-target has been reviewed (see ref. 49). MBD proteins may also be potential targets for epigenetic therapies which would reactivate gene expression by inhibiting the repressive effects of MBD dependent epigenetic silencing. Unlike nucleoside DNMT inhibitors, the reversal of methylation-dependent silencing by an MBD inhibitor would be predicted to be independent of DNA replication and may have a greater level of specificity to transcription of sets of key genes without affecting the protective effect of DNA methylation at nontranscribed regions on genomic integrity.

DNA DEMETHYLASES

One common and frequently occurring feature of autoimmune diseases is the global hypomethylation of T cells and, at least in SLE and RA patients this epigenetic feature might be a disease triggering event.[50,51] The demethylation of DNA can occur through either passive and/or active mechanisms. Passive DNA demethylation usually depends on DNA replication and is due to inactive or reduced active maintenance DNMTs leading to a loss of DNA methylation in the newly synthesized strand. Active DNA demethylation on the other hand can occur independent of DNA replication by demethylating enzymes. Although the identification of enzymes promoting active DNA demethylation has been convincingly confirmed in plants, their existence in mammals is still under debate. It has been hypothesized that the demethylation may be achieved through a base excision repair pathway, where initially a deamination step converts the 5-methylcytosine (5-meC) to thymine before the DNA glycosylase is able to act (see ref. 52). In this scenario the DNA glycosylase would cleave the glycoside bond between the 5-meC base and the deoxyribose, thereby creating a so called AP site. Subsequently, the AP endonuclease could remove the deoxyribose creating a gap which would then be filled by the DNA polymerase and ligase, leading to an unmethylated C. Such activity has been found in vitro for the chicken and the human methyl binding domain protein 4 (MBD4),[53] however it should be emphasized that MBD4 shows a much stronger G/T mismatch repair activity in vitro and that in *mbd4*-knockout mice no DNA demethylation was observed.[54,55]

Direct excision of the methyl group via hydrolysis could be a second possibility how active DNA demethylation is achieved. This would result in the replacement of the methyl group by a hydrogen atom followed by the release of methanol.[52] Such a reaction was reported to be carried out by the methyl binding domain protein MBD2, however from an energetic point of view, this reaction is unfavorable and so far the finding has not been reproduced by others.[56,57] Nevertheless, SLE patients displayed global DNA hypomethylation in CD4+ T cells and two potential DNA demethylases MBD2 and MBD4 were both considerably up-regulated[58] potentially pointing towards a potential drug target. However, these patients also showed a decrease in DNMT1 expression,[59] weakening the argument for a demethylase activity of MBD2 or 4 being responsible for the hypomethylation.

Another member of the MBD family, MBD3, has recently been shown to induce DNA demethylation at specific targets of the genome where it binds. Here, the demethylation seems to be localized to promoter regions with intermediate CpG density and interestingly, promoter having a NF-Y binding site seemed to be significantly affected.[60]

Also an attractive possibility of active DNA demethylation is the enzymatic deamination of 5-meC to T, combined with G/T mismatch repair via DNA glycosylases.[61] This finding seems to be substantiated by experiments performed in cultured breast cancer cells where de novo DNMTs (DNMT3a and DNMT3b) were found to convert 5-meC to thymine, which then was removed via the G/T mismatch base excision repair pathway.[62]

Lastly, 5-meC may also be oxidised to 5-hydroxymethylcytosine (5-hmC).[52] The alpha-ketoglutarate and Fe(II)-dependent enzyme TET1 has been shown to convert 5-meC to 5-hmC in cultured cells.[63] The demethylation might then occur via an active mechanism where e.g., 5-hmC is converted to thymine via a DNA glycosylase-based repair pathway or a passive mechanism since 5-hmC is an unfavourable substrate for the maintenance DNMT1.[63]

Although at this point in mammals no definitive DNA demethylase has been confirmed, it is very likely that active DNA demethylation plays an important role in development and diseases such as cancer and autoimmune diseases. More work will be required to validate demethylases and associated activities as targets in animal or cell line models. While MBDs have been suggested as potential anticancer targets using siRNA and transgenic knock-outs,[64-66] it remains unclear how druggable they will be.[67] However, these models may allow investigation of MBDs as targets in immune diseases.

CONCLUSION

There is growing evidence for a role for epigenetic mechanisms in the development of autoimmune diseases. Small molecule inhibitors of histone modification and DNA methylation maintenance are increasingly becoming available and will be useful chemical biological tools to dissect epigenetic mechanisms in these diseases. However, although epigenetic therapies used in cancer treatment are a promising starting point for the exploration of autoimmune disease treatment, there is a requirement for more specific and less toxic agents. Current epigenetic therapies are not suitable for the treatment of chronic diseases or as chemo-preventative agents. Hopefully a greater understanding of key mechanisms and targets may allow more rational approaches to epigenetic therapies that are disease or target specific and which avoid the unwanted side-effects of current agents.

REFERENCES

1. Hernick M, Fierke CA. Zinc hydrolases: the mechanisms of zinc-dependent deacetylases. Arch Biochem Biophys 2005; 433(1):71-84.
2. de Ruijter AJ, van Gennip AH, Caron HN et al. Histone deacetylases (HDACs): characterization of the classical HDAC family. Biochem J 2003; 370(Pt 3):737-749.
3. Bolden JE, Peart MJ, Johnstone RW. Anticancer activities of histone deacetylase inhibitors. Nat Rev Drug Discov 2006; 5(9):769-784.
4. Xu WS, Parmigiani RB, Marks PA. Histone deacetylase inhibitors: molecular mechanisms of action. Oncogene 2007; 26(37):5541-5552.
5. Warrener R, Beamish H, Burgess A et al. Tumor cell-selective cytotoxicity by targeting cell cycle checkpoints. FASEB J 2003; 17(11):1550-1552.
6. Gui CY, Ngo L, Xu WS et al. Histone deacetylase (HDAC) inhibitor activation of p21WAF1 involves changes in promoter-associated proteins, including HDAC1. Proc Natl Acad Sci USA 2004; 101(5):1241-1246.
7. Blanchard F, Chipoy C. Histone deacetylase inhibitors: new drugs for the treatment of inflammatory diseases? Drug Discov Today 2005; 10(3):197-204.
8. Shuttleworth S, Kerry S. HDAC Inhibitors: New Promise in the Treatment of Immune and Inflammatory Disease. Innovations in Pharmaceutical Technology 2009:16-20.
9. Yamaguchi H, Woods NT, Piluso LG et al. p53 acetylation is crucial for its transcription-independent proapoptotic functions. J Biol Chem 2009; 284(17):11171-11183.
10. Bi G, Jiang G. The molecular mechanism of HDAC inhibitors in anticancer effects. Cell Mol Immunol 2006; 3(4):285-290.
11. Yuan ZL, Guan YJ, Chatterjee D et al. Stat3 dimerization regulated by reversible acetylation of a single lysine residue. Science 2005; 307(5707):269-273.
12. Chen Lf, Fischle W, Verdin E et al. Duration of nuclear NF-kappaB action regulated by reversible acetylation. Science 2001; 293(5535):1653-1657.
13. Gu W, Roeder RG. Activation of p53 sequence-specific DNA binding by acetylation of the p53 C-terminal domain. Cell 1997; 90(4):595-606.
14. Martinez-Balbas MA et al. Regulation of E2F1 activity by acetylation. EMBO J 2000; 19(4):662-671.
15. Luo J, Su F, Chen D et al. Deacetylation of p53 modulates its effect on cell growth and apoptosis. Nature 2000; 408(6810):377-381.
16. Pediconi N, Ianari A, Costanzo A et al. Differential regulation of E2F1 apoptotic target genes in response to DNA damage. Nat Cell Biol 2003; 5(6):552-558.
17. Bandyopadhyay D, Mishra A, Medrano EE. Overexpression of histone deacetylase 1 confers resistance to sodium butyrate-mediated apoptosis in melanoma cells through a p53-mediated pathway. Cancer Res 2004; 64(21):7706-7710.
18. Haggarty SJ, Koeller KM, Wong JC et al. Domain-selective small-molecule inhibitor of histone deacetylase 6 (HDAC6)-mediated tubulin deacetylation. Proc Natl Acad Sci USA 2003; 100(8):4389-4394.
19. Backdahl L, Bushell A, Beck S. Inflammatory signalling as mediator of epigenetic modulation in tissue-specific chronic inflammation. Int J Biochem Cell Biol 2009; 41(1):176-184.
20. Choo QY, Ho PC, Lin HS. Histone deacetylase inhibitors: new hope for rheumatoid arthritis? Curr Pharm Des 2008; 14(8):803-820.
21. Chabane N, Zayed N, Afif H et al. Histone deacetylase inhibitors suppress interleukin-1beta-induced nitric oxide and prostaglandin E2 production in human chondrocytes. Osteoarthritis Cartilage 2008; 16(10):1267-1274.
22. Mahmoodi M, Sahebjam S, Smookler D et al. Lack of tissue inhibitor of metalloproteinases-3 results in an enhanced inflammatory response in antigen-induced arthritis. Am J Pathol 2005; 166(6):1733-1740.
23. Chung YL, Lee MY, Wang AJ et al. A therapeutic strategy uses histone deacetylase inhibitors to modulate the expression of genes involved in the pathogenesis of rheumatoid arthritis. Mol Ther 2003; 8(5):707-717.
24. Jüngel A, Baresova V, Ospelt C et al. Trichostatin A sensitises rheumatoid arthritis synovial fibroblasts for TRAIL-induced apoptosis. Ann Rheum Dis 2006; 65(7):910-912.

25. Nakamura C, Matsushita I, Kosaka E et al. Anti-arthritic effects of combined treatment with histone deacetylase inhibitor and low-intensity ultrasound in the presence of microbubbles in human rheumatoid synovial cells. Rheumatology (Oxford) 2008; 47(4):418-424.
26. Lin HS, Hu CY, Chan HY et al. Anti-rheumatic activities of histone deacetylase (HDAC) inhibitors in vivo in collagen-induced arthritis in rodents. Br J Pharmacol 2007; 150(7):862-872.
27. Nishida K, Komiyama T, Miyazawa S et al. Histone deacetylase inhibitor suppression of autoantibody-mediated arthritis in mice via regulation of p16INK4a and p21(WAF1/Cip1) expression. Arthritis Rheum 2004; 50(10):3365-3376.
28. Manabe H, Nasu Y, Komiyama T et al. Inhibition of histone deacetylase down-regulates the expression of hypoxia-induced vascular endothelial growth factor by rheumatoid synovial fibroblasts. Inflamm Res 2008; 57(1):4-10.
29. Leoni F, Fossati G, Lewis EC et al. The histone deacetylase inhibitor ITF2357 reduces production of pro-inflammatory cytokines in vitro and systemic inflammation in vivo. Mol Med 2005; 11(1-12):1-15.
30. Lührs H, Gerke T, Müller JG et al. Butyrate inhibits NF-kappaB activation in lamina propria macrophages of patients with ulcerative colitis. Scand J Gastroenterol 2002; 37(4):458-466.
31. Vernia P, Annese V, Bresci G et al. Topical butyrate improves efficacy of 5-ASA in refractory distal ulcerative colitis: results of a multicentre trial. Eur J Clin Invest 2003; 33(3):244-248.
32. Glauben R, Batra A, Fedke I et al. Histone hyperacetylation is associated with amelioration of experimental colitis in mice. J Immunol 2006; 176(8):5015-5022.
33. Mishra N, Reilly CM, Brown DR et al. Histone deacetylase inhibitors modulate renal disease in the MRL-lpr/lpr mouse. J Clin Invest 2003; 111(4):539-552.
34. Camelo S, Iglesias AH, Hwang D et al. Transcriptional therapy with the histone deacetylase inhibitor trichostatin A ameliorates experimental autoimmune encephalomyelitis. J Neuroimmunol 2005; 164(1-2):10-21.
35. Gray SG, Dangond F. Rationale for the use of histone deacetylase inhibitors as a dual therapeutic modality in multiple sclerosis. Epigenetics. 2006; 1(2):67-75.
36. Tovar-Castillo LE, Cancino-Díaz JC, García-Vázquez F et al. Under-expression of VHL and over-expression of HDAC-1, HIF-1alpha, LL-37 and IAP-2 in affected skin biopsies of patients with psoriasis. Int J Dermatol. 2007; 46(3):239-246.
37. Dhir M, Montgomery EA, Glöckner SC et al. Epigenetic regulation of WNT signaling pathway genes in inflammatory bowel disease (IBD) associated neoplasia. J Gastrointest Surg 2008; 12(10):1745-1753.
38. Lyko F, Brown R. DNA methyltransferase inhibitors and the development of epigenetic cancer therapies. J Natl Cancer Inst 2005; 97(20):1498-1506.
39. Santi DV, Norment A, Garrett CE. Covalent bond formation between a DNA-cytosine methyltransferase and DNA containing 5-azacytosine. Proc Natl Acad Sci USA 1984; 81(22):6993-6997.
40. Baylin SB. DNA methylation and gene silencing in cancer. Nat Clin Pract Oncol 2005; 2 Suppl 1:S4-11.
41. Yoo CB, Jeong S, Egger G et al. Delivery of 5-aza-2'-deoxycytidine to cells using oligodeoxynucleotides. Cancer Res 2007; 67(13):6400-6408.
42. Brueckner B, Kuck D, Lyko F. DNA methyltransferase inhibitors for cancer therapy. Cancer J 2007; 13(1):17-22.
43. Plummer R, Vidal L, Griffin M et al. Phase I study of MG98, an oligonucleotide antisense inhibitor of human DNA methyltransferase 1, given as a 7-day infusion in patients with advanced solid tumors. Clin Cancer Res 2009; 15(9):3177-3183.
44. Klisovic RB, Stock W, Cataland S et al. A phase I biological study of MG98, an oligodeoxynucleotide antisense to DNA methyltransferase 1, in patients with high-risk myelodysplasia and acute myeloid leukemia. Clin Cancer Res 2008; 14(8):2444-2449.
45. Graham JS, Kaye SB, Brown R. The promises and pitfalls of epigenetic therapies in solid tumours. Eur J Cancer 2009; 45(7):1129-1136.
46. IARC. IARC Monographs on the Evaluation of Carcinogenic Risk of Chemicals to Humans. International Agency for Research on Cancer 1990; 50:415.
47. Jorgensen HF, Bird A. MeCP2 and other methyl-CpG binding proteins. Ment Retard Dev Disabil Res Rev 2002; 8(2):87-93.
48. Unoki M, Kelly JD, Neal DE et al. UHRF1 is a novel molecular marker for diagnosis and the prognosis of bladder cancer. Br J Cancer 2009; 101(1):98-105.
49. Unoki M, Brunet J, Mousli M. Drug discovery targeting epigenetic codes: The great potential of UHRF1, which links DNA methylation and histone modifications, as a drug target in cancers and toxoplasmosis. Biochem Pharmacol 2009; 15:78(10):1279-88.
50. Luo Y, Li Y, Su Y et al. Abnormal DNA methylation in T-cells from patients with subacute cutaneous lupus erythematosus. Br J Dermatol 2008; 159(4):827-833.
51. Richardson B, Scheinbart L, Strahler J et al. Evidence for impaired T-cell DNA methylation in systemic lupus erythematosus and rheumatoid arthritis. Arthritis Rheum 1990; 33(11):1665-1673.

52. Zhu JK. Active DNA demethylation mediated by DNA glycosylases. Annu Rev Genet 2009; 43:143-166.
53. Zhu B, Zheng Y, Angliker H et al. 5-Methylcytosine DNA glycosylase activity is also present in the human MBD4 (G/T mismatch glycosylase) and in a related avian sequence. Nucleic Acids Res 2000; 28(21):4157-4165.
54. Millar CB, Guy J, Sansom OJ et al. Enhanced CpG mutability and tumorigenesis in MBD4-deficient mice. Science 2002; 297(5580):403-405.
55. Wong E, Yang K, Kuraguchi M et al. Mbd4 inactivation increases Cright-arrowT transition mutations and promotes gastrointestinal tumor formation. Proc Natl Acad Sci USA 2002; 99(23):14937-14942.
56. Bhattacharya SK, Ramchandani S, Cervoni N et al. A mammalian protein with specific demethylase activity for mCpG DNA. Nature 1999; 397(6720):579-583.
57. Bird A. DNA methylation patterns and epigenetic memory. Genes Dev 2002; 16(1):6-21.
58. Balada E, Ordi-Ros J, Serrano-Acedo S et al. Transcript overexpression of the MBD2 and MBD4 genes in CD4+ T-cells from systemic lupus erythematosus patients. J Leukoc Biol 2007; 81(6):1609-1616.
59. Lei W, Luo Y, Lei W et al. Abnormal DNA methylation in CD4+ T-cells from patients with systemic lupus erythematosus, systemic sclerosis and dermatomyositis. Scand J Rheumatol 2009:1-6.
60. Brown SE, Suderman MJ, Hallett M et al. DNA demethylation induced by the methyl-CpG-binding domain protein MBD3. Gene 2008; 420(2):99-106.
61. Morgan HD, Dean W, Coker HA et al. Activation-induced cytidine deaminase deaminates 5-methylcytosine in DNA and is expressed in pluripotent tissues: implications for epigenetic reprogramming. J Biol Chem 2004; 279(50):52353-52360.
62. Métivier R, Gallais R, Tiffoche C et al. Cyclical DNA methylation of a transcriptionally active promoter. Nature 2008; 452(7183):45-50.
63. Tahiliani M, Koh KP, Shen Y et al. Conversion of 5-methylcytosine to 5-hydroxymethylcytosine in mammalian DNA by MLL partner TET1. Science 2009; 324(5929):930-935.
64. Bakker J, Lin X, Nelson WG. Methyl-CpG binding domain protein 2 represses transcription from hypermethylated pi-class glutathione S-transferase gene promoters in hepatocellular carcinoma cells. J Biol Chem 2002; 277(25):22573-22580.
65. Auriol E, Billard LM, Magdinier F et al. Specific binding of the methyl binding domain protein 2 at the BRCA1-NBR2 locus. Nucleic Acids Res 2005; 33(13):4243-4254.
66. Berger J, Bird A. Role of MBD2 in gene regulation and tumorigenesis. Biochem Soc Trans 2005; 33(Pt 6):1537-1540.
67. Chapman-Rothe N, Brown R. Approaches to target the genome and its epigenome in cancer. Future Med Chem 2009; 1(8):1481-1495.

CHAPTER 12

PROFILING EPIGENETIC ALTERATIONS IN DISEASE

José Ignacio Martín-Subero* and Manel Esteller

Cancer Epigenetics and Biology Program (PEBC), Bellvitge Biomedical Research Institute (IDIBELL), Barcelona, Spain
Corresponding Author: José Ignacio Martín-Subero—Email: jimartin@idibell.cat

Abstract: Nowadays, epigenetics is one of the fastest growing research areas in biomedicine. Studies have demonstrated that changes in the epigenome are not only common in cancer, but are also involved in the pathogenesis of noncancerous diseases like immunological, cardiovascular, developmental and neurological/psychiatric disorders. At the same time, during the last years, a technological revolution has taken place in the field of epigenomics, which is defined as the study of epigenetic changes throughout the whole genome. Microarray technologies and more recently, the development of next generation sequencing devices are now providing researchers with tools to draw high-resolution maps of DNA methylation and histone modifications in normal tissues and diseases. This chapter will review the currently available high-throughput techniques for studying the epigenome and their applications for characterizing human diseases.

INTRODUCTION

In the last years, it has become evident that genetics alone cannot explain phenotypic manifestations. Instead, it is clear that a given phenotype is rather caused by an interplay between genetic and environmental cues. Exactly in this interface is where epigenetics plays an essential role, as it constitutes the molecular language through which genome and environment communicate with each other.[1,2] Epigenetics is classically defined as the study of chemical modifications at the chromatin level that regulate gene expression without altering the DNA sequence itself,[3] although a more inclusive definition of epigenetic events was recently proposed as "the structural adaptation of chromosomal regions so as to register, signal or perpetuate altered activity states".[4]

Epigenetic Contributions in Autoimmune Disease, edited by Esteban Ballestar.

The most widely studied epigenetic changes are DNA methylation of cytosines within CpG dinucleotides and a growing number of chemical modifications at different aminoacid residues of histone tails (so far over 60 have been identified), e.g., acetylation, methylation, phosphorylation and ubiquitination.[3,5] Although the present chapter will mostly focus on DNA methylation and histone modifications, other epigenetic factors like nuclear positioning, noncoding RNAs and microRNAs, are also associated with gene regulation and chromatin structure.[6-8]

It is beyond doubt that new theories and models in biomedical sciences are not only caused by the creativity of scientists but also to the development of new methods and technologies that provide new facts. In the epigenetics field, the past years have witnessed the introduction of a large number of new techniques that gradually moved from the analysis of few genes to the whole epigenome, giving rise to the term epigenomics.[9-14] Since the development of microarray-based approaches for epigenomics, the number of studies aimed at characterizing the epigenome under normal and altered conditions has grown exponentially. However, the last technical development in the field of epigenomics, which represents an important breakthrough in biomedicine, is the application of next-generation sequencing to obtain whole-genome DNA methylation and histone modification maps.[13,15] The goal of this chapter will be to review the currently available techniques for studying the epigenome and their applications for characterizing human diseases.

DETECTION OF DNA METHYLATION CHANGES

A Historical Perspective

The initial efforts to study the epigenome started in the 1970s. At that time, studies were focused on the measurement of global DNA methylation content and the analysis of particular sequences by Southern blot analyses using methylation-sensitive restriction endonucleases. The limitations of the latter method (e.g., large amounts of high-quality DNA, sequence biases and problems with incomplete digestions) made the study of specific sequences time-consuming and not widely applicable. A real breakthrough took place in 1992 with the introduction of the sodium bisulfite conversion technique, that allowed scientists to easily study DNA methylation.[16] Sodium bisulfite has the property of converting unmethylated cytosine into uracil whereas methylated cytosine remains unmodified. The combination of this chemical modification with genomic sequencing and methylation specific PCR (MSP) made the study of DNA methylation changes widely available and a large number of studies were published from the late 1990s on.[17] However, these PCR based approaches are restricted to the study of few candidate genes and are not suitable as screening techniques to identify novel markers. To overcome this, techniques like Amplification of InterMethylated Sites (AIMS) and Restriction Landmark Genomic Scanning (RLGS), which combine the use of methylation-sensitive restriction endonucleases with 1D or 2D electrophoresis have been established.[18,19] These techniques are time consuming and every new fragment identified as differentially methylated between a control and a test sample has to be cloned and sequenced. Two important steps forward have been made in the recent years with the introduction of the microarray technology[20] and next-generation sequencing,[21] which have provided the basis for a new revolution in epigenetics. These two methods will be explained in detail in the sections below.

DNA Methylation Profiling with DNA Microarrays

Several strategies have been developed to analyze DNA methylation changes with microarrays. (Table 1) These strategies can be classified according to the method applied to differentiate methylated and unmethylated cytosines and according to the type and resolution of the microarray platform.

Basically, there are three different options to prepare the samples for DNA methylation analyses. These are based either on digesting the DNA with methylation-sensitive or -insensitive restriction endonucleases, on isolating the methylated fraction of the genome by affinity–enrichment or on the chemical modification of the DNA by sodium bisulfite.

Examples of methods exploiting the endonuclease digestion approach are Differential Methylation Hybridization (DMH), HpaII tiny fragment Enrichment by Ligation-mediated PCR (HELP) or NotI digestion coupled with BAC arrays.[22-24] The use of methylation-sensitive enzymes is biased by the fact that not all CpG islands contain enzyme recognition sites. Therefore, not all the CpG islands in the genome can be interrogated. To partially overcome this limitation, a recent technical report has applied different combinations of four methylation-sensitive enzymes (i.e., HpaII, Hin6I, AciI and HpyCH4IV), which cover approximately 41% of all CpGs across the genome.[25]

Affinity–enrichment methods are based on the isolation of methylated DNA sequences by applying antibodies or recombinant proteins binding to methylated cytosines, which is less biased towards specific sequences than those methods based on methylation-sensitive endonucleases. Techniques like MeDIP, mDIP and mCIP use an antibody specific for 5-methylcytosine to immunoprecipitate the methylated fraction of the genome.[26,27] Other techniques use recombinant proteins containing methyl-CpG binding domains of proteins like MBD1, MBD2 and MBD3L1 to purify methylated DNA by affinity.[26,28,29] Also, an indirect way of detection methylated regions of the genome is by a classical chromatin immunoprecipitation (ChIP) with antibodies against MBDs.[30] These methods present also some limitations like the low resolution based on the size of immunoprecipitated DNA fragments (~200-1000 bp) and that the level of enrichment of methylated DNA depends on the abundance of CpGs in a given sequence.[31]

The third approach for array-based detection of DNA methylation is the application of bisulfite treatment. As explained above, sodium bisulfite chemically induces a sequence variation by converting unmethylated cytosines into uracil (thymine after a PCR reaction) and leaving methylated cytosines unmodified. This sequence variation allows to use methods already existing for single nucleotide polymorphism (SNP) analysis, which are based on the design of oligonucleotides that specifically bind either to the methylated (C) or to the unmethylated (U/T) allele.[32,33] As compared to the previous two strategies, this method allows to detect methylation changes of individual CpGs.

The methods mentioned above allow a direct detection of DNA methylation patterns. However, there is an additional, but indirect, way for detecting hypermethylated genes. This method applies gene expression profiling before and after treatment with DNA demethylating agents like 5-aza-2'-deoxycytosine (5-AZA), so that hypermethylated genes become reactivated after treatment.[34] Although this technique has allowed the detection of novel cancer-related hypermethylated genes, 5-AZA is highly toxic to the cells and can alter the expression levels of many genes regardless of their methylation status, leading to a high false positive and false negative rate and a thorough and time consuming data validation.[35]

In terms of microarray platforms, there is also a wide range of them available for DNA methylation analysis, which differ in resolution, number and type of genomic regions detected. The initially applied microarrays used spotted CpG island clones.[36] These arrays are biased towards those clones contained in the available libraries and therefore, are not representative for the complete genome. Additionally, regulatory regions of special interest might not be present. Microarrays containing BAC/PAC clones have been also used for epigenomic studies.[23,27,37] Although tiling BAC/PAC arrays containing the complete genome are available, the resolution of BAC/PAC arrays is limited by the size of the inserts (~100-200 Kb). Thus, only a global epigenetic signature for that large DNA stretch can be obtained, rendering the identification of differentially methylated gene promoters difficult.

These arrays have been substituted in the last years by microarrays containing short oligonucleotides (usually ranging from 25 to 75 bp), which can reach a very high resolution, are commercially available and can be easily customized according to the user's needs. Available high-density oligonucleotide arrays for epigenomics include e.g., promoter arrays and CpG island arrays. Also, oligonucleotide tiling arrays have also been also developed, which contain up to several millions of oligonucleotides and virtually cover the whole genome with high resolution. This approach led to the first high-resolution DNA methylation profile of a living organism (*Arabidopsis thaliana*).[38]

One of the limitations of the methods quoted above is that they only provide a blurry picture of the methylome and it is not possible to determine the methylation status of specific CpGs. This problem can be overcome either by bisulfite sequencing of specific CpGs or with CpG-dinucleotide specific microarrays.[32,39] For instance, the technology developed by Bibikova and collaborators (Illumina Inc.) is based on the combination of a bisulfite treatment of the test DNA, oligonucleotide annealing to the methylated or unmethylated specific CpG, oligonucleotide extension, PCR with universal differentially-labeled primers for the methylated or unmethylated allele and hybridization onto a random bead array. This method allows the accurate quantification of the methylation status of up to 1536 individual CpGs located in the promoter regions of selected genes.[32,40] A similar approach has been used to develop the Infinium array (Illumina Inc.), which allows the analysis of the methylation status of 27.578 CpGs located in the promoter regions of 14.475 genes and microRNAs. This assay accomplishes this high multiplexing by combining bisulfite conversion of genomic DNA and whole-genome amplification sample preparation with direct, array-based capture and enzymatic scoring of the CpG loci.[41,42]

Additionally, an alternative approach to microarray hybridization or sequencing has been also developed to measure DNA methylation and is based on matrix-assisted laser desorption ionization time-of-flight (MALDI-TOF) mass spectrometry.[43] This strategy, called EpiTYPER platform, has been developed by Sequenom and relies on the gene-specific amplification of bisulfite treated DNA to quantify methylation of multiple CpG nucleotides for hundreds of genes.

In spite of the development of a wide range of microarray-based technologies to study the epigenome, they all show differences in terms of sample preparation, resolution, type of sequence studied, quantification accuracy and complexity of the bioinformatic tools to analyze the data. Most importantly, none of the microarray-based techniques for DNA methylation profiling can sequence the whole DNA methylome at the single-base-pair resolution.

DNA Methylation Profiling by Next-Generation Sequencing

The complete characterization of the human DNA methylome of a given sample requires the quantification of the methylation status of each of the ~55 million CpG dinucleotides per diploid cell. Although this is far from the abilities of current microarray platforms, the recent development of next-generation sequencing devices is starting to make this achievement possible.[13]

Nowadays, there are different devices that use new technologies to rapidly sequence several gigabases of DNA. These technologies are based e.g., on pyrosequencing using millions of picoliter-scale reactions (454/Roche), sequencing by synthesis either clonal (Genome Analyzer/Illumina) or single-molecule (Helicos/Helicos Bioscience), or sequencing by ligation (SOLiD/ABI, Polonator/Dover Systems, Complete Genomics), and are able to sequence up to 200 gigabases of DNA (and the human genome is made of ~3.1 gigabases) in a single experiment.[21,44]

These next-generation sequencing technologies can be applied to sequence DNA pretreated to obtain the methylated fraction of the genome. (Table 1) For instance, several strategies have been developed to library preparations from methylation-sensitive endonucleases followed next-generation sequencing, like HELP-Seq,[45] Methyl-Seq[46] or methylation-sensitive cut counting (MSCC).[47] In the case of library preparations with material immunoprecipitated with an antibody against 5-methylcytosine, the technique called MeDIP-Seq.[48] However, although these techniques show advantages over their microarray-based counterparts, they cannot provide quantitative information about specific CpG dinucleotides.

Next-generation sequencing approaches have also been used to analyze bisulfite-treated DNA in several variants. For instance, the 454/Roche technology has been used to rapidly sequence 125 amplicons with a mean almost 1700 reads per amplicon.[49] However, the main challenges for a bisulfite sequencing without amplicons is derived from the reduced sequence complexity, as 4 bases are mostly reduced to 3 for unmethylated cytosines. Reduced representation bisulfite sequencing (RRBS) was developed to reduce sequence redundancy by selecting only specific parts of the genome using endonuclease digestions.[50] Other approaches use array-based, solution-based or padlock-based capture of specific DNA sequences before or after bisulfite conversion.[47,51-53] (Table 1)

The techniques mentioned before provide a gradual approximation towards the final goal of sequencing the whole DNA methylome. Whole-genome shotgun bisulfite sequencing (WGSBS) has been recently achieved for small eukaryotic genomes like *A. thaliana*[54,55] and also for human genomes.[56,57] Most interestingly, these studies in humans have surprisingly discovered that stem cells show abundant DNA methylation in nonCG contexts (mCHG and mCHH, where H can be A, C or T). This nonCG methylation seems to be specific for stem cells and disappears upon cell differentiation.[56,57]

GENOME-WIDE DETECTION OF HISTONE MODIFICATIONS

As compared to the variety of methods available to characterize DNA methylation at the genome-wide level, the study of histone modifications is relatively straight-forward. Such analysis is mostly based on a single technique, the so called chromatin immunoprecipitation (ChIP). This technique exploits the availability of antibodies which specifically detect certain histone modifications. Basically, a classical ChIP procedure is based on the following steps: an initial crosslink between histones and DNA by formaldehyde is performed, followed by chromatin shearing and incubation with a highly specific antibody towards a histone modification. Then, the chromatin bound to the antibody is isolated by e.g., agarose or magnetic beads coated with protein A or G and finally the DNA is separated from the proteins by reversing the crosslinks and subsequent DNA extraction. The DNA isolated in this way is enriched for sequences containing the histone modification of interest and can be then used for microarray-based studies.[58,59] The main limitations of ChIP are the necessity of a highly specific antibody for the histone modification of interest, the availability of fresh or frozen material (whole cells are required) and the large amounts of cells required (approximately $\sim 10^7$). Some recent publications have also optimized protocols for ChIP that use a smaller amount of cells (e.g., as little as 100 cells), which are required to study histone modifications in e.g., small subpopulations of cells like stem cells or clinical samples.[60-62]

The immunoprecipitated DNA is then subjected to analysis, either by conventional or quantitative PCR for specific candidate genes, or at the genome-wide scale. To generate genome-wide histone modification maps, there are basically two approaches. One is to use oligonucleotide-based microarrays, that can contain up to millions of oligos located e.g., promoter regions, or CpG islands or the whole-genome for tiling arrays.[63] The second approach, that is gradually substituting the first one, is based on using next-generation sequencing to analyze the immunoprecipitated DNA, technique called ChIP-Seq.[15] This new method has several advantages over the microarrays like higher resolution, less noise and greater coverage. In terms of platforms, the Illumina/Solexa Genome Analyzer has been used in the great majority of the publications on ChIP-Seq, but other next-generation sequencing platforms mentioned previously can also be used for sequencing immunoprecipitated DNA.

PROFILING EPIGENETIC CHANGES IN HUMAN DISEASE

It is known that many essential physiological processes like development, establishment of tissue identity, X-chromosome inactivation, chromosomal stability and gene transcription are regulated by epigenetic mechanisms.[3] Additionally, multiple factors, like aging, nutrition, exposure to metals or maternal behavior in early childhood are able to induce epigenetic changes.[64-66] These environmentally-induced epigenetic modifications are in turn related to susceptibility to malignant and nonmalignant diseases in adulthood.[67] Interestingly, there is evidence showing that monozygotic twins acquire epigenetic and phenotypic changes throughout life,[68,69] which supports the concept that life style influences the phenotype through epigenetic modifications.

Given the importance of epigenetic mechanisms, it is not surprising that alterations in the epigenetic pattern are associated with a wide range of diseases. As different tissues and cell types of our body have different epigenomes (Fig. 1), an essential issue when attempting to characterize the epigenome of human diseases is to use the right test and control samples. For any disease or condition, the target tissue or cell type that is altered with a given disease should be analyzed, e.g., infiltrated tumor biopsies in cancer or brain in neurological diseases. As normal controls, healthy matched tissues must be analyzed to be able to detect disease-associated epigenetic changes and not cell type-specific modifications.[70]

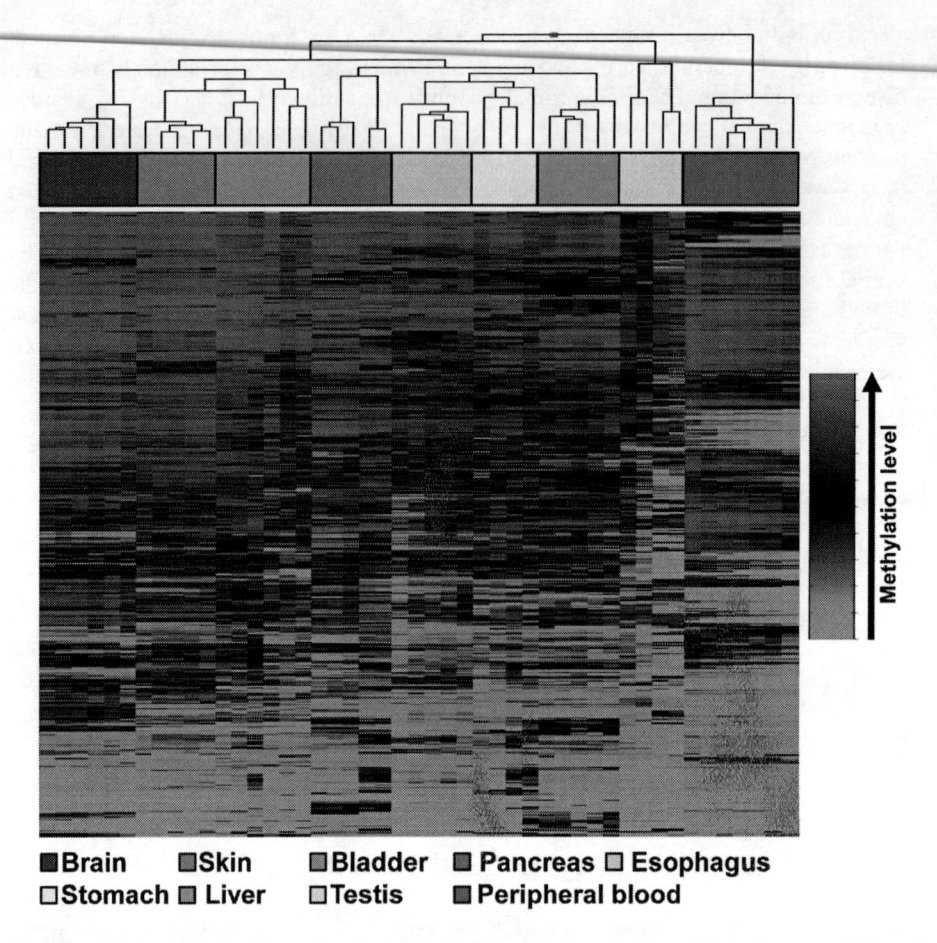

Brain **Skin** **Bladder** **Pancreas** **Esophagus**
Stomach **Liver** **Testis** **Peripheral blood**

Figure 1. Epigenetic profiling of normal tissues. Heatmap from a hierarchical cluster analysis of DNA methylation data generated with the bead-array technology (Illumina Inc.)[32] in different normal tissue samples. A color version of this image is available online at http://www.landesbioscience.com/curie/.

Epigenetics and Cancer

As compared to epigenetic patterns in normal cells, cancer cells are characterized by an intense disruption of the epigenomic machinery, which is reflected into multiple aberrations affecting both content and distribution of DNA methylation and histone modifications.[10,71-73] So far, DNA methylation and especially tumor suppressor gene silencing by hypermethylation, is the best studied epigenetic modification in cancer.[72-76] Over 50 genes have been identified as frequently silenced in cancer by DNA methylation, like *P16/INK4A*, *P14/ARF*, *MLH1* or *MGMT* and DNA methylation patterns allow the differentiation of distinct cancer entities.[76,77] However, with the advent of the science of epigenomics, a more precise and less biased delineation of the cancer cell epigenome is becoming accessible, which is now providing a new generation of genes epigenetically-deregulated in cancer. As shown in a microarray experiment illustrated

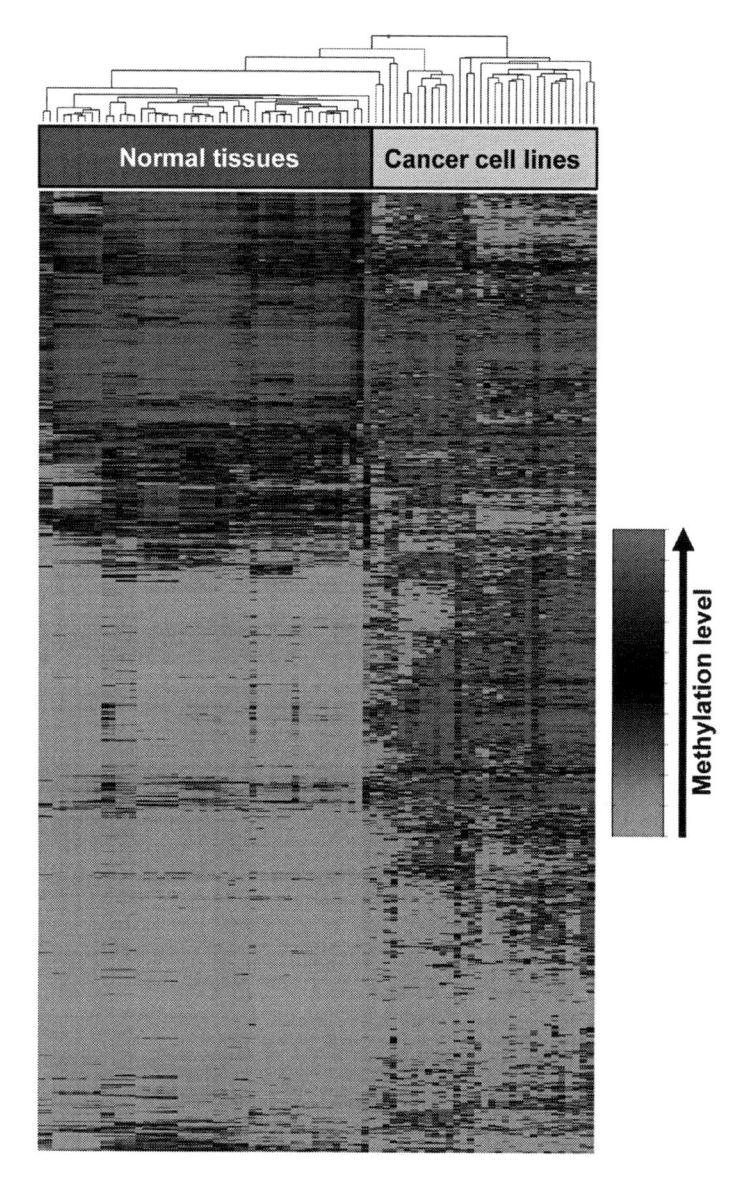

Figure 2. Epigenomic profiling of cancer cells. Heatmap from a hierarchical cluster analysis of DNA methylation data generated with the bead-array technology (Illumina Inc.)[32] in different cancer cell lines and normal controls. Cancer cell lines are characterized by an intense disruption of the DNA methylome. A color version of this image is available online at http://www.landesbioscience.com/curie/.

in Figure 2, cancer cells show a large number of differentially methylated genes as compared to normal cells.

Furthermore, epigenomic studies are now comparing DNA methylation patterns with genome-wide genetic, developmental and transcriptional patterns, which is offering new possibilities for understanding the processes underlying carcinogenesis.[78-82]

Table 1. Techniques used for genome-wide DNA methylation analyses using microarrays and next generation sequencing

Method	Principle	Ref.
Microarray-based		
RLGS	Methylation-sensitive restriction digestion + 2D electrophoresis	19
MCA	Methylation-sensitive restriction digestion + printed membranes/dot-blot analyisis or microarray hybridization	114,115
DMH	Methylation-sensitive restriction digestion + microarray hybridization	22
AIMS	Methylation-sensitive restriction digestion + 1D electrophoresis	18
MSO microarray	Bisulfite conversion + PCR + bead array hybridization	33
ChIP-on-chip	Chromatin immunoprecipitation with antibodies against MBDs + microarray hybridization	30
NotI digestion coupled to BAC array	Methylation-sensitive restriction digestion + microarray hybridization	23
MeDIP-on-chip	Isolation by 5-Methylcytosine antibody + microarray hybridization	27
MCIp-on-chip	Isolation by MBD-Fc beads + microarray hybridization	26
HELP	Methylation-sensitive restriction digestion + microarray hybridization	24
Methylation-specific bead arrays	Bisulfite conversion + allele specific primer extension + bead array hybridization	32
MSNP	Methylation-sensitive restriction digestion + SNP-chip hybridization	116
MMASS	Combinations of methylation-sensitive restriction digestions + microarray hybridization	117
MIRA-assisted microarray analysis	Isolation of methylated DNA by affinity to the MBD2/MBD3L1 complex + microarray hybridization	28
MSDK	Methylation-sensitive restriction digestion + SAGE	118
aPRIMES	Differential restriction and competitive hybridization of methylated and unmethylated DNA	119
Expression profiling after demethylation	Treatment with demethylating agents + expression microarray in cells with and without treatment	120
Next generation sequencing-based		
Methyl–seq	Sequencing-by-synthesis of libraries constructed from size-fractionated HpaII or MspI digests that are compared with randomly sheared fragments	46
HELP–seq	HpaII tiny fragment enrichment by ligation-mediated PCR followed by sequencing	45
MSCC	HpaII digestion followed by the use of a flanking cut with a Type-IIs restriction enzyme (MmeI) and adaptor ligation and then sequencing.	47

continued on next page

Table 1. Continued

Method	Principle	Ref.
MeDIP–seq	Methylated DNA immunoprecipitation followed by sequencing	48
PCR amplicons-Seq	Simultaneous bisulfite sequencing of multiple PCR amplicons	49
RRBS	Selection of only some regions of the genome for sequencing by size-fractionation of DNA fragments after BglII digestion121 or after MspI digestion	50
BC–seq	Selection of only some regions of the genome for sequencing by array or liquid solution capture	121
BSPP	Selection of only some regions of the genome for sequencing by using padlock capture	52
WGSBS	Treatment with sodium bisulfite + sequencing	54-57

Epigenetics and Nonmalignant Diseases

Although most of our knowledge on the association between epigenetics and disease is derived from cancer, nowadays there is increasing interest in understanding the role of epigenetic modifications in the etiology of nonmalignant human diseases. In particular, recent research has detected changes in the epigenetic profile of immunological, cardiovascular, developmental and neurological/psychiatric disorders.

Classical autoimmune disorders, such as systemic lupus erythematosus (SLE) is epigenetically characterized by massive global hypomethylation[83,84] and also the hypomethylation of specific genes, as shown by a recent microarray-based DNA with discordant monozygotic twins.[85]

In the case of cardiovascular diseases, which is one of the most mortal diseases in Western countries, studies have shown that hypomethylation of genomic DNA is present in human atherosclerotic lesions. Furthermore, DNA methylation changes at the promoter region of several genes involved in the pathogenesis of atherosclerosis, such as extracellular superoxide dismutase, estrogen receptor-α, endothelial nitric oxide synthase and 15-lipoxygenase have also been described.[86-88]

The association between epigenetics and developmental disorders is evidenced by the fact that some of these disorders are caused by mutations of genes involved in the epigenetic machinery. For instance, immunodeficiency-centromeric instability-facial anomalies (ICF) syndrome is caused by mutations in the DNA methyltransferase 3A gene (*DNMT3A*),[89] Rett syndrome is caused by mutations in the methyl CpG binding protein 2 gene (*MeCP2*),[90,91] Rubinstein-Taybi syndrome is caused by mutations in the gene encoding the histone acetyltransferase CREB binding protein gene (*CREBBP*)[92] or Sotos syndrome is caused by haploinsufficiency of the histone methyltransferase nuclear receptor-binding SET domain-containing protein 1 gene (*NSD1*).[93]

Also, additional developmental disorders are associated with alterations in the epigenetic phenomenon of imprinting.[94,95] This phenomenon is defined as an epigenetic modification of a specific parental allele, maternal or paternal, of a gene leading to differential expression of the two alleles of the gene in somatic cells of the offspring. Several disorders are caused by genetic (like deletions, uniparental disomies or mutations) changes in imprinted regions of the genome or epigenetic defects. Classical examples of imprinting disorders are the Prader-Willi (PWS) and Angelman syndromes (AS).[96] These two phenotypically-different syndromes are caused by the same genetic defect, but depending on the parental chromosome showing the alteration (paternal or maternal) leads to one phenotype or the other. PWS is caused either deficiency of the paternal copies of the imprinted genes on chromosome region 15q11–q13, while AS affects maternally imprinted genes in the same region.[96]

In neurodegenerative and psychiatric pathologies, several recent reports have started to indicate that they are associated with an epigenetic component.[97] Neurodegenerative disorders like Alzheimer's disease[98,99] and Parkinson's disease[100] have been associated with DNA methylation changes of specific genes, whereas Huntinton's disease seems to be associated with changes in histone mofications like hypoacetylation and gain of histone H3 K9 trimethylation.[101,102] Psychiatric disorders like schizophrenia and bipolar disorder have also been linked with DNA methylation changes as compared to control brain samples.[103] In any case, these studies are still preliminary and future research using genome-wide methods needs to be done to determine the exact role of epigenetics in these diseases and identify the target genes.

CONCLUSION AND FUTURE PERSPECTIVES

The science of epigenomics is one of the most exciting areas in biomedicine today. The detection of epigenetic patterns in health and disease will not only help us to understand the origins and pathobiology of human diseases but also provide a framework for new therapies. After the completion of the human genome, epigeneticists world-wide are now claiming for an international effort to characterize the epigenome.[104-110] This endeavor is indeed a great scale project if one considers the presence of interindividual, tissue-specific and disease-specific epigenomes and that the epigenome is a dynamic system that can be altered throughout life in adaptation to novel environmental cues.[69] To reach that aim, several national and international initiatives have been already started.[111] Such initiatives will certainly take advantage of the rapidly evolving technologies for high-throughput sequencing of the genome-wide DNA methylation and histone modification maps. These technologies are gradually becoming economically more accessible and at the same time are increasing their throughput, both in terms of generating more reads and sequencing larger fragments, which will make subsequent bioinformatic analyses more reliable. Also, these technologies will be able to directly analyze single-molecules after bisulfite treatment, avoiding the biases induced by amplification methods.[56] Finally, the use of Nanopore Sequencing, a novel technology that will be able to differentiate methylated from unmethylated cytosines will certainly herald a new era in DNA methylation analyses, as the entire DNA methylome will be directly sequenced without previous bisultife treatment.[112]

At the pathophysiological level we have to consider that the epigenetic code is only one layer of information. The complete understanding of the cell physiology under normal and altered conditions will require the integration of the genome, epigenome, transcriptome and proteome under the point of view of a systems biology approach. This strategy should also include information about life style and environmental exposures because both health and disease are caused by an interplay between genome and environment. The integration of these different layers, or networks, of cell physiology, into a unified cellular system[113] will be of great importance to understand the mechanisms underlying normal and altered physiology.

ACKNOWLEDGEMENTS

J.I. Martin-Subero's studies on epigenomics are supported by a grant from the Spanish Ministry of Science and Innovation (Project No. SAF2009-08663) and a Ramón y Cajal contract.

REFERENCES

1. Jaenisch R, Bird A. Epigenetic regulation of gene expression: how the genome integrates intrinsic and environmental signals. Nat Genet 2003; 33 Suppl:245-254.
2. Bird A. DNA methylation patterns and epigenetic memory. Genes Dev 2002; 16(1):6-21.
3. Bernstein BE, Meissner A, Lander ES. The mammalian epigenome. Cell 2007; 128(4):669-681.
4. Bird A. Perceptions of epigenetics. Nature 2007; 447(7143):396-398.
5. Kouzarides T. Chromatin modifications and their function. Cell 2007; 128(4):693-705.
6. Chen K, Rajewsky N. The evolution of gene regulation by transcription factors and microRNAs. Nat Rev Genet 2007; 8(2):93-103.
7. Fraser P, Bickmore W. Nuclear organization of the genome and the potential for gene regulation. Nature 2007; 447(7143):413-417.
8. Zaratiegui M, Irvine DV, Martienssen RA. Noncoding RNAs and gene silencing. Cell 2007; 128(4):763-776.
9. Callinan PA, Feinberg AP. The emerging science of epigenomics. Hum Mol Genet 2006; 15 Suppl 1:R95-R101.
10. Esteller M. Cancer epigenomics: DNA methylomes and histone-modification maps. Nat Rev Genet 2007; 8(4):286-298.
11. Fazzari MJ, Greally JM. Epigenomics: beyond CpG islands. Nat Rev Genet 2004; 5(6):446-455.
12. Laird PW. The power and the promise of DNA methylation markers. Nat Rev Cancer 2003; 3(4):253-266.
13. Laird PW. Principles and challenges of genome-wide DNA methylation analysis. Nat Rev Genet 2010; 11(3):191-203.
14. Beck S, Olek A, Walter J. From genomics to epigenomics: a loftier view of life. Nat Biotechnol 1999; 17(12):1144.
15. Park PJ. ChIP-seq: advantages and challenges of a maturing technology. Nat Rev Genet 2009; 10(10):669-680.
16. Frommer M, McDonald LE, Millar DS et al. A genomic sequencing protocol that yields a positive display of 5-methylcytosine residues in individual DNA strands. Proc Natl Acad Sci USA 1992; 89(5):1827-1831.
17. Herman JG, Graff JR, Myohanen S et al. Methylation-specific PCR: a novel PCR assay for methylation status of CpG islands. Proc Natl Acad Sci USA 1996; 93(18):9821-9826.
18. Frigola J, Ribas M, Risques RA et al. Methylome profiling of cancer cells by amplification of inter-methylated sites (AIMS). Nucleic Acids Res 2002; 30(7):e28.
19. Kawai J, Hirotsune S, Hirose K et al. Methylation profiles of genomic DNA of mouse developmental brain detected by restriction landmark genomic scanning (RLGS) method. Nucleic Acids Res 1993; 21(24):5604-5608.
20. Ramsay G. DNA chips: state-of-the art. Nat Biotechnol 1998; 16(1):40-44.
21. Metzker ML. Sequencing technologies—the next generation. Nat Rev Genet 2010; 11(1):31-46.
22. Huang TH, Perry MR, Laux DE. Methylation profiling of CpG islands in human breast cancer cells. Hum Mol Genet 1999; 8(3):459-470.
23. Ching TT, Maunakea AK, Jun P et al. Epigenome analyses using BAC microarrays identify evolutionary conservation of tissue-specific methylation of SHANK3. Nat Genet 2005; 37(6):645-651.
24. Khulan B, Thompson RF, Ye K et al. Comparative isoschizomer profiling of cytosine methylation: the HELP assay. Genome Res 2006; 16(8):1046-1055.

25. Schumacher A, Kapranov P, Kaminsky Z et al. Microarray-based DNA methylation profiling: technology and applications. Nucleic Acids Res 2006; 34(2):528-542.

26. Gebhard C, Schwarzfischer L, Pham TH et al. Genome-wide profiling of CpG methylation identifies novel targets of aberrant hypermethylation in myeloid leukemia. Cancer Res 2006; 66(12):6118-6128.

27. Weber M, Davies JJ, Wittig D et al. Chromosome-wide and promoter-specific analyses identify sites of differential DNA methylation in normal and transformed human cells. Nat Genet 2005; 37(8):853-862.

28. Rauch T, Li H, Wu X et al. MIRA-assisted microarray analysis, a new technology for the determination of DNA methylation patterns, identifies frequent methylation of homeodomain-containing genes in lung cancer cells. Cancer Res 2006; 66(16):7939-7947.

29. Jorgensen HF, Adie K, Chaubert P et al. Engineering a high-affinity methyl-CpG-binding protein. Nucleic Acids Res 2006; 34(13):e96.

30. Ballestar E, Paz MF, Valle L et al. Methyl-CpG binding proteins identify novel sites of epigenetic inactivation in human cancer. EMBO J 2003; 22(23):6335-6345.

31. Weber M, Hellmann I, Stadler MB et al. Distribution, silencing potential and evolutionary impact of promoter DNA methylation in the human genome. Nat Genet 2007; 39(4):457-466.

32. Bibikova M, Lin Z, Zhou L et al. High-throughput DNA methylation profiling using universal bead arrays. Genome Res 2006; 16(3):383-393.

33. Gitan RS, Shi H, Chen CM et al. Methylation-specific oligonucleotide microarray: a new potential for high-throughput methylation analysis. Genome Res 2002; 12(1):158-164.

34. Karpf AR. Epigenomic reactivation screening to identify genes silenced by DNA hypermethylation in human cancer. Curr Opin Mol Ther 2007; 9(3):231-241.

35. Shames DS, Minna JD, Gazdar AF. Methods for detecting DNA methylation in tumors: from bench to bedside. Cancer Lett 2007; 251(2):187-198.

36. Yan PS, Chen CM, Shi H et al. Applications of CpG island microarrays for high-throughput analysis of DNA methylation. J Nutr 2002; 132(8 Suppl):2430S-2434S.

37. Wilson IM, Davies JJ, Weber M et al. Epigenomics: mapping the methylome. Cell Cycle 2006; 5(2):155-158.

38. Zhang X, Yazaki J, Sundaresan A et al. Genome-wide high-resolution mapping and functional analysis of DNA methylation in arabidopsis. Cell 2006; 126(6):1189-1201.

39. Adorjan P, Distler J, Lipscher E et al. Tumour class prediction and discovery by microarray-based DNA methylation analysis. Nucleic Acids Res 2002; 30(5):e21.

40. Bibikova M, Chudin E, Wu B et al. Human embryonic stem cells have a unique epigenetic signature. Genome Res 2006; 16(9):1075-1083.

41. Bibikova M, Le J, Barnes B et al. Genome-wide DNA methylation profiling using Infinium assay. Epigenomics 2009; 1(1):177-200.

42. Kanduri M, Cahill N, Goransson H et al. Differential genome-wide array-based methylation profiles in prognostic subsets of chronic lymphocytic leukemia. Blood 2010; 115(2):296-305.

43. Ehrich M, Turner J, Gibbs P et al. Cytosine methylation profiling of cancer cell lines. Proc Natl Acad Sci USA 2008; 105(12):4844-4849.

44. von Bubnoff A. Next-generation sequencing: the race is on. Cell 2008; 132(5):721-723.

45. Oda M, Glass JL, Thompson RF et al. High-resolution genome-wide cytosine methylation profiling with simultaneous copy number analysis and optimization for limited cell numbers. Nucleic Acids Res 2009; 37(12):3829-3839.

46. Brunner AL, Johnson DS, Kim SW et al. Distinct DNA methylation patterns characterize differentiated human embryonic stem cells and developing human fetal liver. Genome Res 2009; 19(6):1044-1056.

47. Ball MP, Li JB, Gao Y et al. Targeted and genome-scale strategies reveal gene-body methylation signatures in human cells. Nat Biotechnol 2009; 27(4):361-368.

48. Ruike Y, Imanaka Y, Sato F et al. Genome-wide analysis of aberrant methylation in human breast cancer cells using methyl-DNA immunoprecipitation combined with high-throughput sequencing. BMC Genomics 2010; 11:137.

49. Taylor KH, Kramer RS, Davis JW et al. Ultradeep bisulfite sequencing analysis of DNA methylation patterns in multiple gene promoters by 454 sequencing. Cancer Res 2007; 67(18):8511-8518.

50. Meissner A, Mikkelsen TS, Gu H et al. Genome-scale DNA methylation maps of pluripotent and differentiated cells. Nature 2008; 454(7205):766-770.

51. Hodges E, Smith AD, Kendall J et al. High definition profiling of mammalian DNA methylation by array capture and single molecule bisulfite sequencing. Genome Res 2009; 19(9):1593-1605.

52. Li JB, Gao Y, Aach J et al. Multiplex padlock targeted sequencing reveals human hypermutable CpG variations. Genome Res 2009; 19(9):1606-1615.

53. Mamanova L, Coffey AJ, Scott CE et al. Target-enrichment strategies for next-generation sequencing. Nat Methods 2010; 7(2):111-118.

54. Cokus SJ, Feng S, Zhang X et al. Shotgun bisulphite sequencing of the Arabidopsis genome reveals DNA methylation patterning. Nature 2008; 452(7184):215-219.
55. Lister R, O'Malley RC, Tonti-Filippini J et al. Highly integrated single-base resolution maps of the epigenome in Arabidopsis. Cell 2008; 133(3):523-536.
56. Lister R, Pelizzola M, Dowen RH et al. Human DNA methylomes at base resolution show widespread epigenomic differences. Nature 2009; 462(7271):315-322.
57. Laurent L, Wong E, Li G et al. Dynamic changes in the human methylome during differentiation. Genome Res 2010; 20(3):320-331.
58. Bernstein BE, Humphrey EL, Liu CL et al. The use of chromatin immunoprecipitation assays in genome-wide analyses of histone modifications. Methods Enzymol 2004; 376:349-360.
59. Huebert DJ, Kamal M, O'Donovan A et al. Genome-wide analysis of histone modifications by ChIP-on-chip. Methods 2006; 40(4):365-369.
60. Kiermer V. Embryos and biopsies on the ChIP-ing forecast. Nat Methods 2006; 3(8):583.
61. O'Neill LP, VerMilyea MD, Turner BM. Epigenetic characterization of the early embryo with a chromatin immunoprecipitation protocol applicable to small cell populations. Nat Genet 2006; 38(7):835-841.
62. Attema JL, Papathanasiou P, Forsberg EC et al. Epigenetic characterization of hematopoietic stem cell differentiation using miniChIP and bisulfite sequencing analysis. Proc Natl Acad Sci USA 2007; 104(30):12371-12376.
63. Lee TI, Jenner RG, Boyer LA et al. Control of developmental regulators by Polycomb in human embryonic stem cells. Cell 2006; 125(2):301-313.
64. Christensen BC, Houseman EA, Marsit CJ et al. Aging and environmental exposures alter tissue-specific DNA methylation dependent upon CpG island context. PLoS Genet 2009; 5(8):e1000602.
65. Jirtle RL, Skinner MK. Environmental epigenomics and disease susceptibility. Nat Rev Genet 2007; 8(4):253-262.
66. Weaver IC, Cervoni N, Champagne FA et al. Epigenetic programming by maternal behavior. Nat Neurosci 2004; 7(8):847-854.
67. Weidman JR, Dolinoy DC, Murphy SK et al. Cancer susceptibility: epigenetic manifestation of environmental exposures. Cancer J 2007; 13(1):9-16.
68. Kaminsky ZA, Tang T, Wang SC et al. DNA methylation profiles in monozygotic and dizygotic twins. Nat Genet 2009; 41(2):240-245.
69. Fraga MF, Ballestar E, Paz MF et al. Epigenetic differences arise during the lifetime of monozygotic twins. Proc Natl Acad Sci USA 2005; 102(30):10604-10609.
70. Martin-Subero JI, Ammerpohl O, Bibikova M et al. A comprehensive microarray-based DNA methylation study of 367 hematological neoplasms. PLoS One 2009; 4(9):e6986.
71. Baylin SB, Ohm JE. Epigenetic gene silencing in cancer—a mechanism for early oncogenic pathway addiction? Nat Rev Cancer 2006; 6(2):107-116.
72. Esteller M. Epigenetics in cancer. N Engl J Med 2008; 358(11):1148-1159.
73. Laird PW. Cancer epigenetics. Hum Mol Genet 2005; 14 Spec No 1:R65-76.
74. Feinberg AP, Tycko B. The history of cancer epigenetics. Nat Rev Cancer 2004; 4(2):143-153.
75. Jones PA, Baylin SB. The epigenomics of cancer. Cell 2007; 128(4):683-692.
76. Paz MF, Fraga MF, Avila S et al. A systematic profile of DNA methylation in human cancer cell lines. Cancer Res 2003; 63(5):1114-1121.
77. Costello JF, Fruhwald MC, Smiraglia DJ et al. Aberrant CpG-island methylation has nonrandom and tumour-type-specific patterns. Nat Genet 2000; 24(2):132-138.
78. Keshet I, Schlesinger Y, Farkash S et al. Evidence for an instructive mechanism of de novo methylation in cancer cells. Nat Genet 2006; 38(2):149-153.
79. Martin-Subero JI, Kreuz M, Bibikova M et al. New insights into the biology and origin of mature aggressive B-cell lymphomas by combined epigenomic, genomic and transcriptional profiling. Blood 2009; 113(11):2488-2497.
80. Ohm JE, Baylin SB. Stem cell chromatin patterns: an instructive mechanism for DNA hypermethylation? Cell Cycle 2007; 6(9):1040-1043.
81. Schlesinger Y, Straussman R, Keshet I et al. Polycomb-mediated methylation on Lys27 of histone H3 premarks genes for de novo methylation in cancer. Nat Genet 2007; 39(2):232-236.
82. Widschwendter M, Fiegl H, Egle D et al. Epigenetic stem cell signature in cancer. Nat Genet 2007; 39(2):157-158.
83. Ballestar E, Esteller M, Richardson BC. The epigenetic face of systemic lupus erythematosus. J Immunol 2006; 176(12):7143-7147.
84. Corvetta A, Della Bitta R, Luchetti MM et al. 5-Methylcytosine content of DNA in blood, synovial mononuclear cells and synovial tissue from patients affected by autoimmune rheumatic diseases. J Chromatogr 1991; 566(2):481-491.

85. Javierre BM, Fernandez AF, Richter J et al. Changes in the pattern of DNA methylation associate with twin discordance in systemic lupus erythematosus. Genome Res 2010; 20(2):170-179.

86. Lund G, Andersson L, Lauria M et al. DNA methylation polymorphisms precede any histological sign of atherosclerosis in mice lacking apolipoprotein E. J Biol Chem 2004; 279(28):29147-29154.

87. Turunen MP, Aavik E, Yla-Herttuala S. Epigenetics and atherosclerosis. Biochim Biophys Acta 2009; 1790(9):886-891.

88. Gluckman PD, Hanson MA, Buklijas T et al. Epigenetic mechanisms that underpin metabolic and cardiovascular diseases. Nat Rev Endocrinol 2009; 5(7):401-408.

89. Ehrlich M. The ICF syndrome, a DNA methyltransferase 3B deficiency and immunodeficiency disease. Clin Immunol 2003; 109(1):17-28.

90. Amir RE, Van den Veyver IB, Wan M et al. Rett syndrome is caused by mutations in X-linked MECP2, encoding methyl-CpG-binding protein 2. Nat Genet 1999; 23(2):185-188.

91. Esteller M. Rett syndrome: the first forty years: 1966-2006. Epigenetics 2007; 2(1):1.

92. Bartsch O, Schmidt S, Richter M et al. DNA sequencing of CREBBP demonstrates mutations in 56% of patients with Rubinstein-Taybi syndrome (RSTS) and in another patient with incomplete RSTS. Hum Genet 2005; 117(5):485-493.

93. Tatton-Brown K, Rahman N. Sotos syndrome. Eur J Hum Genet 2007; 15(3):264-271.

94. Horsthemke B, Buiting K. Genomic imprinting and imprinting defects in humans. Adv Genet 2008; 61:225-246.

95. Reik W, Walter J. Genomic imprinting: parental influence on the genome. Nat Rev Genet 2001; 2(1):21-32.

96. Nicholls RD, Saitoh S, Horsthemke B. Imprinting in Prader-Willi and Angelman syndromes. Trends Genet 1998; 14(5):194-200.

97. Urdinguio RG, Sanchez-Mut JV, Esteller M. Epigenetic mechanisms in neurological diseases: genes, syndromes and therapies. Lancet Neurol 2009; 8(11):1056-1072.

98. Chen KL, Wang SS, Yang YY et al. The epigenetic effects of amyloid-beta(1-40) on global DNA and neprilysin genes in murine cerebral endothelial cells. Biochem Biophys Res Commun 2009; 378(1):57-61.

99. Wang SC, Oelze B, Schumacher A. Age-specific epigenetic drift in late-onset Alzheimer's disease. PLoS One 2008; 3(7):e2698.

100. Pieper HC, Evert BO, Kaut O et al. Different methylation of the TNF-alpha promoter in cortex and substantia nigra: Implications for selective neuronal vulnerability. Neurobiol Dis 2008; 32(3):521-527.

101. Ryu H, Lee J, Hagerty SW et al. ESET/SETDB1 gene expression and histone H3 (K9) trimethylation in Huntington's disease. Proc Natl Acad Sci USA 2006; 103(50):19176-19181.

102. Sadri-Vakili G, Bouzou B, Benn CL et al. Histones associated with downregulated genes are hypo-acetylated in Huntington's disease models. Hum Mol Genet 2007; 16(11):1293-1306.

103. Mill J, Tang T, Kaminsky Z et al. Epigenomic profiling reveals DNA-methylation changes associated with major psychosis. Am J Hum Genet 2008; 82(3):696-711.

104. Jones PA, Martienssen R. A blueprint for a Human Epigenome Project: the AACR Human Epigenome Workshop. Cancer Res 2005; 65(24):11241-11246.

105. Esteller M. The necessity of a human epigenome project. Carcinogenesis 2006; 27(6):1121-1125.

106. Rauscher FJ, 3rd. It is time for a Human Epigenome Project. Cancer Res 2005; 65(24):11229.

107. Jeltsch A, Walter J, Reinhardt R et al. German human methylome project started. Cancer Res 2006; 66(14):7378.

108. Garber K. Momentum building for human epigenome project. J Natl Cancer Inst 2006; 98(2):84-86.

109. Eckhardt F, Beck S, Gut IG et al. Future potential of the Human Epigenome Project. Expert Rev Mol Diagn 2004; 4(5):609-618.

110. Bradbury J. Human epigenome project—up and running. PLoS Biol 2003; 1(3):E82.

111. Jones PA, Archer TK, Baylin SB et al. Moving AHEAD with an international human epigenome project. Nature 2008; 454(7205):711-715.

112. Branton D, Deamer DW, Marziali A et al. The potential and challenges of nanopore sequencing. Nat Biotechnol 2008; 26(10):1146-1153.

113. van Steensel B. Mapping of genetic and epigenetic regulatory networks using microarrays. Nat Genet 2005; 37 Suppl:S18-24.

114. Toyota M, Ho C, Ahuja N et al. Identification of differentially methylated sequences in colorectal cancer by methylated CpG island amplification. Cancer Res 1999; 59(10):2307-2312.

115. Estecio MR, Yan PS, Ibrahim AE et al. High-throughput methylation profiling by MCA coupled to CpG island microarray. Genome Res 2007; 17(10):1529-1536.

116. Yuan E, Haghighi F, White S et al. A single nucleotide polymorphism chip-based method for combined genetic and epigenetic profiling: validation in decitabine therapy and tumor/normal comparisons. Cancer Res 2006; 66(7):3443-3451.

117. Ibrahim AE, Thorne NP, Baird K et al. MMASS: an optimized array-based method for assessing CpG island methylation. Nucleic Acids Res 2006; 34(20):e136.
118. Hu M, Yao J, Polyak K. Methylation-specific digital karyotyping. Nat Protoc 2006; 1(3):1621-1636.
119. Pfister S, Schlaeger C, Mendrzyk F et al. Array-based profiling of reference-independent methylation status (aPRIMES) identifies frequent promoter methylation and consecutive downregulation of ZIC2 in pediatric medulloblastoma. Nucleic Acids Res 2007; 35(7):e51.
120. Suzuki H, Gabrielson E, Chen W et al. A genomic screen for genes upregulated by demethylation and histone deacetylase inhibition in human colorectal cancer. Nat Genet 2002; 31(2):141-149.
121. Hodges E, Smith AD, Kendall J et al. High definition profiling of mammalian DNA methylation by array capture and single molecule bisulfite sequencing. Genome Res 2009; 19(9):1593-605.

INDEX